HOT TOPICS IN ENDOCRINE AND ENDOCRINE-RELATED DISEASES

Edited by **Monica Fedele**

Hot Topics in Endocrine and Endocrine-Related Diseases
http://dx.doi.org/10.5772/46124
Edited by Monica Fedele

Contributors

Carmen Sanz, Veronica Hurtado, Isabel Roncero, Enrique Blazquez, Elvira Alvarez, Imre Zoltan Kun, Zsuzsanna Szanto, Jozsef Balazs, Anisie Nasalean, Camelia Gliga, Cristina Carnovale, Paola Ingaramo, Daniel Francés, M. Teresa Ronco, Ebe D'Adamo, Benjamin U. Nwosu, Vania Maria Correa Da Costa, Antongiulio Faggiano, Manuel Estrada, Carla Basualto-Alarcón, Enrique Jaimovich, Rodrigo Maass, Marie-Lise Jaffrain-Rea, Emrah Yerlikaya, Fulya Akin

Published by InTech

Janeza Trdine 9, 51000 Rijeka, Croatia

Publishing Process Manager Oliver Kurelic
Technical Editor InTech DTP team
Cover InTech Design team

Additional hard copies can be obtained from orders@intechopen.com

Hot Topics in Endocrine and Endocrine-Related Diseases, Edited by Monica Fedele
p. cm.
ISBN 978-953-51-1080-4

For EU product safety concerns:
IN TECH d.o.o., Prolaz Marije Krucifikse Kozulić 3, 51000 Rijeka, Croatia,
info@intechopen.com or visit our website at intechopen.com.

Meet the editor

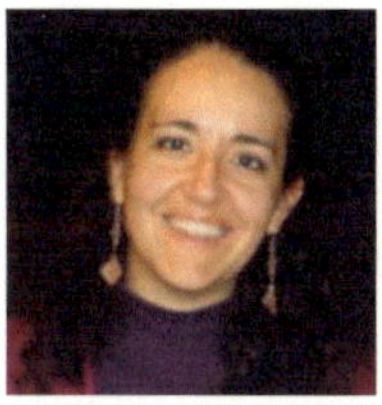

Dr. Monica Fedele is lead researcher at the Institute of Experimental Endocrinology and Oncology of the National Research Council in Italy. She graduated in Biological Sciences at the University of Naples, receiving her PhD in Cellular and Molecular Biology and Pathology, and residency in Clinical Pathology, at the Medical School of the same University. Dr. Fedele trained in molecular oncology and was a postdoctoral investigator in USA, focusing on the development of transgenic and knockout mice for the HMGA genes. Her main scientific achievements are the isolation and characterization of the cancer-related gene PATZ, the demonstration of the oncogenic activity of the chromatin proteins HMGA1 and HMGA2, and the discovery of their critical role in the development of pituitary adenomas.

Contents

Preface

The endocrine system plays a vital role in whether or not you develop a wide range of diseases, not only including strictly endocrine-diseases.

This book includes selected contemporary topics representing exciting recent developments in the field of endocrine and endocrine-related diseases. It is the result of a collaboration among eminent scientists and clinicians coming from eight different countries, including Argentina, Brazil, Chile, Italy, Romania, Spain, Turkey and United States.

Basic and advanced recent trends and research studies in a number of endocrine and endocrine-related disorders are covered by the different chapters of the book. We will read about hereditary neuroendocrine tumors, with emphasis on their still poorly defined natural history and clinical course; pituitary tumors, with a comprehensive overview of the recent advances in their pathogenesis; thyroid dysfunctions, including those related to aging and iodine deficiency; diabetes, with its hepatic complications, and double diabetes, a new definition that summarizes the coexistence of features of both type 1 and type 2 diabetes in the same individual, with a comprehensive discussion of the various aspects of this disorder and a focus on the search for a treatment paradigm in children and adolescents. Moreover, we will read about the testosterone as a new player in metabolic disorders and as a potential drug to counteract skeletal muscle diseases; the glucagon-like peptide type 1 and its multiple actions for which it can be considered an anti-diabetogenic agent and may have important implications in pathophysiological states such as obesity; the-insulin-like-growth-factor role in different human pathologies, including cancer; and the pediatric nonalcoholic fatty liver disease.

I hope that, at the end, the reader will have a critic and advanced overview of selected hot pathologies related to the endocrine field.

Dr. Monica Fedele
Institute of Experimental Endocrinology and Oncology,
National Research Council,
Naples, Italy

Chapter 1

Hereditary Neuroendocrine Tumor Syndromes

Antongiulio Faggiano, Valeria Ramundo,
Luisa Circelli and Annamaria Colao

Additional information is available at the end of the chapter

http://dx.doi.org/10.5772/53841

1. Introduction

Neuroendocrine tumours (NETs) are rare and heterogeneous neoplasms with variable biological behaviour. The estimated incidence of NETs is about 1-5 cases/100,000/year. The most recent data show a progressive increase of the incidence in the last years and a high increase of their prevalence and survival [1]. NETs can be sporadic or can arise in complex hereditary endocrine disorders such as Multiple Endocrine Neoplasias (MENs), Familial Paragangliomatosis (FPGLs), Neurofibromatosis type 1 (NF1), von Hippel-Lindau Disease (VHL), Tuberous Sclerosis (TSC) [1]. It has been estimated that hereditary NETs occurrence varies with site of origin of the tumour, ranging 5 to 30% of cases [1]. Due to the recent advances in the knowledge of biology and genetics of NETs, these rates seems to be an underestimation and novel mutations of well known oncogenes or tumour suppressor genes as well as new genes and molecular pathways responsible for unknown syndromes are expected to be characterized.

Patients with hereditary NET syndromes inherit the susceptibility to develop multiple endocrine neoplasias which can be associated with non-endocrine tumours and/or non-tumour lesions. They are characterized by germline mutations usually inherited as an autosomal dominant disease according to the Knudson's "two-hits hypothesis" [2].

Compared to the sporadic forms, hereditary NETs generally present an earlier age at onset, multiple tumour localizations, higher secretory activity. Diagnosis is made around sixth decade of life in sporadic NETs while it is anticipated of about three decades in hereditary tumours [3]. The identification of hereditary NET syndromes is relevant to achieve a precocious diagnosis and this may be important to prevent severe complications and unfavourable outcome. For this reason, the genetic screening is nowadays a well established procedure in many tumor types allowing to reclassify as carrier of specific hereditary NET syndromes, a number of patients with an apparently sporadic tumours [4]. Some studies, focusing in particular on MEN type 1, highlighted that the genetic screening impacts on the management and clinical outcome of NETs, because it allows to detect tumours at an early stage or even before their development [5-7].

In spite of these recent advances, at now, clinical pictures of most of the hereditary NET syndromes are incomplete or not updated. In addition, follow-ups of these patients are not standardized. Furthermore, although in the last years it has been possible to identify a lot of genes and molecular pathways responsible for the development of hereditary NETs, many other molecular pathways responsible for apparently sporadic NETs or influencing the phenotype of well known hereditary NETs remain to be detected and characterized.

In summary, the genetic origin influences the natural history of NETs, however, natural history and clinical course of hereditary NETs is not well defined for most of the actually known hereditary NET syndromes and other syndromes remained to be discovered.

In this chapter two hereditary endocrine syndromes (Multiple Endocrine Neoplasias and Familial Paragangliomatosis) will be discussed.

2. Epidemiology and clinical characteristics

2.1. Multiple Endocrine Neoplasias

Multiple Endocrine Neoplasias (MENs) are rare hereditary autosomal dominant syndromes with complete penetrance and variable expressivity, characterized by the onset of various endocrine and non endocrine tumors with different localization. We distinguish the MEN type 1 (MEN1) and MEN type 2 (MEN2) that are two distinct syndromes.

2.1.1. MEN1

MEN1 or Wermer's Syndrome (OMIM #131100) is characterized by high penetrance (more than 95% of carriers develop disease within 50 years of age), variable inter- and intra-familial expressivity and genetic anticipation [3, 8]. It has been estimated that the prevalence of MEN1 is 2-3:100,000 individuals, with the same distribution between males and females [9]. MEN1 is characterized by the occurrence of tumors of the parathyroid glands, the anterior pituitary, the pancreatic islets and the adrenal glands, as well NETs in the foregut (thymic, bronchial and gastric carcinoids). Other non-endocrine tumors can associate in the skin (angiofibromas, lipomas, collagenomas) and in the central nervous system (ependimoma, meningioma) (Table 1). According to the MEN Consensus published in 2001, the clinical diagnosis of this syndrome is based on the concomitant occurrence of at least two of the three MEN1-related endocrine tumors (parathyroid adenoma, pituitary adenoma, duodeno-pancreatic-NET). Familial MEN1 is defined as at least one MEN1-related NET plus at least one first-degree relative with at least one of the three classical tumors or a known germline *MEN1* mutation [10].

http://dx.doi.org/10.5772/53841

Endocrine tumors	**%**
Parathyroid glands	75-95
Pancreatic islets	55
Gastrinomas	45
Insulinomas	10
Non-functioning	10
Other (VIPomas, etc.)	2
Pituitary	47
PRLomas	30
Non-functioning	10
ACTHomas	1
GH-omas	3-6
Adrenal cortical	20
Foregut	18
Thymus	8
Lungs	8
Stomach	5
Non-endocrine tumors	
Skin	80
Angiofibromas	75
Collagenomas	5
Lipomas	30
Leiomyomas	5
CNS (meningiomas)	25

ACTH: adrenocorticotrophic hormone; CNS: central nervous system; GH: growth hormone; PRL: prolactin; VIP: vasoactive intestinal peptide.

Table 1. Endocrine and non-endocrine tumors associated to Multiple Endocrine Neoplasia type 1

Typically, NETs associated to MEN1 rise up two decades before the sporadic ones. They are generally benign; however, both duodeno-pancreatic NETs and carcinoids can be malignant.

Hyperparathyroidism, caused by parathyroid adenoma/hyperplasia, is often the first manifestation of MEN1. About 75-95% of MEN1 patients develop parathyroid adenomas [10]. Usually parathyroid adenomas are multiple and benign. The main clinical manifestations of primary hyperparathyroidism and the resulting hypercalcemia are represented by renal diseases (dehydration, hypercalciuria, nephrolithiasis and, in advanced cases, kidney failure), bone changes (early osteopenia/osteoporosis), neurological manifestations (drowsiness, depression, confusion), gastrointestinal disturbances (anorexia, constipation, nausea, vomiting) and cardiovascular alterations (hypertension, short QT-trait).

Laboratory investigation to detect primary hyperparathyroidism consist of measurement of (ionized) calcium, phosphate and parathyroid hormone in blood and the 24-hour calcium excretion in the urine. Bone densitometry can be used to detect bone mass reduction. Parathyroid adenomas can be localized by neck ultrasonography (US) and Tc-99m sestamibi scintigraphy (useful to detect also ectopic parathyroid glands).

Pancreatic endocrine tumors develop in about 55% of MEN1 patients [11]. Pancreatic tumor in the context of MEN1 is, generally, multicentric with considerable variability in size (micro-and macro-tumors) and clinical behavior (lesion localized, invasive or metastatic). Multicentric microadenomas are present in 90% of MEN1 patients [12]. It is common to detect functioning NETs associated with non-functioning NETs. The main locations of occurrence are represented by the pancreas in toto and the duodenal submucosa. In order of frequency, the duodeno-pancreatic NETs associated with the syndrome of gastrin hypersecretion are the most frequent and are responsible for the Zollinger-Ellison syndrome. Functioning syndromes and related symptoms are shown in Table 2.

Hormonal syndromes often occur late and may indicate metastases in 50% of MEN1 patients [13].

Laboratory investigation to detect duodeno-pancreatic NETs includes specific markers (such as gastrin, insulin, glucose, glucagon) and the aspecific marker cromogranin-A. Duodeno-pancreatic NETs can be detected by US and echo-endoscopy, magnetic resonance imaging (MRI), computed tomography (CT) and functional imaging techniques such as somatostain receptor scintigraphy.

Pituitary adenomas are found in about 50% of MEN1 patients and evidence of MEN1 is found in approximately 2.7% of patients with pituitary adenomas [10]. Pituitary tumors in MEN1, compared to sporadic tumors, are larger in size and more aggressive. Since childhood MEN1 subjects need to be evaluated for pituitary tumors [14].

The diagnosis of functioning pituitary adenoma is confirmed by determining a specific hormone excess on blood or urinary samples. Pituitary adenomas can be detect visually by MRI with gadolinium contrast.

Syndrome	Symptoms
Zollinger-Ellison syndrome (gastrin hypersecretion)	Pain or burning sensation in the abdomen Nausea Vomiting Diarrhea Fatigue Weakness Weight loss
Insulinoma syndrome	Anxiety Behavior changes Clouded vision Confusion Convulsions Dizziness Headache Hunger Loss of consciousness Rapid heart rate Sweating Tremor Weight gain
Verner-Morrison syndrome (VIP hypersecretion)	Abdominal pain and cramping Diarrhea (watery, and often in large amounts) Flushing or redness of the face Nausea Weight loss
Somatostatinoma syndrome	Mild diabetes mellitus Steatorrhoea Gall stones
Glucagonoma syndrome	Anemia Diarrhea Weight loss Necrolytic migratory erythema Diabetes mellitus

Table 2. Functioning syndromes and related symptoms associated to Multiple Endocrine Neoplasia type 1

2.1.2. MEN2

MEN2 or Sipple's Syndrome (OMIM #171400) is an autosomal dominant disease resulting from germline mutations of the RET proto-oncogene, with an estimated prevalence of 1:30,000 subjects [10]. It is divided in three clinical variants: a) MEN2A (medullary thyroid cancer, pheochromocytoma, primary hyperparathyroidism and cutaneous lichen amyloidosis or Hirschsprung disease); b) familial medullary thyroid cancer (FMTC); c) MEN2B (medullary thyroid cancer, pheochromocytoma, mucosal and intestinal ganglioneuromatosis, marfanoid habitus) [10, 15, 16]. Although these variants have medullary thyroid cancer as a common denominator, they differ for the aggressiveness of this cancer, in a decreasing order MEN2B>MEN2A>FMTC [15]. In patients with FMTC, medullary thyroid cancer (MTC) is the only clinical manifestation. According to the "International RET Mutation Consostium", to make the diagnosis of FMTC is required the onset of medullary thyroid cancer (MTC) in at least four family members [17]. About 56% of cases belong to the subtype 2A, while the subtype 2B is the most aggressive with an elevated morbidity and mortality [15, 16, 18].

Plasma free metanephrines have the highest sensitivity and specificity for detecting pheochromocytoma. However, measurement of 24-hour urine catecholamines and metanephrines, and serum catecholamines are also frequently used [19, 20]. Imaging techniques include abdomen CT-scan and/or MRI. Functional imaging techniques include somatostatin receptor scintigraphy and metaiodobenzylguanidine (MIBG) scintigraphy.

2.2. Familial paragangliomatosis

Familial Paragangliomatosis (FPGLs) are hereditary syndromes of susceptibility to multiple neuroectodermal tumors characterized by high vascularisation and slow growth that arise from the medullar of adrenal glands (pheochromocytomas, PCCs) or from extra-adrenal ganglia (paragangliomas, PGLs).

PCCs and PGLs occur as sporadic tumors and in 10-50% of cases the tumors were associated with hereditary syndromes, mainly MEN2, von Hippel–Lindau disease (VHL), and neurofibromatosis type 1 (NF1) [21]. A small fraction is associated with other syndromes, including Carney triad, Carney–Stratakis syndrome, and, very rarely, MEN1.

There are four subtypes of FPGLs. PGLs can found in all three types of FPGL while phaeochromocytomas are very rare in the FPGL3 [22].

Hereditary PCCs/PGLs, in comparison to sporadic ones, arise more prematurely, can be bilateral or multifocal and can more frequently relapse.

About 10% of the PCCs/PGLs is malignant. FPGL4 is characterized by an increase chance of malignant paragangliomas; in this disorder, then, renal cell cancers and thyroid cancers can be found [22].

Pheochromocytomas and sympathetic paragangliomas result in hypersecretion of catecholamines, which can cause headache, palpitations, hypertension, tachycardia and excessive perspiration, as well as many other nonspecific symptoms. Although most pheochromocytomas and paragangliomas are benign, they can cause major morbidity and death due to uncontrolled hypertension precipitated by stressful events such as anesthesia and pregnancy. Parasympathetic paraganglioma are typically located within the head and neck and usually do not secrete excess catecholamines. They generally do not present symptomatically unless there is a mass effect causing a visible or palpable mass.

Laboratory tests include plasma free metanephrines, 24-hour urine catecholamines and metanephrines.

Imaging techniques include neck, skull base and abdomen/pelvis CT-scan and/or MRI. Functional imaging techniques include somatostatin rceptor scintigraphy and MIBG scintigraphy.

3. Genetic pathways and pathophysiology of mutations

The genetic origin influences the natural history of NETs. This is particularly evident in MEN1 where the diagnosis is made around the sixth decade of life in sporadic tumors while it is anticipated of about three decades in hereditary tumors [3, 10]. The identification of hereditary NET syndromes is relevant to achieve a precocious diagnosis of the tumors and this may be important to prevent severe complications and unfavourable outcome. In the last years, it has been possible to identify a number of genes and molecular pathways involved in the development of NETs. Of consequence, some patients with apparently sporadic tumor have been reclassified as carriers of hereditary NET with relevant implications on the clinical course of disease and quality of life.

3.1. Multiple Endocrine Neoplasias

3.1.1. MEN1

MEN1 is an autosomal dominant syndrome resulting from an inactivating germline mutation of the *MEN1* gene located on chromosome 11q13 [23].

Up to 80% of MEN1-associated tumors exhibit loss of heterozigosity (LOH) of 11q13, indicating that *MEN1* functions as a tumor suppressor gene.

Approximately 21% of sporadic pancreatic neuroendocrine tumors (PNETs) harbour mutations in *MEN1*, but there is substantial variation across different tumor subtypes. Whereas only 8% of insulinomas and non-functioning PNETs have identifiable MEN1 mutations, they are more frequent in gastrinomas [37%), VIPomas (44%) and glucagonomas (67%) [24-31].In contrast to the relatively low frequency of MEN1 mutations in sporadic PNETs, up to 68% display LOH at chromosome 11q13 [32].

This raises the possibility there may be other, yet to be identified, tumor suppressor genes on the long arm of chromosome 11. Similarly, LOH of chromosome 11 is present in up to 78% of gastrointestinal carcinoids, but the frequency of MEN1 mutations is much lower. Gortz et al. reported MEN1 mutations in 2/11 (18%) gastrointestinal carcinoids and 2/11 [18%) lung carcinoids [26] and Debelenko et al identified MEN1 mutations in 4/11 (36%) lung carcinoids [33]. The MEN1 gene product, menin, is a nuclear protein that binds to many transcription factors, including the AP1 component JunD. Upon binding to JunD, menin represses JunD-mediated transcription to inhibit cellular proliferation. Inactivating mutations of MEN1 disrupt the binding to JunD to enhance transcription and augment cellular proliferation [34, 35]. More recently, menin was also identified in a complex with the MLL histone methyltransferase that associates with regulatory elements in the promoters of the cell cycle inhibitors p27KIP1 and p18Ink4c to methylate histone H3 and enhance gene transcription [36]. In mouse models, the absence of Men1 results in down-regulation of p27KIP1 and p18Ink4c and a phenotype resembling the MEN1 syndrome, including islet-cell hyperplasia [37, 38].

Of note, a similar phenotype was also observed in p27KIP1/p18Ink4c double-mutant mice suggesting that deregulation of the cell cycle may be the critical consequence of MEN1 mutations and a necessary feature of NET pathogenesis in general [39]. Recently, the telomerase (hTERT) gene was identified as a menin target gene. The end of chromosome in a cell, shorten after DNA replication. Eventually, after several cell divisions, the DNA loses its stability and the cell is subjected to apoptosis. Telomerase is an enzyme that maintains the length of the telomeres and is not expressed in normal cells, but it is active in stem cells and tumor cells. Menin is a suppressor of the expression of the telomerase gene. Possibly, inactivation of menin could lead to cell immortalization by telomerase expression, which could allow a cell to develop into a tumor cell [40].

In approximately 10-15% of patients with a clinical diagnosis of MEN1 is not possible to identify a known mutation, due to the presence of regulatory sequences inactivated. In such cases the genetic analysis of first-degree relatives of patients with apparently negative family history can be helpful in identifying possible new mutations [41].

3.1.2. MEN2

MEN2 is dominantly inherited, and its genetic cause, mutations of the REarranged during Transfection (RET) protooncogene, was first recognized nearly 20 years ago [10, 42-44].

Since then, the range of mutations identified, their potential for predicting clinical course, and the underlying functional effects have been explored. Detection of RET mutations in MEN2 represents a paradigm for genetically guided patient management, and genotype–phenotype correlations in this disease now inform recommended interventions, patient and family screening, and long-term follow-up [10, 45].

The RET proto-oncogene encodes a receptor tyrosine kinase that is required for the development of neural-crest derived cells, the urogenital system, and the central and peripheral nervous systems, notably the enteric nervous system [46, 47].

The RET protein has a large extracellular domain containing a cysteine-rich region and a series of cadherin homology domains, a transmembrane domain, and an intracellular tyrosine kinase domain, required for RET phosphorylation and downstream signalling [48, 49].

The RET kinase is structurally similar to other tyrosine kinases, sharing many conserved functional motifs and regulatory residues that have been shown to have importance for kinase enzyme function [50]. RET is activated by binding of a multi-protein ligand complex. RET binds a soluble ligand of the glial cell-line-derived neurotrophic factor (GDNF) family but also requires a co-receptor of the GDNF family receptors a (GFRa), which is tethered to the cell membrane via glycosylphosphatidylinositol linkage [51, 52]. Initially, GDNF binds to GFRa, and these complexes are then able to recruit RET to form heterohexamers that are concentrated in regions of the cell membrane called lipid rafts These are membrane domains enriched in glycosylphosphatidylinositol-linked proteins and signaling molecules that provide a platform not only for enhanced cell signaling, but also for regulation of receptor kinase activity and down-regulation [53].

Activation of RET leads to stimulation of multiple downstream pathways, including mitogen-activated protein kinase and extracellular signal-regulated kinase, phosphoinositide 3-kinase and protein kinase B, signal transducer and activator of transcription 3, proto-oncogene tyrosine-protein kinase Src1, and focal adhesion kinase that promote cell growth, proliferation, survival, and/or differentiation [54, 55].

MEN2 is associated with point mutations of RET, predictably leading to its activation in the absence of ligands and co-receptors. Mutations are primarily amino acid substitutions affecting a very small number of RET codons in either the extracellular domain or within the kinase domain.

Mutations are dominant, requiring only a single mutant allele to confer the disease phenotype. MEN2 RET mutation occurrence [56-59] are available online (http://www.arup.utah.edu/database/MEN2/MEN2_welcome.php). Together, these data suggest strong overall themes as to functional effects of these mutations, but also as to their clinical significance.

Together, these data suggest strong overall themes as to functional effects of these mutations, but also as to their clinical significance. Strong associations of disease subtype, and also specific disease phenotypes, with individual RET mutations have made it possible to stratify risk of MEN2 by genotype [10, 45].

The management guidelines of the American Thyroid Association base the recommendations for initial diagnosis, therapeutic intervention, and long-term follow-up on patient genotype and the current understanding of the natural history of the disease associated with each RET mutation. Mutations of cysteine residues (primarily cysteines 609, 611, 618, 620, 630, and 634] in the RET extracellular domain account for the majority of MEN2A cases, and are also common in patients with FMTC. Intracellular kinase domain mutations are mainly associated with FMTC and MEN2B. Mutations in the intracellular codons 768, 790, 791, 804, and 891 underlie FMTC, and occur less commonly in patients with MEN2A [60] while specific mutations of codon 918 (M918T) or 883 (A883F) account for the vast majority of MEN2B cases, and are exclusive to the subtype [61].

In addition to association with disease subtype, significant correlations of specific mutations with disease features are reported. For example, RET codon 634 mutations carry a greater patient risk for pheochromocytoma and parathyroid hyperplasia [62-64] and are associated with a higher frequency of detection of MTC at the time of early thyroidectomy [65].

Variation in clinical presentation has even been observed with different codon 634 substitutions. The specific substitution of an arginine at codon 634 (C634R) is strongly associated with increased risk of parathyroid hyperplasia increased frequency of distant metastases, earlier onset of both lymph node and distant metastases, and bilaterality of pheochromocytoma [66, 67].

3.2. Hereditary pheochromocytoma/paraganglioma syndromes

During the last decade, mutations in the genes encoding different subunits of the succinate dehydrogenase (SDH) complex have been linked to familial PCC/PGL syndrome, and subsequent genetic screenings have revealed that about 30% of PCCs and PGLs are caused by hereditary mutations [68, 69]. In addition, several novel susceptibility genes, such as kinesin family member 1B (KIF1Bb) [70], EGL nine homolog 1, also termed PHD2 (EGLN1/PHD2) [71], transmembrane protein 127 (TMEM127) [72], and MYC-associated factor X (MAX) [73], have recently been added to the list. The predisposing genes that have been identified seem at a first glance to have entirely different functions but, in spite of this, malfunction of their different gene products can give rise to clinically and histologically undistinguishable tumors. Nevertheless, some clinical features may be quite different, e.g. patients with SDHB mutations have considerably higher risk of malignancy than many other PCC/PGL patients [74].

The feature of RET gene and MEN2 syndrome were previously described, we want to remember that activating RET mutations predispose to PCCs, which are often recurrent and bilateral, but typically have a low risk of malignancy.

Familial paragangliomatosis are associated to known germline mutations of the genes encoding subunits of succinate dehydrogenase (SDH).

SDH is a mitochondrial enzyme complex consisting of four subunits: SDHA, SDHB, SDHC, and SDHD, which are all encoded by the nuclear genome [75]. The enzyme, also known as mitochondrial complex II, is involved both in the tricarboxylic acid cycle, where it catalyzes the oxidation of succinate to fumarate, and in the respiratory electron transfer chain, where it transfers electrons to coenzyme Q. The gene SDHA is located on chromosome 5p15.33 and consists of 15 exons. It encodes a protein that functions as a part of the catalytic core and contains the binding site for succinate. The other part of the catalytic domain, which also forms an interface with the membrane anchor, is encoded by SDHB, a gene of eight exons located on chromosome 1p36.13. SDHC on chromosome 1q23.3 and SDHD on chromosome 11q23.1 contain six and four exons, respectively, and encode two hydrophobic proteins that anchor the complex to the mitochondrial inner membrane. The link between SDH and neuroendocrine tumors was first established in the year 2000, when germline mutations in SDHD were discovered in patients withfamilial PGLs [76]. SDHD mutations were subsequently found also in apparently sporadic PCCs [77] and PGLs [78] as well as in familial PCCs [79]. Shortly after, germline mutations were also identified in SDHB in both PCCs and PGLs [80]. SDHC mutations were reported in PGLs in 2000 [81] and were also recently found in PCCs [82]. During several years, homozygous and compound heterozygous mutations in the gene encoding the fourth subunit, SDHA, were associated with a rare early-onset.

Germline mutations in the SDHx genes give rise to familial PCC–PGL syndrome, sometimes only referred to as familial PGL. The syndrome can be divided into PGL1, PGL2, PGL3, and PGL4, which are caused by mutations in SDHD, SDHAF2, SDHC, and SDHB respectively. They are all inherited in an autosomal dominant manner but with varying penetrance.

SDHD is putatively maternally imprinted and PGL1 is thus only passed on to children by their father [83], although one exception of maternal transmission has been reported [84]. To date, PGL2 has also only been diagnosed in individuals with an affected father, suggesting a similar parent-of-origin-specific inheritance for SDHAF2 [85]. No specific PCC/PGL syndrome has yet been described for SDHA mutations, but they seem to have a low penetrance of PCC/PGL and do not seem to be associated with a familial presentation [86, 87]. The prevalence of PCC/PGL syndrome is unknown, but a summary of the cases reviewed here (about 13% of all PCC/PGL cases) gives an estimate of 1:50 000 to 1:20 000, the majority represented by PGL1 and PGL4. Apart from PCCs and PGLs, SDHB mutations have been associated with renal cell carcinoma [88]. One SDHD mutation carrier with a renal cell tumor has also been described, as well as a few cases of SDHB and SDHD patients with thyroid carcinoma [88, 89]. In addition, mutations in SDHB, SDHC, and SDHD can give rise to the Carney–Stratakis syndrome, characterized by the dyad of PGLs and gastrointestinal stromal tumors. Very recently, SDHA mutations were also reported in two patients with gastrointestinal stromal tumors but without PGLs [90].

SDHD mutations (PGL1) predispose most frequently to parasympathetic, often multifocal PGLs, but also to sympathetic PGLs and PCCs. Several national and multinational studies have gathered information about tumor characteristics in patients with PCC/PGL syndrome [69, 88-92].

4. New susceptibility genes in hereditary PCC/PGLs

4.1. Transmembrane protein 127(TMEM127)

TMEM127 is a gene of four exons located on 2q11.2, a locus identified as a PCC susceptibility locus in 2005 [93]. The transmembrane protein was recently revealed to function as a tumor suppressor, and germline mutations in TMEM127 were detected in PCCs [72]. Qin et al. also demonstrated that TMEM127 is a negative regulator of mechanistic target of rapamycin, formerly mammalian target of rapamycin (mTOR), thus linking a critical signalling pathway for cell proliferation and cell death to the initiation and development of PCC. Both missense and nonsense mutations in TMEM127 have been reported. LOH of the gene was detected in tumors of all tested mutation carriers, suggesting a classical two-hit model of inactivation.

So far, no specific syndrome has been described for TMEM127. Other tumors, including MTC, breast cancer, and myelodysplasia, have been identified in carriers of TMEM127 mutations, but a causal relationship between the tumors and the mutations remains to be established [94]. A clear family history in only a fourth of the patients suggests an incomplete penetrance, and in a single family, the penetrance of PCC was 64% by the age of 55 years [95].

Among 990 patients with PCC or PGL, negative for RET, VHL, and SDHB/C/D mutations, TMEM127 mutations were identified in 20 (2.0%) of the cases, all of which had PCC [95]. Another study revealed one additional PCC patient with a TMEM127 mutation [96]. No

TMEM127 mutations were detected in 129 sympathetic and 60 parasympathetic PGLs [93], but in a recent study, germline missense variants were detected in two out of 48 patients with multiple PGLs [97], one of which also displayed bilateral PCC. Summarizing the 23 reported patients, all but one (96%) had PCC and 39% had bilateral PCC.Two (9%) had PGL, of which one had sympathetic and the other multiple parasympathetic PGLs. The mean age at presentation was 43 years, and one patient (4%) displayed a malignant tumor.

4.2. MYC-associated factor X (MAX)

MAX is a gene of five exons, located on chromosome 14q23.3. It encodes a transcription factor, MAX, that belongs to the basic helix–loop–helix leucine zipper (bHLHZip) family and plays an important role in regulation of cell proliferation, differentiation, and death as a part of the MYC/MAX/MXD1 network [98]. Members of the MYC family are proto-oncoproteins and their expression correlates with growth and proliferation, whereas expression of MXD1 (also known as MAD) is associated with differentiation. Heterodimerization of MAX with MYC family members results in sequence-specific DNA-binding complexes that act as transcriptional activators. In contrast, heterodimers of MAX with MXD1 family member repress transcription of the same target genes by binding to the same consensus sequence and thus antagonize MYC–MAX function. Interestingly, PC12 cells, derived from a rat PCC, express only a mutant form of MAX incapable of dimerization, and a reintroduction of normal MAX in these cells resulted in a repressed transcription and inhibited growth [99]. This suggests that some tumors can grow in the absence of MYC–MAX dimers and may imply that MAX can function as a tumor suppressor. A tumor suppressor role of MAX was most recently confirmed when germline MAX mutations were discovered in PCC patients by next-generation exome sequencing [73]. The mutations were missense, nonsense, splice site, or altering the start codon, and immunohistochemical analysis confirmed the lack of full-length MAX in the tumors. LOH of 14q, caused either by uniparental disomy or by chromosomal loss, was seen in investigated tumors in agreement with classical tumor suppressor behaviour.

MAX mutations segregate with the disease in families with PCC [73], but no specific syndrome has been described yet. A paternal origin of the mutated allele in investigated cases, together with the absence of PCC in persons who inherited a mutated allele from their mother, may suggest a paternal transmission of disease similar to that of PGL1 (SDHD) and PGL2 (SDHAF2). MAX-associated PCCs and PGLs. Comino-Mendez et al. [73] reported 12 PCC patients with MAX mutations, of which three were discovered with exome sequencing and four were relatives of those. The remaining five were found in a subsequent screening of 59 PCC patients lacking mutations in other known susceptibility genes but suspected to have hereditary disease (due to bilateral tumors, early age of onset, and/or familial antecedents with the disease). Of the 12 patients, eight (67%) had bilateral PCC and the mean age at presentation was 32 years. Notably, 25% of the patients (38% of the probands) showed metastasis at diagnosis, suggesting that MAX mutations are associated with a high risk of malignancy. So far, no studies on PGLs have been reported.

5. Therapy of hereditary NETs

5.1. Multiple Endocrine Neoplasias

5.1.1. MEN1

The therapeutic management of MEN1-related hyperparathyroidism, as the only curative therapy, is a surgical approach designed to remove all hyperfunctioning parathyroid tissue. This approach consists of the sub-total or total parathyroidectomy followed by autotransplantation of parathyroid tissue in a normal forearm. This approach is clearly different surgery for sporadic hyperparathyroidism. The main consequence of a radical intervention is a severe hypoparathyroidism, which requires treatment with high doses of calcium and vitamin D. This condition often leads to a difficulty in controlling the homeostasis of calcium and a reduced quality of life for the possible occurrence of gastro-intestinal disorders. It is not rare, in addition, the recurrence of hyperparathyroidism even after an apparently total parathyroidectomy. Studies are in progress to evaluate the efficacy of calcium-mimetic agents in the treatment of primary hyperparathyroidism in patients MEN1. Also somatostatin analogues, used in MEN1 subjects for the treatment of duodeno-pancreatic NETs, can have a role in reducing the levels calcium and PTH [6, 10, 100, 101]. The therapy of duodeno-pancreatic NETs in MEN1 patients varies depending on the type and number of tumors. Drug therapy involves the use of biologic therapy such as somatostatin analogues. For all pancreatic tumors MEN1-dependent, the standard surgical treatment involves the distal pancreatectomy combined with ultrasonography and intraoperative manual palpation. In the case of tumors located in the head of the pancreas a duodeno-cephalo-pancreatectomy second Whipple should be practiced. The treatment of choice of a solitary gastrinoma is enucleation. However, in MEN1patients gastrinomas are often multiple and/or metastatic and the role of surgery, in these cases, it is debated [6, 10].

Several studies are ongoing to evaluate the efficacy of new drugs such as tyrosine kinase and mTOR inhibitors for the treatment of metastatic pancreatic NETs.

The treatment of pituitary adenomas in MEN1 patients varies depending on the type of adenoma and is the same treatment applied to the sporadic counterpart. Finally, even in the case of a successful therapy, MEN1-related pituitary adenomas require a careful follow-up because these neoplasms can easily recur [6, 10].

At the moment there is no known preventive surgical approach that can significantly improve outcomes in MEN1 patients, with the exception of prophylactic thymectomy to prevent the occurrence of the rare thymic carcinoid tumor, a tumor frequently malignant and aggressive. This further supports the need to identify quite early the presence of malignancies, with a view to a better clinical management [10].

5.1.2. MEN2

The therapeutic strategy for MEN2 patients should be adapted to the clinical variant and the type of mutation in the *RET* gene according to the risk levels.

Subjects with the highest risk level have the most aggressive MTC and should have thyroidectomy with a central node dissection within the first six months of life and preferably within the first month of life. In subjects classified as risk 2 level, thyroidectomy with removal of the posterior capsule should be performed before the age of five years. For subjects with the lowest risk level (risk level 1) at this moment there are differing opinions on when thyroidectomy should be performed. According to some authors, in fact, total thyroidectomy with lymph node dissection of the central compartment should be practiced within the fifth year of life, according to others such intervention should be performed later, but within the tenth year of life. Other authors finally suggest to periodically perform the pentagastrin stimulation test for calcitonin and to perform the surgery at the first positive test. In all cases, if a pheochromocytoma is present, total thyroidectomy should be performed after surrenectomy to avoid a catecholaminergic crisis during the surgery [10].

Several studies are ongoing to evaluate the efficacy of new drugs such as tyrosine kinase inhibitors for the treatment of metastatic MTC.

The treatment of choice in unilateral pheochromocytoma in MEN2 is laparoscopic adrenalectomy [10].

The treatment for hyperparathyroidism in MEN2 includes the same surgical strategy as provided in other syndromes associated with multiple parathyroid adenomas [10].

5.2. Familial paragangliomatosis

The treatment of choice for FPGL is surgical removal of paraganglioma / pheochromocytoma, after preparation with α-and β-adrenergic blocking drugs in order to improve the perioperative hemodynamic stability. In the case of benign pheochromocytomas/paragangliomas the percentage of full resolution with surgery is approximately 100% [102]. Early intervention and timely manner helps to minimize the morbidity and mortality of this disease.For malignant pheochromocytomas/paragangliomas are available chemo- and radiotherapic approaches. Studies are in progress to evaluate the efficacy of tyrosine kinase inhibitors, such as sunitinib, for the treatment of malignancies. At the moment, there is no specific treatment prior to the onset of hereditary pheochromocytomas/paragangliomas [103, 104].

Early diagnosis and a periodic follow-up are the best approaches for the management and better outcome because of the possible malignant degeneration, especially in the forms associated with *SDHB* gene mutations [105].

6. Impact of genetic screening on natural history and clinical management

In the last years, the growing number of subjects with hereditary NET who is diagnosed at a pre-clinical stage is changing the clinical picture of these tumors. Until now the clinical features and natural history of hereditary NETs were based on data from patients with clinical evidence of disease. With the identification of specific genes responsible for the development of hereditary NETs, more and more subjects are recognized to be carriers of NET-related gene mutations. Pre-clinical genetic screening in asymptomatic first-degree relatives of patients with hereditary NET syndromes leads to detect these neoplasias at an early stage, even when subjects are still asymptomatic.

The genetic risk assessment can provide crucial information on the patient's future risk for tumors and the assessed risk to their family members. An early genetic diagnosis in asymptomatic subjects is recommended to identify subjects at risk to develop one of the above mentioned hereditary NET syndromes as early as possible before the occurrence of clinical manifestations, in order to improve their long-term outcome and to ensure a survival and quality of life similar to that observed in the general population [5].

Since the screening for early symptoms starts, parents should be given counseling in the process of considering the test for their child. Support by a psychosocial worker may be a valuable part of the counseling.

Early detection of tumors in patients with hereditary NETs could encourage the use of cytostatic drugs for blocking the development of lesions in early stage or even in a pre-clinical phase, before that they are developed. Several studies are underway to demonstrate the anti-proliferative effect of these drugs.

7. Clinical, biochemical and instrumental monitoring of patients with hereditary NETs

Periodical evaluations in reference health centers are necessary in subjects with hereditary NETs in a pre-clinical phase (before the appearance of tumors), especially young subjects, to early detect tumors and prevent complications and risk of malignant transformation.

7.1. Multiple Endocrine Neoplasias

MEN1 patients and MEN1 carriers have to be monitored periodically.

The new guidelines for periodic clinical, biochemical and morphological monitoring of MEN1 patients is shown in Table 3 [106].

7.2. Familial paragangliomatosis

Patients with FPGL and SDHx carriers have to be monitored periodically to detect the presence of new lesions and to rule out a malignancy. Periodic clinical examination, laboratory tests measuring plasma free metanephrines, 24-hour urine catecholamines and metanephrines, imaging techniques including neck, skull base and abdomen/pelvis CT-scan and/or MRI and functional imaging techniques including somatostatin receptor scintigraphy and MIBG scintigraphy are mandatory in all patients with FPGL.

Tumor	Age to begin (yrs)	Biochemical tests annually	Imaging tests (time interval)
Parathyroid adenoma	8	Calcium, PTH	-
Gastrinoma	20	Gastrin	-
Insulinoma	5	Glucose, insulin	-
Other enteropancreatic NETs	10	CgA, PP, VIP, glucagon	MRI, CT or EUS (annually)
Anterior pituitary	5	PRL, IGF-1	MRI (every 3 yrs)
Foregut carcinoid	20	-	CT or MRI (every 1-2 yrs)

PTH: parathyroid hormone; CgA: chromogranin-A; PP: pancreatic polypeptide; VIP: vasoactive intestinal peptide; PRL: prolactin; IGF-1: insulin-like growth factor 1; MRI: magnetic resonance imaging; CT: computed tomography; EUS: echoendoscopy ultrasonography.

Table 3. Periodic clinical, biochemical and morphological monitoring of MEN1 patients

Author details

Antongiulio Faggiano[1,2], Valeria Ramundo[1], Luisa Circelli[2] and Annamaria Colao[1]

1 Department of Molecular and Clinical Endocrinology and Oncology, "Federico II" University of Naples, Italy

2 Endocrinology Unit, National Cancer Institute, Fondazione G. Pascale, Naples, Italy

References

[1] Karges. W, Adler G. [Clinical genetics of neuroendocrine tumors]. Med Klin (Munich). 2003 Dec 15;98(12):712-6

[2] Knudson AG Jr. Mutation and cancer: statistical study of retinoblastoma. Proc Natl Acad Sci U S A. 1971 Apr;68(4):820-3

[3] Marx S, Spiegel AM, Skarulis MC, Doppman JL, Collins FS, Liotta LA. Multiple endocrine neoplasia type 1: clinical and genetic topics. Ann Intern Med. 1998 Sep 15;129(6):484-94

[4] Ramundo V, Ercolino T, Faggiano A, Giachè V, Ragghianti B, Rapizzi E, Colao A, Mannelli M. Genetic-clinical profile of subjects with apparently sporadic extra-adrenal paragangliomas. Front Endocrinol (Lausanne). 2012;3:65.

[5] Ramundo V, Milone F, Severino R, Savastano S, Di Somma C, Vuolo L, De Luca L, Lombardi G, Colao A, Faggiano A. Clinical and prognostic implications of the genet-

ic diagnosis of hereditary NET syndromes in asymptomatic patients. Horm Metab Res. 2011 Oct;43(11):794-800

[6] Lourenco Jr DM, Toledo RA, Coutinho FL, Margarido LC, Siqueira SAC, Cortina MA, Montenegro FL, Machado MC, Toledo SP. The impact of clinical and genetic screenings on the management of the multiple endocrine neoplasia type 1. CLINICS 2007;62(4):465-76

[7] Pieterman CR, Schreinemakers JM, Koppeschaar HP, Vriens MR, Rinkes IH, Zonnenberg BA, van der Luijt RB, Valk GD. Multiple endocrine neoplasia type 1 (MEN1): its manifestations and effect of genetic screening on clinical outcome. Clin Endocrinol (Oxf). 2009 Apr;70(4):575-81.

[8] WERMER P. Genetic aspects of adenomatosis of endocrine glands. Am J Med. 1954 Mar;16(3):363-71

[9] Busygina V, Bale AE. Multiple Endocrine Neoplasia Type 1 (MEN1) as a Cancer Predisposition Syndrome: Clues into the Mechanisms of MEN1-related Carcinogenesis. Yale J Biol Med. 2006 Dec;79(3-4):105-14

[10] Brandi ML, Gagel RF, Angeli A, Bilezikian JP, Beck- Peccoz P, Bordi C, Conte-Devolx B, Falchetti A, Gheri RJ, Libroia A, Lips CJM, Lombardi G, Mannelli M, Pacini F, Ponder BAJ, Raue F, Skogseid B, Tamburano G, Thakker RH, Thompson NW, Tomassetti P, Tonelli F, Wells SA, Marx SJ. Guidelines for Diagnosis and Therapy of MEN Type 1 and Type 2. J Clin Endocrinol Metab 2001; 86:5658-5671

[11] Kouvaraki MA, Shapiro SE, Cote GJ, Lee JE, Yao JC, Waguespack SG, Gagel RF, Evans DB, Perrier ND. Management of pancreatic endocrine tumors in multiple endocrine neoplasia type 1. World J Surg. 2006 May;30(5):643-53.

[12] Anlauf M, Schlenger R, Perren A, Bauersfeld J, Koch CA, Dralle H, Raffel A, Knoefel WT, Weihe E, Ruszniewski P, Couvelard A, Komminoth P, Heitz PU, Klöppel G. Microadenomatosis of the endocrine pancreas in patients with and without the multiple endocrine neoplasia type 1 syndrome. Am J Surg Pathol. 2006 May;30(5):560-74.

[13] Akerström G, Hessman O, Hellman P, Skogseid B. Pancreatic tumours as part of the MEN-1 syndrome. Best Pract Res Clin Gastroenterol. 2005 Oct;19(5):819-30.

[14] Ciccarelli A, Daly AF, Beckers A. The epidemiology of prolactinomas. Pituitary. 2005;8(1):3-6.

[15] Raue F, Frank-Raue K. Multiple endocrine neoplasia type 2: 2007 update. Horm Res. 2007;68 Suppl 5:101-4.

[16] Romei C, Mariotti S, Fugazzola L, Taccaliti A, Pacini F, Opocher G, Mian C, Castellano M, degli Uberti E, Ceccherini I, Cremonini N, Seregni E, Orlandi F,Ferolla P, Puxeddu E, Giorgino F, Colao A, Loli P, Bondi F, Cosci B, Bottici V,Cappai A, Pinna G, Persani L, Verga U, Boscaro M, Castagna MG, Cappelli C,Zatelli MC, Faggiano A, Francia G, Brandi ML, Falchetti A, Pinchera A, Elisei R; ItaMEN network. Multiple

endocrine neoplasia type 2 syndromes (MEN2): resultsfrom the ItaMEN network analysis on the prevalence of different genotypes and phenotypes. Eur J Endocrinol. 2010 Aug;163(2):301-8.

[17] Mulligan LM, Marsh DJ, Robinson BG, Schuffenecker I, Zedenius J, Lips CJ, Gagel RF, Takai SI, Noll WW, Fink M, et al. Genotype-phenotype correlation in multiple endocrine neoplasia type 2: report of the International RET Mutation Consortium. J Intern Med. 1995 Oct;238(4):343-6

[18] Frank-Raue K, Rondot S, Raue F. Molecular genetics and phenomics of RET mutations: Impact on prognosis of MTC. Mol Cell Endocrinol. 2010 Jun30;322(1-2):2-7.

[19] Lenders JW, Pacak K, Eisenhofer G. New advances in the biochemical diagnosis of pheochromocytoma: moving beyond catecholamines. Ann N Y Acad Sci. 2002 Sep; 970:29-40.

[20] Sawka AM, Jaeschke R, Singh RJ, Young WF Jr. A comparison of biochemical tests for pheochromocytoma: measurement of fractionated plasma metanephrines compared with the combination of 24-hour urinary metanephrines and catecholamines. J Clin Endocrinol Metab. 2003 Feb;88(2):553-8.

[21] Maher ER, Eng C. The pressure rises: update on the genetics of phaeochromocytoma. Hum Mol Genet. 2002 Oct 1;11(20):2347-54

[22] Boedeker CC, Neumann HP, Offergeld C, Maier W, Falcioni M, Berlis A, Schipper J. Clinical features of paraganglioma syndromes. Skull Base. 2009 Jan;19(1):17-25

[23] Chandrasekharappa SC, Guru SC, Manickam P et al. Positional cloning of the gene for multiple endocrineneoplasia-type 1. Science 1997; 276(5311): 404–407.

[24] Zhuang Z, Vortmeyer AO, Pack S et al. Somatic mutations of the MEN1 tumor suppressor gene in sporadicgastrinomas and insulinomas. Cancer Research 1997; 57(21): 4682–4686.

[25] Moore PS, Missiaglia E, Antonello D et al. Role of disease-causing genes in sporadic pancreatic endocrine tumors: MEN1 and VHL. Genes, Chromosomes & Cancer 2001; 32(2): 177–181.

[26] Gortz B, Roth J, Krahenmann A et al. Mutations and allelic deletions of the MEN1 gene are associated with a subset of sporadic endocrine pancreatic and neuroendocrine tumors and not restricted to foregut neoplasms. The American Journal of Pathology 1999; 154(2): 429–436.

[27] Cupisti K, Hoppner W, Dotzenrath C et al. Lack of MEN1 gene mutations in 27 sporadic insulinomas. European Journal of Clinical Investigation 2000; 30(4): 325–329.

[28] Wang EH, Ebrahimi SA, Wu AY et al. Mutation of the MENIN gene in sporadic pancreatic endocrine tumors. Cancer Research 1998; 58(19): 4417–4420.

[29] Shan L, Nakamura Y, Nakamura M et al. Somatic mutations of multiple endocrine neoplasia type 1 gene in the sporadic endocrine tumors. Laboratory Investigation 1998; 78(4): 471–475.

[30] Yu F, Jensen RT, Lubensky IA et al. Survey of genetic alterations in gastrinomas. Cancer Research 2000; 60(19): 5536–5542.

[31] Goebel SU, Heppner C, Burns AL et al. Genotype/phenotype correlation of multiple endocrine neoplasia type 1 gene mutations in sporadic gastrinomas. The Journal of Clinical Endocrinology and Metabolism 2000; 85(1): 116–123.

[32] Perren A, Komminoth P & Heitz PU. Molecular genetics of gastroenteropancreatic endocrine tumors. Annals of the New York Academy of Sciences 2004; 1014: 199–208.

[33] Debelenko LV, Brambilla E, Agarwal SK et al. Identification of MEN1 gene mutations in sporadic carcinoidtumors of the lung. Human Molecular Genetics 1997; 6(13): 2285–2290.

[34] Agarwal SK, Guru SC, Heppner C et al. Menin interacts with the AP1 transcription factor JunD andrepresses JunD-activated transcription. Cell 1999; 96(1): 143–152.

[35] Gobl AE, Berg M, Lopez-Egido JR et al. Menin represses JunD-activated transcription by a histone deacetylase-dependent mechanism. Biochimica et Biophysica Acta 1999; 1447(1): 51–56.

[36] Milne TA, Hughes CM, Lloyd R et al. Menin and MLL cooperatively regulate expression of cyclin-dependent kinase inhibitors. Proceedings of the National Academy of Sciences of the United States of America 2005; 102(3):749–754.

[37] Karnik SK, Hughes CM, Gu X et al. Menin regulates pancreatic islet growth by promoting histone methylation and expression of genes encoding p27Kip1 and p18INK4c. Proceedings of the National Academy of Sciences of the United States of America 2005; 102(41): 14659–14664.

[38] Crabtree JS, Scacheri PC, Ward JM et al. A mouse model of multiple endocrine neoplasia, type 1, develops multiple endocrine tumors. Proceedings of the National Academy of Sciences of the United States of America 2001; 98(3): 1118–1123

[39] Franklin DS, Godfrey VL, O'Brien DA et al. Functional collaboration between different cyclin-dependent kinase inhibitors suppresses tumor growth with distinct tissue specificity. Molecular and Cellular Biology 2000; 20(16): 6147–6158.,

[40] MANABU HASHIMOTO1, SATORU KYO1, XIANXIN HUA3, HIDETOSHI TAHARA4, MIKI NAKAJIMA2 MASAHIRO TAKAKURA1, JUNKO SAKAGUCHI1, YOSHIKO MAIDA1, MITSUHIRO NAKAMURA1, TOMOMI IKOMA1, YASUNARI MIZUMOTO1 and MASAKI INOUE1 Role of menin in the regulation of telomerase activity in normal and cancer cells Int J Oncol2008 Aug;33(2):333-40

[41] Nuzzo V, Tauchmanová L, Falchetti A, Faggiano A, Marini F, Piantadosi S, Brandi ML, Leopaldi L, Colao A. MEN1 family with a novel frameshift mutation. J Endocrinol Invest. 2006 May;29(5):450-6

[42] Mulligan LM, Eng C, Healey CS, Clayton D, Kwok JBJ, Gardner E, et al. Specific mutations of the RET proto-oncogene are related to disease phenotype in MEN2A and FMTC. Nature Genet. 1994;6:70-4

[43] Mulligan LM, Kwok JBJ, Healey CS, Elsdon MJ, Eng C, Gardner E, et al. Germ-line mutations of the RET proto-oncogene in multiple endocrine neoplasia type 2A. Nature. 1993;363:458-60,

[44] Donis-Keller H, Dou S, Chi D, Carlson KM, Toshima K, Lairmore TC,et al. Mutations in the RET proto-oncogene are associated with MEN2A and FMTC. Hum Mol Genet. 1993;2(7):851-6,

[45] Kloos RT, Eng C, Evans DB, Francis GL, Gagel RF, Gharib H, et al. Medullary thyroid cancer: management guidelines of the American Thyroid Association. Thyroid. 2009;19(6):565-612

[46] Pachnis V, Mankoo B, Costantini F. Expression of the c-ret protooncogene during mouse embryogenesis. Development. 1993;119:1005-17.

[47] Attie-Bitach T, Abitbol M, Gerard M, Delezoide AL, Auge J, Pelet A, et al. Expression of the RET proto-oncogene in human embryos. Am J Med Genet. 1998;80(5):481-6

[48] Takahashi M, Cooper G. ret transforming gene encodes a fusion protein homologous to tyrosine kinases. Mol Cell Biol. 1987;7:1378-85.

[49] Takahashi M, Buma Y, Iwamoto T, Inaguma Y, Ikeda H, Hiai H. Cloning and expression of the ret proto-oncogene encoding a tyrosine kinase with two potential transmembrane domains. Oncogene. 1988;3:571-8

[50] Hanks SK, Quinn AM, Hunter T. The protein kinase family: conservedfeatures and deduced phylogeny of the catalytic domains. Science.1988;241(4861):42-52

[51] Parkash V, Leppanen VM, Virtanen H, Jurvansuu JM, Bespalov MM, Sidorova YA, et al. The structure of the glial cell line derived neurotrophic factor-coreceptor complex: insights into RET signalling and heparin binding. J Biol Chem. 2008;283(50):35164-72

[52] Schlee S, Carmillo P, Whitty A. Quantitative analysis of the activation mechanism of the multicomponent growth-factor receptor Ret. Nat Chem Biol. 2006;2(11):636-44

[53] Staubach S, Hanisch FG. Lipid rafts: signaling and sorting platforms of cells and their roles in cancer. Expert Rev Proteomics. 2011;8(2):263-77

[54] Arighi E, Borrello MG, Sariola H. RET tyrosine kinase signaling in development and cancer. Cytokine and Growth Factor Reviews. 2005;16:441-67

[55] Plaza-Menacho I, Morandi A, Mologni L, Boender P, Gambacorti- Passerini C, Magee AI, et al. Focal adhesion kinase (FAK) binds RET kinase via its FERM domain, pri-

ming a direct and reciprocal RET-FAK transactivation mechanism. J Biol Chem. 2011;286(19):17292-302

[56] Margraf RL, Crockett DK, Krautscheid PM, Seamons R, Calderon FR, Wittwer CT, et al. Multiple endocrine neoplasia type 2 RET protooncogene database: repository of MEN2-associated RET sequence variation and reference for genotype/phenotype correlations. HumMutat. 2009;30(4):548-56

[57] Machens A, Dralle H. Familial prevalence and age of RET germline mutations: implications for screening. Clin Endocrinol (Oxf). 2008;69(1):81-7

[58] Raue F, Frank-Raue K. Update multiple endocrine neoplasia type 2. Fam Cancer. 2010;9(3):449-57

[59] Richards ML. Thyroid cancer genetics: multiple endocrine neoplasia type 2, non-medullary familial thyroid cancer, and familial syndromes associated with thyroid cancer. Surg Oncol Clin N Am. 2009;18(1):39-52

[60] Berndt I, Reuter M, Saller B, Frank-Raue K, Groth P, Grussendorf M, et al. A new hot spot for mutations in the ret protooncogene causing familial medullary thyroid carcinoma and multiple endocrine neoplasia type 2A. J Clin Endocrinol Metab. 1998;83(3): 770-4

[61] Machens A, Dralle H. Pheochromocytoma penetrance varies by RET mutation in MEN2A. Surgery. 2008;143(5):696

[62] Eng C, Clayton D, Schuffenecker I, Lenoir G, Cote G, Gagel RF, et al. The relationship between specific RET proto-oncogene mutations and disease phenotype in multiple endocrine neoplasia type 2: International RET Mutation Consortium. JAMA. 1996;276:1575-9

[63] Yip L, Cote GJ, Shapiro SE, Ayers GD, Herzog CE, Sellin RV, et al. Multiple endocrine neoplasia type 2: evaluation of the genotypephenotype relationship. Arch Surg. 2003;138(4):409-16.

[64] Quayle FJ, Fialkowski EA, Benveniste R, Moley JF. Pheochromocytoma penetrance varies by RET mutation in MEN2A. Surgery. 2007;142(6):800- 5

[65] Szinnai G, Meier C, Komminoth P, Zumsteg UW. Review of multiple endocrine neoplasia type 2A in children: therapeutic results of early thyroidectomy and prognostic value of codon analysis. Pediatrics. 2003;111(2):E132-9

[66] Punales MK, Graf H, Gross JL, Maia AL. RET codon 634 mutations in multiple endocrine neoplasia type 2: variable clinical features and clinical outcome. J Clin Endocrinol Metab. 2003;88(6):2644-9

[67] Rodriguez JM, Balsalobre M, Ponce JL, Rios A, Torregrosa NM, Tebar J, et al. Pheochromocytoma in MEN2A syndrome. Study of 54 patients. World J Surg. 2008;32(11): 2520-6

[68] Amar L, Bertherat J, Baudin E, Ajzenberg C, Bressac-de Paillerets B, Chabre O, Chamontin B, Delemer B, Giraud S, Murat A, Niccoli-Sire P, Richard S, Rohmer V, Sadoul JL, Strompf L, Schlumberger M, Bertagna X, Plouin PF, Jeunemaitre X, Gimenez-Roqueplo AP. Genetic testing in pheochromocytoma or functional paraganglioma. J Clin Oncol. 2005 Dec 1;23(34):8812-8

[69] Mannelli M, Castellano M, Schiavi F, Filetti S, Giacchè M, Mori L, Pignataro V, Bernini G, Giachè V, Bacca A, Biondi B, Corona G, Di Trapani G, Grossrubatscher E, Reimondo G, Arnaldi G, Giacchetti G, Veglio F, Loli P, Colao A, Ambrosio MR, Terzolo M, Letizia C, Ercolino T, Opocher G; Italian Pheochromocytoma/Paraganglioma Network. Clinically guided genetic screening in a large cohort of italian patients with pheochromocytomas and/or functional or nonfunctional paragangliomas. J Clin Endocrinol Metab. 2009 May;94(5):1541-7

[70] Schlisio S, Kenchappa RS, Vredeveld LC, George RE, Stewart R, Greulich H, Shahriari K, Nguyen NV, Pigny P, Dahia PL, Pomeroy SL, Maris JM, Look AT, Meyerson M, Peeper DS, Carter BD, Kaelin WG Jr. The kinesin KIF1Bbeta acts downstream from EglN3 to induce apoptosis and is a potential 1p36 tumor suppressor. Genes Dev. 2008 Apr 1;22(7):884-93

[71] Ladroue C, Carcenac R, Leporrier M, Gad S, Le Hello C, Galateau-Salle F, Feunteun J, Pouysségur J, Richard S, Gardie B. PHD2 mutation and congenital erythrocytosis with paraganglioma. N Engl J Med. 2008 Dec 18;359(25):2685-92.

[72] Qin Y, Yao L, King EE, Buddavarapu K, Lenci RE, Chocron ES, Lechleiter JD, Sass M, Aronin N, Schiavi F, Boaretto F, Opocher G, Toledo RA, Toledo SP, Stiles C, Aguiar RC, Dahia PL. Germline mutations in TMEM127 confer susceptibility to pheochromocytoma. Nat Genet. 2010 Mar;42(3):229-33.

[73] Comino-Méndez I, Gracia-Aznárez FJ, Schiavi F, Landa I, Leandro-García LJ, Letón R, Honrado E, Ramos-Medina R, Caronia D, Pita G, Gómez-Graña A, de Cubas AA, Inglada-Pérez L, Maliszewska A, Taschin E, Bobisse S, Pica G, Loli P, Hernández-Lavado R, Díaz JA, Gómez-Morales M, González-Neira A, Roncador G, Rodríguez-Antona C, Benítez J, Mannelli M, Opocher G, Robledo M, Cascón A. Exome sequencing identifies MAX mutations as a cause of hereditary pheochromocytoma. Nat Genet. 2011 Jun 19;43(7):663-7

[74] Gimenez-Roqueplo AP, Favier J, Rustin P, Rieubland C, Crespin M, Nau V, Khau Van Kien P, Corvol P, Plouin PF, Jeunemaitre X; COMETE Network. Mutations in the SDHB gene are associated with extra-adrenal and/or malignant phaeochromocytomas. Cancer Res. 2003 Sep 1;63(17):5615-21

[75] Rutter J, Winge DR, Schiffman JD Succinate dehydrogenase - Assembly, regulation and role in human disease.Mitochondrion. 2010 Jun;10(4):393-401.

[76] Baysal BE, Ferrell RE, Willett-Brozick JE, Lawrence EC, Myssiorek D, Bosch A, van der Mey A, Taschner PE, Rubinstein WS, Myers EN, Richard CW 3rd, Cornelisse CJ,

Devilee P, Devlin B. Mutations in SDHD, a mitochondrial complex II gene, in hereditary paraganglioma. Science. 2000 Feb 4;287(5454):848-51

[77] Gimmo O, Armanios M, Dziema H, Neumann HP, Eng C. Somatic and occult germline mutations in SDHD, a mitochondrial complex II gene, in nonfamilial pheochromocytoma. Cancer Res. 2000 Dec 15;60(24):6822-5.

[78] Dannenberg H, Dinjens WN, Abbou M, Van Urk H, Pauw BK, Mouwen D, Mooi WJ, de Krijger RR. Frequent germ-line succinate dehydrogenase subunit D gene mutations in patients with apparently sporadic parasympathetic paraganglioma. Clin Cancer Res. 2002 Jul;8(7):2061-6.

[79] Astuti D, Latif F, Dallol A, Dahia PL, Douglas F, George E, Sköldberg F, Husebye ES, Eng C, Maher ER. Gene mutations in the succinate dehydrogenase subunit SDHB cause susceptibility to familial pheochromocytoma and to familial paraganglioma. Am J Hum Genet. 2001 Jul;69(1):49-54.

[80] Astuti D, Douglas F, Lennard TW, Aligianis IA, Woodward ER, Evans DG, Eng C, Latif F, Maher ER. Germline SDHD mutation in familial phaeochromocytoma. Lancet. 2001 Apr 14;357(9263):1181-2.

[81] Niemann S, Müller U. Mutations in SDHC cause autosomal dominant paraganglioma, type 3. Nat Genet. 2000 Nov;26(3):268-70

[82] Peczkowska M, Cascon A, Prejbisz A, Kubaszek A, Cwikła BJ, Furmanek M, Erlic Z, Eng C, Januszewicz A, Neumann HP. Extra-adrenal and adrenal pheochromocytomas associated with a germline SDHC mutation. Nat Clin Pract Endocrinol Metab. 2008 Feb;4(2):111-5

[83] van der Mey AG, Maaswinkel-Mooy PD, Cornelisse CJ, Schmidt PH, van de Kamp JJ. Genomic imprinting in hereditary glomus tumours: evidence for new genetic theory. Lancet. 1989 Dec 2;2(8675):1291-4

[84] Pigny P, Vincent A, Cardot Bauters C, Bertrand M, de Montpreville VT, Crepin M, Porchet N, Caron P. Paraganglioma after maternal transmission of a succinate dehydrogenase gene mutation. J Clin Endocrinol Metab. 2008 May;93(5):1609-15

[85] Kunst HP, Rutten MH, de Mönnink JP, Hoefsloot LH, Timmers HJ, Marres HA, Jansen JC, Kremer H, Bayley JP, Cremers CW. SDHAF2 (PGL2-SDH5) and hereditary head and neck paraganglioma. Clin Cancer Res. 2011 Jan 15;17(2):247-54

[86] Burnichon N, Brière JJ, Libé R, Vescovo L, Rivière J, Tissier F, Jouanno E, Jeunemaitre X, Bénit P, Tzagoloff A, Rustin P, Bertherat J, Favier J, Gimenez-Roqueplo AP. SDHA is a tumor suppressor gene causing paraganglioma. Hum Mol Genet. 2010 Aug 1;19(15):3011-20

[87] Korpershoek E, Favier J, Gaal J, Burnichon N, van Gessel B, Oudijk L, Badoual C, Gadessaud N, Venisse A, Bayley JP, van Dooren MF, de Herder WW, Tissier F, Plouin PF, van Nederveen FH, Dinjens WN, Gimenez-Roqueplo AP, de Krijger RR. SDHA

immunohistochemistry detects germline SDHA gene mutations in apparently sporadic paragangliomas and pheochromocytomas. J Clin Endocrinol Metab. 2011Sep; 96(9):E1472-6

[88] Neumann HP, Pawlu C, Peczkowska M, Bausch B, McWhinney SR, Muresan M, Buchta M, Franke G, Klisch J, Bley TA, Hoegerle S, Boedeker CC, Opocher G, Schipper J, Januszewicz A, Eng C; European-American Paraganglioma Study Group. Distinct clinical features of paraganglioma syndromes associated with SDHB and SDHD gene mutations. JAMA. 2004 Aug 25;292(8):943-51

[89] Ricketts CJ, Forman JR, Rattenberry E, Bradshaw N, Lalloo F, Izatt L, Cole TR, Armstrong R, Kumar VK, Morrison PJ, Atkinson AB, Douglas F, Ball SG, Cook J, Srirangalingam U, Killick P, Kirby G, Aylwin S, Woodward ER, Evans DG, Hodgson SV, Murday V, Chew SL, Connell JM, Blundell TL, Macdonald F, Maher ER. Tumor risks and genotype-phenotype-proteotype analysis in 358 patients with germline mutations in SDHB and SDHD. Hum Mutat. 2010 Jan;31(1):41-51

[90] Pantaleo MA, Astolfi A, Indio V, Moore R, Thiessen N, Heinrich MC, Gnocchi C, Santini D, Catena F, Formica S, Martelli PL, Casadio R, Pession A, Biasco G. SDHA loss-of-function mutations in KIT-PDGFRA wild-type gastrointestinal stromal tumors identified by massively parallel sequencing. J Natl Cancer Inst. 2011 Jun 22;103(12):983-7

[91] Benn DE, Robinson BG. Genetic basis of phaeochromocytoma and paraganglioma. Best Pract Res Clin Endocrinol Metab. 2006 Sep;20(3):435-50

[92] Burnichon N, Rohmer V, Amar L, Herman P, Leboulleux S, Darrouzet V, Niccoli P, Gaillard D, Chabrier G, Chabolle F, Coupier I, Thieblot P, Lecomte P, Bertherat J, Wion-Barbot N, Murat A, Venisse A, Plouin PF, Jeunemaitre X, Gimenez-Roqueplo AP; PGL.NET network. The succinate dehydrogenase genetic testing in a large prospective series of patients with paragangliomas. J Clin Endocrinol Metab. 2009 Aug; 94(8):2817-27

[93] Dahia PL, Hao K, Rogus J, Colin C, Pujana MA, Ross K, Magoffin D, Aronin N, Cascon A, Hayashida CY, Li C, Toledo SP, Stiles CD; Familial Pheochromocytoma Consortium. Novel pheochromocytoma susceptibility loci identified by integrative genomics. Cancer Res. 2005 Nov 1;65(21):9651-8

[94] Jiang S, Dahia PL. Minireview: the busy road to pheochromocytomas and paragangliomas has a new member, TMEM127. Endocrinology. 2011 Jun;152(6):2133-40

[95] Yao L, Schiavi F, Cascon A, Qin Y, Inglada-Pérez L, King EE, Toledo RA, Ercolino T, Rapizzi E, Ricketts CJ, Mori L, Giacchè M, Mendola A, Taschin E, Boaretto F, Loli P, Iacobone M, Rossi GP, Biondi B, Lima-Junior JV, Kater CE, Bex M, Vikkula M, Grossman AB, Gruber SB, Barontini M, Persu A, Castellano M, Toledo SP, Maher ER, Mannelli M, Opocher G, Robledo M, Dahia PL. Spectrum and prevalence of FP/TMEM127 gene mutations in pheochromocytomas and paragangliomas. JAMA. 2010 Dec 15;304(23):2611-9

[96] Burnichon N, Lepoutre-Lussey C, Laffaire J, Gadessaud N, Molinié V, Hernigou A, Plouin PF, Jeunemaitre X, Favier J, Gimenez-Roqueplo AP. A novel TMEM127 mutation in a patient with familial bilateral pheochromocytoma. Eur J Endocrinol.2011 Jan;164(1):141-5

[97] Neumann HP, Sullivan M, Winter A, Malinoc A, Hoffmann MM, Boedeker CC, Bertz H, Walz MK, Moeller LC, Schmid KW, Eng C. Germline mutations of the TMEM127 gene in patients with paraganglioma of head and neck and extraadrenal abdominal sites. J Clin Endocrinol Metab. 2011 Aug;96(8):E1279-82

[98] Grandori C, Cowley SM, James LP, Eisenman RN. The Myc/Max/Mad network and the transcriptional control of cell behavior. Annu Rev Cell Dev Biol. 2000;16:653-99

[99] Hopewell R, Ziff EB. The nerve growth factor-responsive PC12 cell line does not express the Myc dimerization partner Max. Mol Cell Biol. 1995 Jul;15(7):3470-8

[100] Faggiano A, Tavares LB, Tauchmanova L, Milone F, Mansueto G, Ramundo V, De Caro ML, Lombardi G, De Rosa G, Colao A. Effect of treatment with depot somatostatin analogue octreotide on primary hyperparathyroidism (PHP) in multiple endocrine neoplasia type 1 (MEN1) patients. Clin Endocrinol (Oxf). 2008 Nov;69(5):756-62

[101] Falchetti A, Cilotti A, Vaggelli L, Masi L, Amedei A, Cioppi F, Tonelli F, Brandi ML. A patient with MEN1-associated hyperparathyroidism, responsive to cinacalcet. Nat Clin Pract Endocrinol Metab. 2008 Jun;4(6):351-7

[102] Young WF Jr. Paragangliomas: clinical overview. Ann N Y Acad Sci. 2006 Aug; 1073:21-9

[103] Erlic Z, Neumann HP. Familial pheochromocytoma. Hormones (Athens). 2009 Jan-Mar;8(1):29-38

[104] Joshua AM, Ezzat S, Asa SL, Evans A, Broom R, Freeman M, Knox JJ. Rationale and evidence for sunitinib in the treatment of malignant paraganglioma/ pheochromocytoma. J Clin Endocrinol Metab. 2009 Jan;94(1):5-9

[105] Boedeker CC, Neumann HP, Offergeld C, Maier W, Falcioni M, Berlis A, Schipper J. Clinical features of paraganglioma syndromes. Skull Base. 2009 Jan;19(1):17-25

[106] Thakker RV, Newey PJ, Walls GV, Bilezikian J, Dralle H, Ebeling PR, Melmed S, Sakurai A, Tonelli F, Brandi ML. Clinical Practice Guidelines for Multiple Endocrine Neoplasia Type 1 (MEN1). J Clin Endocrinol Metab. 2012 Sep;97(9):2990-3011

Chapter 2

New Insights in the Pathogenesis of Pituitary Tumours

Marie-Lise Jaffrain-Rea, Sandra Rotondi and
Edoardo Alesse

Additional information is available at the end of the chapter

http://dx.doi.org/10.5772/56028

1. Introduction

Pituitary adenomas (PA) are frequent and typically benign endocrine neoplasia, which clinical prevalence is estimated around 1/1000 inhabitants [1]. The vast majority are sporadic. PA are endowed with significant clinical morbidity related to hormonal hypersecretion, neurological symptoms due to intracranial mass effects or invasion of the surrounding structures and/or secondary hypopituitarism. Their evolution is quite variable, ranging from indolent tumours with an extremely slow growing potential, to recurrent, aggressive, and exceptionally malignant tumours. Their current clinical management is based on pharmacological treatment, mainly dopamine-agonists (DA) and somatostatin analogues (SSA), surgery and radiotherapy [2]. Despite considerable progress in the management of PA, a significant subset of patients are not satisfactorily controlled. Long-term uncontrolled pituitary hormone hypersecretion, leading to potential severe systemic diseases, and tumour recurrence or aggressiveness still represent a difficult clinical challenge. Understanding the mechanisms involved in the pathogenesis of PA is essential for the development of new therapeutic strategies. In this chapter, we will summarize current concepts in pituitary tumorigenesis and focus our attention on the most recent insights and new perspectives in this field.

2. Pituitary tumours

Primary pituitary tumours in human are mainly represented by PA arising from endocrine cells in the anterior lobe and craniopharyngiomas. These latter are divided into adamanti-nomatous, which derive from the Rathke's pouch, and papillary craniopharyngiomas.

Additional tumour types deriving from non-endocrine cells of the anterior pituitary and the neurophypohysis can be found [3], which pathogenesis is poorly known and will not be considered in this review.

2.1. Classification

PA may be classified according to their macroscopic characteristics into micro- (< 1 cm) or macro-adenomas (≥ 1 cm), and enclosed or invasive adenomas. Invasion of the surrounding structures (cavernous sinuses, bone, sphenoidal sinus) is generally defined according to neuroradiological imaging – especially magnetic resonance imaging -, although intra-operative findings may introduce some correction to the pre-operative radiological classification or reveal macroscopic dural invasion. Of note, microscopic evidence of dural invasion is rarely present on surgical samples. The functional classification of PA is based on their hormone-secreting potential, which may be associated with bio-clinical evidence of hormone hypersecretion or recognized by immunohistochemistry (IHC) for pituitary hormones and/or by specific ultrastructural features. From an epidemiological point of view, prolactinomas are by far the most frequent (50-60%), followed by clinically non-functioning PA (NFPA) (20-30%), somatotrophinomas (10-15%), corticotrophinomas (5-10%) and thyreotrophinomas (1-2%) [1,2,4]. Recruitment bias are frequently encountered in pathological series, since most prolactinomas are treated by DA only. Clinico-pathological correlations in PA have been recently reviewed [4]. In the large majority of PA associated with bio-clinical evidence of hormone secretion, except functional hyperprolactinemia, pathological examination will confirm the diagnosis of PRL, GH, ACTH or TSH-secreting tumours and potentially identify bi- or multi-hormonal secretion. This is especially true for GH-secreting PA, which may also secrete PRL, less frequently glycoprotein hormones, or both (multihormonal). TSH-secreting adenomas are rare and frequently multihormonal. Ultrastructural studies of secreting PA may disclose a "densely granulated" (DG) or "sparsely granulated" (SG) pattern, which may reflect significant differences in hormone secretion and tumour behaviour. This has been well studied in somatotrophinomas, where IHC for cytokeratin can be used to disclose the typical "dot-like" staining pattern of SG adenomas. Although a continuum exists between the SG and DG types, pure SG are typically more aggressive than DG somatotrophinomas [5]. Pathological examination of NFPA may show negative immunostaining for all pituitary hormones (the "null cell" or endocrine inactive histotype), positive immunostaining for FSH and/or LH (gonadotrophinomas) or reveal silent secretion of other pituitary hormones, in particular ACTH and GH ("silent" secreting PA). Cell lineage may also be identified by the expression of specific transcription factors (see "pituitary ontogenesis") [4]. It is generally accepted that most NFPA derive from the gonadotroph lineage, since data obtained from primary cultures or molecular analysis of these tumours frequently reveal a silent expression of gonadotropins or their subunits, including α–subunit only. Also, transgenic mice overexpressing SV40 under the control of the βFSH promoter develop gonadotroph hyperplasia and PA with reduced gonadotropin immunoreactivity and ultrastructural characteristics similar to human null cell PA [6]. Silent corticotroph adenomas are commonly aggressive and different subtypes have been described. Pituitary carcinomas are strictly defined by the presence of extra-pituitary dissemination (see "pituitary carcinomas"). Therefore, no diagnosis of pituitary carcinoma can be made on a surgical pituitary sample. Considerable efforts have been made to recognize the aggressive potential of PA according to pathological criteria. However, mitoses are generally rare and the percentage of cells immunopositive for the Ki67 antigen (which is expressed throughout the cell cycle and detected with the MIB1 monoclonal antibody) is currently considered as the best marker of cell proliferation. A Ki67 index ≥3% is commonly associated with invasiveness [4], although it can be reduced by pre-operative pharmacological treatment in secreting PA [7]. Immunostaining for p53 is also frequently associated with invasiveness and is typically present in carcinomas [4]. For these reasons, the 2004 WHO conference has proposed to define as "atypical adenomas" a subset of invasive PA characterized by Ki67 labelling ≥ 3% and extensive p53 nuclear staining [8]. However, many criticisms remain and search for reliable markers of aggressiveness or malignancy is going on. Gene expression profiling comparing non-invasive adenomas with their invasive counterpart [9, 10] or with pituitary carcinomas [11] represents a promising approach.

2.2. Origin

The pathogenesis of PA is multifactorial. Traditionally, two theories have been proposed: the primary pituitary origin, and the hypothalamic origin of PA or, more generally speaking, the concept that PA may derive from abnormal pituitary regulation. Acromegaly or Cushing's disease resulting from ectopic secretion of GHRH or CRH by neuroendocrine tumours, respectively, or estrogen-induced prolactinomas, represent the main evidence for the second theory. However, the chief lesion in such conditions is hyperplasia, with PA developing in a very minority of cases, whereas hyperplasia is exceptionally observed surrounding the tumoral tissue in human PA. Although hyperplasia may be difficult to identify (reticulin staining is not routinely proposed), there is accumulating evidence supporting the primary pituitary origin of PA. Indeed, PA are essentially monoclonal in origin, and a number of genetic abnormalities have been identified these tumours, which include somatic events and inherited predisposition. The relatively low rate of recurrences following complete surgical removal of enclosed PA, especially microadenomas, also favours a primary pituitary hypothesis. However, polyclonality can also be observed on PA, and different clones may develop in a synchronous or delayed pattern, possibly accounting for tumour progression or regrowth [12]. A unifying view is that pituitary tumorigenesis is a multistep and multifactorial process, which includes early initiating genetic events, growth promotion by extracellular factors (including the extracellular matrix, growth factors, cytokines, neuropeptides and peripheral hormones) and additional genetic events contributing to a further progression of the tumour in terms of invasiveness, recurrences and, exceptionally, metastasis [13,14].

3. Pituitary developmental pathways and their potential alterations in pituitary tumours

Because the expanding knowledge about the molecular mechanisms involved in pituitary ontogenesis is providing new clues in the understanding of pituitary tumorigenesis, relevant findings in this field will be summarized.

3.1. Ontogenesis of the pituitary gland

The anterior pituitary lobe (AP) derives from an invagination of the oral ectoderm forming the Rathke's pouch (RP), which cells proliferate and subsequently undergo progressive terminal differentiation into the 5 adult pituitary cell types (corticotrophs; somatotrophs, lactotrophs, gonadotrophs and thyreotrophs), whereas the posterior lobe (or neurohypophysis) derives from a specialized region of the neuroectoderm, the infundibulum. The intermediate lobe also arises from the RP and contains melanotrophs in rodents but is virtually absent in humans. The molecular mechanisms of pituitary ontogenesis have been mainly studied in the mouse and, in addition to genetic models which have contributed to elucidate the role of single proteins [6], analysis of transcriptomes obtained from cDNA libraries in the developing embryo represents a promising tool to identify new genes involved in this process [15,16]. Complex interactions between signalling molecules (in particular opposite signals coming from the diencephalon and the ventral ectoderm) and pituitary transcriptions factors (TFs) are involved and tightly regulated in a spatially and temporally organised manner. Extensive reviews are available on this topic [17,18]. Genetic defects in pituitary TFs are responsible for inherited abnormalities in pituitary development, spanning from syndromic diseases due to defects in early factors (*eg*. Pitx2, Lhx3/4, Hesx1) to multiple pituitary hormone deficiency (*eg* Prop-1, *Pit-1*) or single hormone deficiency (*eg*. Tpit) [16]. Noteworthy, some of these defects are associated with transient pituitary hyperplasia. On the other hand, abnormal signalling from developmental molecules such as FGFs, BMPs, and master developing pathways (Wnt Hedgehog, Notch) is being increasingly recognized in PA. Table 1 summarizes the potential involvement of developmental TFs and signalling molecules in PA. Overall, the expression of TFs involved in the terminal differentiation of pituitary cells (*eg*. Pit-1, Tpit) is maintained in functioning PA and may contribute to identify the original cell lineage in NFPA [4,19]. However, a phenotypic marker may not be fully specific, as reported for NeuroD1, which is frequently expressed in NFPA in addition to corticotrophinomas [20]. Early to intermediate pituitary TFs such as Hesx1, Pitx1 and PROP1 are expressed in the adult pituitary gland and in all PA [21-23]. PROP1 represses *Hesx1* expression while up-regulating that of *Pit-1* and *SF1* and *Prop-1* transgenic mice develop different PA phenotypes, except corticotrophinomas [24]. Pitx2, which is required at different stages of pituitary development, is expressed in the normal pituitary, in PRL- and TSH-secreting PA and selectively overexpressed in NFPA [22]. FOXL2 is also expressed in the adult pituitary and overexpressed in gonadotroph and NFPA [25].

Gene	Expression during ontogenesis	Function	Expression in pituitary tumours
Early signalling molecules in pituitary development			
BMPs (BMP 2 and 4)	VD	BMP4: essential for the invagination of Rathke's pouch; BMP2*:* involved in opposing gradients with FGF8 that generate distinct patterns of transcription factors expression	BMP4: overexpressed in prolactinomas, underexpressed in corticotrophinomas
FGFs (FGF 8 and 10)	VD/RP	FGF10 : essential for cell survival FGF8: involved in the maintenance of RP cells proliferation opposing gradients with BMP2	NA
WNT4 and 5A/ β-catenin	VD/RP	Involved in pituitary development and in the induction of *Pit-1*	Wnt4 : expressed in GH/PRL/TSH-secreting PA
Shh/*Gli2*	VD; oral ectoderm except RP	Involved in early proliferation and cell type determination as well as in the control of adult pituitary cell function and proliferation	Shh: underexpressed in PA, including corticotrophinomas
Notch 2 and 3	VD/RP	Required for early lineage commitment and the terminal differentiation of distinct cell lineages	Notch3: overexpressed in NFPA
Sox2	VD/RP	Required for pituitary development and the maintenance or proliferation of pituitary progenitor cells	Expressed in adamantinomatous craniopharyngiomas
Transcriptional factors that control pituitary development			
Hesx1	VD/RP	Involved in early pituitary development	Expressed in all PA phenotypes
Otx2	RP	Involved in RP development, in particular in the expression of *Hesx1*	NA
Lhx3-4	RP	Required for cell survival and prevention of apoptosis	NA
Isl1	RP	Required for the proliferation and differentiation of pituitary progenitors	NA
Six 1, 3 and 6	RP	Six1 regulates cell proliferation; Six6 is required for pituitary development and cell proliferation; Six3 interacts with Hesx1	NA
Pitx 1 and 2	RP	Pitx1 e Pitx2 activate the early transcription of the *aGSU* gene, while promoting cell proliferation, then they	Pitx1: expressed in all PA phenotypes Pitx2: overexpressed in NFPA

Gene	Expression during ontogenesis	Function	Expression in pituitary tumours
		activate *LHβ, FSHβ, GnRH, PRL* and *GH* gene transcription, while promoting cell differentiation Pitx1 also binds the *POMC* promoter	
FOXL2	AP	A transcriptional activator of *αGSU*	Overexpressed in NFPA
Corticotroph differentiation			
NeuroD1	RP	A transcriptional activator of *POMC,* involved in corticotroph differentiation	Expressed in corticotrophinomas and a subset of NFPA
Tpit	POMC precursor	A transcriptional activator of *POMC,* essential for the specification and terminal differentiation of corticotrophs and melanotrophs,	Expressed in secreting and silent corticotrophinomas
Differentiation of Pit-1 lineages: somatotroph, lactotroph and thyreotroph differentiation			
Prop1	RP	A transcriptional activator of *Pit-1* and a trascriptional repressor of *Hesx1*	Expressed in all PA phenotypes
Gata2	RP	Interacts and cooperates with *Pit-1* for the activation of *TSHβ*	Expressed essentially in gonadotroph and thyreotroph PA
Pit-1	Pit-1 lineages	Essential for the terminal differentiation and expansion of GH/PRL/TSH-secreting cells; an enhancer of *GH, PRL, TSHβ* e *GHRHR* gene expression and a repressor of *Gata2*	Expressed in GH/PRL/TSH-secreting PA (including NFPA with silent secretion)
CREB	Pit-1 lineages	Required in somatotrophs	Expressed in all somatotrophinomas
Gonadotroph differentiation			
Gata2	RP/pituitary	A promoter of *SF1* gene expression	See above
SF1	Gonadotrope	A promoter of *αGSU, FSHβ, GnRHR* gene expression, it also interacts with Egr1 and Pitx1 for the activation of LHβ	Expressed in the majority of gonadotroph/ NFPA, not in GH/PRL-secreting PA
Egr1	Gonadotrope	Required for *LHβ* gene expression	NA

Table 1. Expression of pituitary developmental signalling molecules and TFs

3.2. Developmental pathways in pituitary adenomas

Three master developmental pathways – Wnt, Hedgehog and Notch – have been involved in several human diseases, in particular in cancer. We will attempt to summarize current knowledge about their role in pituitary development and tumorigenesis, which is likely to expand significantly in the next years.

3.2.1. *The Wnt/beta-catenin pathway*

The canonical Wnt/β-catenin signalling pathway plays a role in the specification of pituitary progenitor/stem cells and β-catenin modulates the transcriptional activity of several pituitary TFs, in particular Pitx2, PROP-1 (thereby promoting the activation of *Pit-1* and the repression of *Hesx1*) and SF1 [26]. Wnt4 and Wnt5a have been involved in pituitary development and growth, respectively. Wnt signalling has also been recently involved in the pathogenesis of craniopharyngiomas [27-30] and PA [26]. Briefly, secreted Wnt proteins bind the Frizzled (Fz)/ Lipoprotein low-density receptor (LPR) membrane complex on the cell surface of target cells, inducing an intracellular reponse mediated by Dishevelled (Dsh), the glycogen synthase kinase 3β (GSK-3β), Adenomatous Polypous Coli (APC), axin and β-catenin. In the absence of Wnt ligands, the GSK-3/APC/axin complex drives phosphorylated β–catenin to proteasome-mediated degradation and Wnt signalling is repressed. In the presence of Wnt ligands, the inhibition of β–catenin phosphorylation leads to its cytoplasmic accumulation, nuclear localization and activation of Wnt target genes (*eg cyclin D, c-myc, survivin*). Wnt signalling is modulated by several secreted Wnt inhibitors and further regulated by adhesion molecules (*eg.* E-cadherin) and extra-cellular signalling pathways (*eg.* FGF). Beta-catenin mutants lacking phosphorylation sites are able to activate Wnt signalling in a constitutive manner. Activating mutations of the β–catenin gene (*cadherin-associated protein β1/CTNNB1*) have been reported in several human neoplasias and in adamantinomatous craniopharyngiomas (ACPs) [27]. Although the prevalence of *CTNNB1* mutations has been variably appreciated in craniopharyngiomas, they are specific for the ACP phenotype and consist of amino acid substitution of GSK-3β phosphorylation site or flanking residues [28, 29]. Their causative role in the development of ACPs has been recently proven in a transgenic mice model [30]. *CTNNB1* mutations are exceptional in PA, but several members of the Wnt signalling pathway have been detected at a transcriptional level [26]. Studies on β-catenin expression and localization in PA have lead to conflicting results, some studies reporting a nuclear accumulation in a variable proportion of cases (0-57%) and others a predominant membrane staining with a frequent cytoplasmic immunopositivity [26]. A reduced expression of several Wnt inhibitors has been reported in PA [31]. Among them, WIF1 is a tumour suppressor, which reduced protein expression was predominantly reported in NFPA, although transcriptional down-regulation is common in all histotypes [31].

3.2.2. *Sonic hedgehog*

Sonic hedgehog (Shh) is involved in pituitary ontogenesis and regulates pituitary hormone release. Shh signalling is mediated by Patched receptors (Ptc1, Ptc2) and the Gli family of TFs. During ontogenesis, Shh is expressed by the ventral diencephalon and by the oral ectoderm immediately adjacent to RP. There is recent evidence that Shh signalling is of particular importance before the RP detachs from the oral ectoderm, and that Gli2 is responsible for the proliferation of early pituitary progenitors and for the diencephalic induction of FGF8 and

BMP4 [32]. This is consistent with reports of human inactivating Gli2 germline mutations associated with severe pituitary developmental defects and different degrees of craniofacial abnormalities [33]. In the adult pituitary Shh/Ptc2/Gli1 signalling is active in corticotrophs and stimulates POMC transcription and ACTH release; Gli1 is necessary for CRF signalling [34]. Contrasting with the corticotroph specificity of Shh, Ptc receptors are also expressed in other pituitary secreting cells, although in a phenotype-specific manner [34]. Shh immunostaining was found low or absent in a large series of PA, including corticotrophinomas, whereas the expression of Ptch receptors was retained [35]. Shh was also found to stimulate ACTH, GH and PRL secretion by normal and tumorous pituitary cells *in vitro* and to inhibit cell proliferation in pituitary cell lines [35]. Thus, Shh may exert differential effects on pituitary cell growth (with stimulating effects on progenitor cells and inhibiting effects in differentiated cells) and is able to differentially modulate secretion and proliferation in PA.

3.2.3. Notch/Hes1

Notch signalling regulates progenitor cell differentiation during embryogenesis. Notch is a cell-to-cell signalling network composed by transmembrane ligands (in mammals Delta-like 1,3,4 and Jagged 1,2), the transmembrane Notch receptors (Notch 1-4), and a transcription factor (in mammals RBPJ), which is activated by the intracellular fragment of Notch after ligand-induced Notch cleavage has occurred. Notch target genes encode beta-helix loop-helix (bHLH) TFs, in particular the *Hairy Enhancer of Split (Hes)* family. A peculiarity of Notch signalling is lateral inhibition, with intracellular signalling being inactive in cells expressing Notch ligands. After the Notch pathway was shown to be oncogenic in haematological malignancies, it has been involved in several solid tumours, with either oncogenic or tumour suppressing functions, depending on the tissue and the expression of the different components of the Notch pathway. Notch is also involved in angiogenesis and participates in tumour angiogenesis through interactions with the VEGF pathway [36]. Genes encoding Notch signalling molecules are temporally and spatially regulated in the developing pituitary. During rodent pituitary ontogenesis, expression of the *Notch2, Notch 3* and *Delta-like 1 (Dll1)* genes was observed in the RP, whereas *Delta-like 3 (Dll3)* gene expression was restricted to the melanotrophs and early corticotrophs [37]. PROP-1 has been shown to specifically induce Notch2, with *Prop1* ablation inducing a dramatic reduction in *Notch2* and a concomitant increase in *Dll1* [37]. Expression of the *Hes1* and *Hes6* genes was also observed in the RP [37]. HES1 was subsequently shown to repress the expression of different cell cycle inhibitors and mediate the balance between pituitary progenitors proliferation and differentiation [38]. At the moment, few data are available on the possible role of the Notch pathway in the pituitary tumorigenesis. Overexpression of Notch3 has been recently reported in NFPA [39], and several elements of the Notch pathways have been identified in the transcriptome of prolactinomas [40] and multihormonal PA [41], suggesting that new data will be available in the future.

3.3. Pituitary stem cells

The pituitary gland is characterized by a high degree of plasticity, which is involved in pituitary function changes through life and adaptation to physiological and pathological

http://dx.doi.org/10.5772/56028

variations in peripheral hormone feed-back. Several conditions require a re-organization of pituitary cell composition, with an expansion of a specific cell pool (*eg.* lactotrophs during pregnancy and lactation). This may theoretically result from an increased proliferation of already differentiated cells, a transdifferentiation from a pre-existing cell population or a recruitment of putative adult pituitary stem/progenitor cells [42,43]. The presence of post-natal pituitary progenitor/stem cells able to self-renew and differentiate into hormone-secreting cells has now been recognized by several groups. Five potential pituitary stem cells or progenitor cell populations have been characterized in the mouse and reported as side population (SP), pituitary colony-forming cells, nestin-expressing cells, $Sox2^+/Sox9^-$ cells and GFR-α2-Prop1-Stem cell marker-expressing (GPS) cells, respectively [42,43]. The best characterized are SP cells, $Sox2^+/Sox9^-$ and GPS cells [42,43]. These cell populations represent <1% to 3-5% of anterior pituitary cells, are localized mainly along the Rathke's cleft (the proposed pituitary stem cells niche) and are able to form pituispheres *in vitro*. The question arises whether these cells may contribute to pituitary tumorigenesis. Cancer stem cells have been reported in a number of human malignancies and derive their name from their ability to develop tumours, in the same way by which normal stem cells lead to organ development. Their origin is not fully understood and they may derive from normal stem cells, re-differentiation/dedifferentiation of progenitor or differentiated cells, or both [42]. A possible role for pituitary progenitor/stem cells in pituitary tumorigenesis has been recently proposed. Conditional deletion of RB in *Pax7* precursors was sufficient to generate NFPA in mice [44]. In addition, floating clonal spheres have been isolated from two human PA [45]. These putative 'pituitary adenoma stem-like cells' (PASCs) overexpressed several stem cells-related genes, including components of the Notch and Wnt/β-catenin pathways and were tumorigenic *in vivo*. Tumours from the mice craniopharyngioma model cited hitherto also contained cells with phenotypic characteristics of progenitor/stem cells and *Sox2*/*Sox9* expression [30]. Similar findings have been reported in human ACP, with a subset of samples also expressing RET or GFRα [46]. Further work is warranted to clarify the possible contribution of stem cells in PA, especially in those showing an aggressive behavior.

4. Genetics of pituitary tumours

PA are triggered by a variety of genetic abnormalities [13,14,47]. The vast majority occur at a somatic level, but inherited predisposition is being increasingly recognized.

4.1. Inherited predisposition to pituitary tumours

Although inherited predisposition to PAs is often recognized in a familial setting, a sporadic presentation may occur. In addition to their implications for familial screening, genes involved in hereditary tumours may provide important clues in the comprehension of the molecular basis of tumorigenesis. We have recently reviewed this topic and proposed an algorithm for genetic screening in patients with PA [48].

4.1.1. Multiple Endocrine Neoplasia type 1 (MEN1)

MEN1 is an autosomal dominant condition defined by the presence, in a single subject or within a single family, of two or more hyperplastic and/or adenomatous lesions of the parathyroid glands (~90%), the gastro-entero-pancreatic (GEP) tract (30-80%) and/or the anterior pituitary (~40%). The clinical characteristics of MEN1-related PA have been recently reviewed elsewhere [48,49]. Briefly, their phenotypic distribution is unremarkable when compared to sporadic PA, with a predominance of prolactinomas (~60%), but they are more frequently invasive and resistant to pharmacological treatment. Pediatric onset is not uncommon, especially for PRL- and ACTH-secreting PA, and carcinomas have been reported. Peritumoral hyperplasia is rare, but multiple and plurihormonal adenomas are more frequent than in sporadic PA [50]. Since the identification of the *MEN1* gene in 11q13, direct sequencing has been developed in many laboratories worldwide and more than 600 mutations have been identified. Molecular defects in the *MEN1* gene have been reported in details [51] and consist of insertions/deletions with frameshift (40%), non-sense (>20%) and missense (<20%) mutations, scattered throughout the entire coding region and splice sites of the gene. Large deletions (1%) may occur and escape direct sequencing, requiring additional molecular techniques such as Multiple Ligase Probe Amplification (MLPA) for their identification. Most mutations are supposed to lead to a truncated protein (>70%). Although no clear genotype-phenotype association has been established, aberrant familial expression of *MEN1*-related tumours and reports of severe phenotypes associated with mutations that completely abolish menin function suggest that this aspect may currently be underestimated [52]. However, in an increasing proportion of cases, especially in the presence of a sporadic association of *MEN1*–related tumours, no MEN1 gene mutations are found (up to 10-30%). In particular, the relatively common association between PA and primary hyperparathyroidism has been ascribed to MEN1 in <10% of the cases [53]. *MEN1* is a tumour suppressor gene encoding a 610 amino-acid protein, menin, with somatic inactivation of the wild-type allele in *MEN1* tumours occurring mostly through LOH. Different MEN1 mouse models have been generated, including conditional tissue-specific models, which have largely confirming the role of *MEN1* inactivation in endocrine tumorigenesis [51]. Recently, pituitary tumour targeting in a $MEN1^{+/-}$ mice model through *in situ* injection of the *MEN1* gene in adenoviral vectors has proven to restore menin expression and significantly reduce cell proliferation [54]. Menin is an ubiquitous nuclear protein, which has been involved in a complex network of protein-protein interactions and implicated in the regulation of gene transcription, DNA repair and cell division. Menin suppresses PRL transcription and participates in cell cycle control through the induction of the cyclin-dependent kinases inhibitor (CKI) genes encoding $p27^{Kip1}$ and $p18^{Ink4c}$. It also interacts with nuclear receptors involved in the control of pituitary function and/or proliferation such as ERα and PPARγ and with Smad proteins, involved in TGFβ signalling. A role for menin as a general co-regulator of transcription involved in epigenetic changes on histone proteins has emerged during the last decade (see "epigenetics") [55]. Alterations in the *MEN1* gene play a limited role in sporadic pituitary tumorigenesis, and <3% of patients presenting with apparently sporadic PA have germline *MEN1* mutations. However, contrasting with the expression of menin in all normal pituitary cell types, variable degrees of underexpression have been reported in all human PA histotypes, with complete loss occurring in a PRL-secreting carcinoma [56]. Although LOH in 11q13 may account for reduced menin expression in a subset of PA, post-transcriptional and post-translational mechanisms are also likely.

4.1.2. Carney Complex (CNC)

The "complex of myxomas, spotty skin pigmentation, and endocrine overactivity" is a rare and heterogeneous condition, characterized by the association of endocrine overactivity and tumors - Primary Pigmented Nodular Adrenocortical Disease (PPNAD), acromegaly, thyroid and gonadal tumors – with cardiac myxomas, schwannomas and skin pigmented lesions [57]. Primary pituitary presentation is rare and pituitary abnormalities are mainly represented by an hyperplasia of GH/PRL-secreting cells, which frequently translates into mild hyperprolactinemia and/or subclinical alterations of GH/IGF1 secretion. Early onset GH/IGF1 hypersecretion may induce gigantism, but acromegaly and somatotrophinomas develop in a minority of patients (15%). Up to 70% of CNC patients present in a familial setting, with an autosomal dominant transmission. Germline heterozygote mutations in the *regulatory subunit type 1A of cAMP-dependent protein kinase* (*PKRAR1A*) gene in 17q22-24 can be identified in ~60% of the cases, especially in familial forms (80%), with recent evidence for some genotype-phenotype correlation [58]. Most *PKRAR1A* mutations are distributed through the coding sequence, 20% are intronic and affect splicing and two short deletions have been identified as hot spots [57,58]. LOH at the corresponding locus may be observed in CNC-related PA and conditional pituitary heterozygous knockout of the *PKRAR1A* gene is associated with an increased prevalence of PA arising from the Pit-1 dependent lineage [59], supporting a tumour suppressor function for PKRAR1A. CNC tumours show increased protein kinase A (PKA) activity and abnormal activation of the cAMP pathway. A second locus for Carney complex (CNC2) has been mapped in 2p16 by linkage analysis in CNC kindreds and confirmed by FISH analysis. Because most alterations were amplifications, undisclosed oncogenes may be involved [57,58]. A missense mutation in the *MYH8* gene, encoding the myosin heavy polypeptide 8, has been exceptionally reported in a CNC variant co-segregating with the trismus-pseudocamptodactyly syndrome [60]. An increased prevalence of point mutations in the phosphodiesterase *PDE11A* gene has also been reported in CNC patients affected by *PKRAR1A* mutations [61]. However, these variants were associated with an increased prevalence of adrenal and testicular tumours but did not impact the prevalence of PA.

4.1.3. McCune Albright Syndrome (MAS)

MAS is a rare sporadic disease due to post-zygotic activating mutations in the *α subunit of the stimulatory G protein* (*GNAS1)* gene on 20q13 leading to mosaicism. It is typically characterized by the clinical triad of café-au-lait skin spots, polyostotic fibrous dysplasia and autonomous endocrine overactivity syndromes, including peripheral precocious puberty, hyperthyroidism and GH/IGF-1 and/or PRL hypersecretion [62]. Due to mosaicism, *GNAS1* sequencing on leukocyte DNA is disappointing, since less than 50% can be detected even in the presence of a typical MAS triad [63]. Pituitary abnormalities are similar to those observed in CNC patients, with a typical hyperplasia of GH/PRL-secreting cells and somatotrophinomas developing in a minority of patients. This can be explained by constitutive activation of the cAMP pathway as a common molecular hallmark of MAS-and CNC-related cellular abnormalities. In MAS patients, increased cAMP signalling only occurs in cells affected by activating mutations of *GNAS1*, which typically affect the Arginine 201 residue [63].

4.1.4. MEN-4 and other CDKI-related disorders

Inactivating mutations in the *CDKN1B* gene encoding $p27^{Kip1}$ have been involved in atypical multiple endocrine neoplasia syndromes called MENX in the rat and MEN4 in humans, respectively, where a familial association of acromegaly, hyperparathyroidism, testicular cancer and angiomyolipomas was reported [64]. In this kindred, both the proband and his father had acromegaly and a germline heterozygous W76X truncating mutation was found. Subsequently, additional *CDKN1B* mutations were reported in MEN1-like patients by different groups, with hyperparathyroidism appearing as a constant feature and the presence of additional PA phenotypes being confirmed in some cases (one ACTH-secreting and one micro-NFPA) [65]. Associated tumours in these patients included gastro-entero-pancreatic endocrine tumours, carcinoids and papillary thyroid cancer. In most cases, functional studies *in vitro* have revealed decreased protein expression, cellular mislocalization in the cytoplasm, or a defective interaction with protein partners [65]. Search for mutations in *CDKN1B* and genes encoding additional CKIs has also been performed in 196 patients with MEN1-like syndromes. In addition to common benign polymorphisms, mutations in the *CDKN1B/* $p27^{Kip1}$ gene were the most frequently encountered (1.5%), followed by genes encoding $p15^{Ink4b}$ (1.0%), $p18^{Ink4c}$ (0.5%) and $p21^{WAF1}$ (0.5%) [66]. However, PA were associated only with mutations in the *CDKN1B/*$p27^{Kip1}$ and *CDKN1A/*$p21^{Cip1}$ genes [66]. Of note, the association between primary hyperparathyroidism and PA does not appear to be explained by *CDKN1B/* $p27^{Kip1}$mutations [67]. Overall, human *CDKI*-related conditions are very rare but appear to be inherited in a dominant manner.

4.1.5. The pituitary adenoma-paraganglioma/pheochromocytoma association: A new syndrome?

Succinate dehydrogenase (SDH) is a mitochondrial enzyme composed of four functionally different subunits A,B,C,D. Mutations in genes encoding the SDH B,C and D subunits predispose to pheochromocytomas/ paragangliomas and additional tumours, including thyroid cancer. Recently, a germline mutation in the *SDHD* gene leading to a truncated protein was reported in an acromegalic patient affected by a pheochromocytoma occurring in a familial context. LOH at the corresponding locus in 11q23 was found in the pituitary GH-secreting macroadenoma, suggesting a role for SDHD loss in pituitary tumorigenesis [68]. Because the association between PA and pheochromocytomas/paragangliomas has been reported in the literature, further search for inactivating mutations in *SDH* genes is warranted.

4.1.6. Familial Isolated Pituitary Adenomas (FIPA) and the Aryl hydrocarbon receptor Interacting Protein (AIP) gene

Familial Isolated Pituitary Adenomas (FIPA) are defined by the familial presentation of PA in the absence of syndromic features. In 2006, 64 European FIPA kindreds were reported, including patients affected by prolactinomas (55%), somatotrophinomas (~30%), non-secreting PA (~15%) and corticotrophinomas (<5%) [69]. The prevalence of FIPA among PA was estimated about 2-3% and kindreds were almost equally divided into homogeneous and heterogeneous, as defined by the familial association of PA with a single or multiple phenotypes, respectively. Familial homogeneous somatotrophinomas, previously reported as "Isolated Familial Somatotrophinomas", accounted for ~20% of the whole series. In the same year, the *Aryl hydrocarbon receptor Interacting Protein (AIP)* gene was identified as a predisposition gene in two large Finnish pedigrees with GH- and/or PRL-secreting adenomas [70]. The *AIP* gene was located in 11q13.3 and its causative role in FIPA was soon supported by the identification of germline *AIP* mutations in 11/73 FIPA kindreds (15%), including 50% of those presenting with homogeneous somatotrophinomas and ~10% of heterogenous kindreds [71]. Since this date, *AIP*-related FIPA have been further identified worldwide [48]. These findings and the expanding knowledge about the implications of germline *AIP* mutations and the potential role of AIP in the pathogenesis of PA have been recently reviewed [48,72] and will be summarized and updated. Because *AIP* was originally reported as a "Pituitary Adenoma Predisposition" (PAP) gene with a low penetrance, and on the basis of accumulating evidence for an incomplete penetrance of PA in AIP^{mut}-FIPA kindreds, screening for *AIP* mutations in patients with an apparently sporadic presentation of the disease was then performed by several groups. Although *AIP* mutations were very rarely observed in unselected patients, they could be identified in 12% of patients presenting with pituitary macroadenomas before the age of 30 [73] and up to 23% of pediatric PA patients [74]. The highest prevalence was found in patients presenting with gigantism and/or early onset GH/PRL-secreting PA. The phenotype of AIP^{mut} PA has now been well characterised. Most AIP^{mut} PA are somatotrophinomas (up to 80%), followed by prolactinomas (13.5%) and any other phenotype, with a male predominance and a frequent early onset of the disease [75]. Compared to their non-AIP^{mut} counterpart, AIP^{mut} somatotrophinomas are more aggressive and resistant to SSA [74]. AIP^{mut} prolactinomas are also frequently aggressive and resistant to DA. From a molecular point of view, more than 50 *AIP* mutations have been identified so far and distributed through the entire coding sequence. Most are truncating (60-70%) - including the Finnish AIP^{Q14X} founding mutation –, more than 20% are missense and a few hotspots have been reported. Large deletions (10%) and exceptional promoter mutations may also be encountered, in addition to changes of uncertain biological significance (polymorphisms and non-splicing intron variants). The molecular pathways involved in AIP-related pathogenesis have not been elucidated yet, but an $AIP^{+/-}$ mice model has been developed [76]. Interestingly, the wild type strain of mice used for the generation of the $AIP^{+/-}$ model spontaneously develops prolactinomas, and heterozygous $AIP^{+/-}$ ablation lead to a full penetrance of PA, with a shift toward a GH-secreting phenotype and an earlier onset of the disease. While further supporting the tumour suppressing function of AIP in somatotrophs, these findings highlight the importance of the genetic background and the contribution of genetic modifiers in the development of AIP^{mut} PA, which have also been recognized in humans [77]. Pituitary tissue surrounding AIP^{mut} PA has been rarely described, but hyperplasia was recently reported [78]. The *AIP* gene encodes a 330 amino-acids cytoplasmic protein (AIP/XAP2/ARA9), which is abundantly expressed by normal somatotrophs and to a lesser extent by lactotrophs. It is frequently down-regulated in AIP^{mut} PA, due to somatic

AIP hemizygosity, but also in invasive sporadic somatotrophinomas and in prolactinomas, whereas it appears to be upregulated in a subset of NFPA [reviewed in 48]. Loss of AIP expression has been recently proposed as a marker of aggressiveness in sporadic somatotrophinomas [79]. Accordingly GH_3 cell proliferation was increased by *AIP* gene silencing or inactivation and decreased by overexpression of wild-type *AIP*, respectively [reviewed in 48,72]. The AIP protein presents a N-terminal immunophilin-like domain (FKBP-52), but its functional properties appear to be mediated essentially through three tetratricopeptide repeats (TPR) and a C-terminal α-helix, which are involved in multiple protein-protein interactions. Identified partners of AIP include: 1) the Aryl Hydrocarbon Receptor (AHR or "dioxin receptor"), a transcription factor involved in cell response to polycyclic aromatic hydrocarbons but also in developmental processes and the regulation of cell cycle and differentiation, which is stabilized in the cytoplasm in a multimeric AIP/AHR/Hsp90 complex; 2) the phosphodiesterases PDE4A5 and PDE2A, both implicated in cAMP signalling ; 3) the anti-apoptotic factor survivin and RET, which prevents the stability of the AIP/survivin complex; 4) members of the steroid receptor superfamily (*eg.* PPARα, ERα); 5) viral proteins [48,72]. Most *AIP* mutations reported so far may theoretically disrupt one or more functional interactions of AIP and defective interactions with PDE4A5 have been proven *in vitro* [72]. An emerging field of research is the potential role of AIP as a mediator of SSA in the treatment of somatotrophinomas, which would explain the frequent pharmacological resistance of AIP^{mut} tumours. Indeed, AIP immunostaining was recently reported to be higher in somatotrophinomas treated with SSA pre-operatively than in untreated tumours [80] and proposed as a predictive factor for the post-operative response to SSA in these tumours [81] Accordingly, octreotide treatment was found to increase AIP expression in GH_3 cells [80].

4.2. Somatic events in pituitary tumours

Somatic events in pituitary tumours include genetic and epigenetic changes. Intragenic mutations are less frequently encountered than in other solid tumours. Indeed, oncogene activation is mainly triggered by the overexpression of genes involved in extracellular signalling and cell cycle progression, with a few gain-of-function mutations and occasional rearrangements being reported. Inactivation of tumour suppressor genes is very common and occurs through epigenetic changes more frequently than through loss-of-function mutations and/or allelic deletions. MicroRNAs (miRs) have also recently emerged as important regulators of gene/protein expression in pituitary tumours.

4.2.1. Chromosome and DNA alterations in PA

Several chromosome abnormalities have been reported in PA, although on limited series of tumours, and include aneuploidy and evidence for intrachromosomal gain or loss of DNA. For example, trisomies involving chromosomes 5, 8 and 12 appear to be very frequent in prolactinomas [82], whereas trisomies involving chromosomes 7, 9 and 20 were reported in NFPA [83]. Conversely, monosomy of chromosome 11 was observed in an aggressive MEN1-related prolactinoma [84] and LOH with single or multiple allelic deletions at different loci have been reported, which also appear to be more frequent in invasive PA. For instance, the frequency of LOH in 11q13, 13q12-14 and/or 10q26 was found to increase from <10% in low grade to nearly 75% in high grade PA, according to a modified Hardy's classification [85]. As compared to other solid tumours, classical somatic oncogenic mutations are relatively rare in PA [reviewed in 13,47]. The most frequent oncogenic mutation is represented by activating missense mutations in the *GNAS1* gene, the so-called *Gsp* oncogene, which has been reported in up to 40% of somatotrophinomas and occasionally in other phenotypes (<10% NFPA, <5% corticotrophinomas) [86]. A single B-Raf mutation (V600E) was reported in a NFPA sample [87]. Other activating mutations have been reported in aggressive tumours, such as activating H-Ras point mutations in pituitary carcinomas, PKCα in invasive PA and more recently PIK3CA in pituitary carcinomas and invasive secreting PA [88]. A pituitary specific truncated form of the FGFR4 (ptFGFR4) endowed with constitutive phosphorylation was also reported in prolactinomas, and a truncated activin receptor (Alk4), devoided of growth suppressing activity, has been observed in NFPA [19]. More frequently, overexpression of oncogenic proteins has been reported in the absence of mutations and ascribed to gene amplification or transcriptional upregulation. These include overexpression of growth factors and cytokines (*eg.* TGFα,VEGF) and their receptors (*eg.* EGFR), proteins involved in the control of cell cycle and proliferation (*eg.* cyclins, HMGAs, PTTG, c-myc), cell survival (*eg.*Bcl2, survivin, BAG1), intracellular signalling (*eg.* GNAS1, PIK3CA, Akt) and tumour invasion (*eg.* MMPs). Somatic inactivating mutations in TSGs are even less common. Although p53 frequently accumulates in aggressive PA and especially in pituitary carcinomas, rare mutations have been reported in carcinomas only [89]. Homozygous deletions in the protein-binding pocket of pRB have been reported in a minority of PA showing a complete loss of pRb expression [90]. However, downregulation of TSGs occurs very frequently in PA, due to LOH, epigenetic silencing or microRNAs dysregulation. Pituitary TSGs have been recognized among proteins involved in cell cycle control (*eg.* CKIs, pRb, Zac1), extracellular signalling (*eg.* TGFβ, BMP4, FGFR2), DNA repair (*eg.* p53, GADD45γ) or apoptosis (*eg.* PTAG, DAPK1), which will be discussed further on. Current studies on gene expression profiling in PA are giving an important contribution to the identification of new genes, which expression is dysregulated in PA [10,13,91,92]. It should be kept in mind, however, that a subset of proteins involved in pituitary tumorigenesis may be downregulated regardless of gene expression, since increased protein degradation through the proteasome pathway may in some cases play a prevalent role, as reported for $p27^{Kip1}$ or Reprimo [93] and miRs may impact the stability and translation of target mRNAs (see "microRNAs").

4.2.2. Epigenetics in PA

Epigenetic changes are mainly characterized by DNA methylation and histone modifications, leading to chromatin remodelling and regulation of gene expression through a modulation of DNA accessibility to TFs. Epigenetic changes may coexist with genetic events (*eg.* inactivating mutations, LOH). Methylation of cytosine residues in CpG islands of gene promoters is associated with gene silencing and is inheritable through successive divisions, with *de novo* methylation being carried out by the DNA methyltransferase DNMT3, whereas histone modifications, such as methylation, acetylation, or phosphorylation, are reversible upon specific enzymatic modifications and their effect on gene transcription can be predicted through a "histone code" [94]. For instance, acetylation and trimethylation on specific Lysine residues (K) on histone 3 (H3K9Ac and H3K4me3, respectively) are associated with an open chromatin configuration and active gene transcription, whereas other modifications on histones 3 and 4 (*eg.* H3K9me3, H3K27me3, H4K12Ac) are associated with a closed chromatin configuration and gene silencing. Aberrant gene expression due to epigenetic changes can be involved at all stages of tumourigenesis and is very frequently encountered in PA [95]. An early event in pituitary tumorigenesis is silencing of the *CDKN2A/p16*^{INK4a} gene by promoter methylation, which has been reported in all PA histotypes, though it may be less frequent in somatotrophinomas. Down-regulation of additional TSGs may be at least partially explained by gene promoter methylation, including other cell cycle regulators (*eg.* p15^{INK4b}, pRB, p14^{ARF}, GADD45γ, neuronatin/NTTA, *MEG3*), developmental and growth factor signalling molecules (*eg.* FGFR2, WIF1, RASSF1A), pro-apoptotic genes (*eg.* PTAG, DAP kinase, Zac1), genes involved in cell adhesion (*eg.* E-cadherin, H-cadherin) and TFs (*eg.* Ikaros 6) [13,47,95]. Of note, a minority of these genes are normally imprinted (*eg. MEG3, Zac1, NNTA*). In contrast, promoter hypomethylation can induce overexpression of pituitary oncogenes. For instance, loss of imprinting of the *GNAS1* gene may be responsible for an overexpression of the wild-type gene, mimicking the effects of the *Gsp* oncogene. Abnormal expression of MAGE-A3, an X-chromosome linked gene silenced by thorough promoter methylation in normal pituitary cells, has been explained by promoter hypomethylation in PA [96]. Further characterization of DNA methylome by specific array techniques appears as a promising tool for the identification of new genes modified by abnormal methylation patterns [97]. Histone modifications may contribute either to transcriptional repression, as reported for *FGFR2* [96] and *BMP4* [98], or to increased gene expression, as reported for the estrogen-induced *MAGE-3A* expression [96] or for *DNMT3* [95]. An interesting function of menin as a co-regulator of transcription though histone changes has also been proposed to explain several alterations in gene expression observed in *MEN1*-related tumours [55]. Menin is able to tether histone deacetylase activity to genes, thereby repressing gene expression, as reported for JunD- or NF-kB-dependent transcription. On the other hand, as a part of Mixed Lineage Leukemia (MLL) protein-containing complexes which specifically triggers H3K4me3 trimethylation, menin has been involved in the activation of several genes, including homeobox genes *(Hox)*, *CDKN1B/p27*^{Kip1}, *CDKN2C/p18*^{Ink4} and nuclear hormone receptor sensitive genes. These functions of menin and their final effects on cell proliferation depend on the cellular context and may explain why menin acts as a TSG in endocrine cells and a co-oncogenic protein in leukemias [99].

4.2.3. The emerging role of microRNAs and other non-coding RNAs

MicroRNAs (miRs) are small non-coding RNA molecules (18-25 nucleotides) involved in the post-transcriptional regulation of mRNAs stability. More than 600 miRs have been reported in the human genome and up to 30% of genes are believed to be regulated by miRs. Briefly, miRs derive from the intracellular processing of precursors called pri- and pre-miRNAs, and mature miRs bind to the 3' untranslated sequence of mRNA target molecules, leading to the formation of miRs duplexes. MiRs duplexes are incorporated into protein containing RNA-induced silencing complexes (RISC) and, according to their degree of complementarity with miRs, target mRNAs can be cleaved (perfect complementarity) or undergo partial degradation and translational inhibition (imperfect complementarity, which is the most common figure). MiRs have been involved in the control of pituitary development [100] and function [101]. Alterations in miRs expression profile, including loss or gain of expression, have been increasingly involved in pituitary tumorigenesis. Since the first report on miR15a and miR16-1 downregulation in GH- and PRL-secreting macroadenomas [102], more than 100 dysregulated miRs have been identified in PA, with phenotype-specific expression profiles being reported in GH- and/or PRL-secreting, ACTH-secreting or NFPA [103-112]. Although in most cases their biological significance is not fully understood, several miRs have been involved in the control of pituitary cell cell proliferation, differentiation, apoptosis, cell adhesion and metabolism, and a subset has been linked to a more aggressive behavior or even to malignant transformation [103, 104, 110]. Target mRNAs are also being increasingly recognized. For instance, *Bcl2* mRNA is a target for miR-16-1 and the expression of *Bcl2* can be upregulated as a consequence of miR-16-1 down-regulation, contributing to promote cell survival. In somatotrophinomas, loss of miR-126 contributes to cell proliferation through an upregulation of the PI3K regulatory subunit β (which amplificates PI3K signalling) [104], whereas upregulation of miR-107 has been recently involved in AIP silencing [105]. Overexpression of PTTG and HMGAs in PA may also be partially explained by specific miRs dysregulation [104, 106,107]. Another interesting aspect is the potential role of LOH in the dysregulation of miRs expression, as reported for miR-15a and miR-16-1 which may be underexpressed as a consequence of LOH in 13q14. There is also recent evidence that the miRs profile in PA may be influenced by their pre-operative pharmacological treatment, as reported in somatotrophinomas treated by lanreotide [106] and in prolactinomas treated by bromocriptine [108]. A non exhaustive list of miRs involved in pituitary tumorigenesis is shown in Table 2. Other non-coding RNAs may also be implicated. The *Maternally Expressed Gene 3 (MEG3)*, a large non-coding RNA molecule expressed by normal pituitary cells and selectively lost in NFPA, suppresses cell proliferation through p53-mediated/p21 independent and pRB-mediated pathways [113]. *MEG3* is part of the imprinted *DLK1/MEG* locus, where maternally expressed genes (*eg MEG3*) are non-coding RNAs and paternally expressed genes (*eg DLK1*) encode proteins. Interestingly, silencing of the *DLK1/MEG* locus in NFPA is responsible for the underexpression of additional non-coding RNAs, including several miRs [114].

MicroRNA	**Cromosome map (h)**	**Molecular defect**	**Histotype**	**Function**	**Ref.**
miR-128a	2q21.3	Overexpression	NFPA	Target gene: *Wee1* (↓)	109
		Down-regulation	All PA GH	Target gene: *BMI1** (↑)	103 111
miR-26a/b	3p21 (a) 2q35 (b)	Overexpression	NFPA (miR-26a) GH (miR-26a/b)	Potential target genes: *Hox-A5, PLAG1* Target gene (miR26b): *PTEN* (↓)	103 111
		Down-regulation	GH/PRL/NFPA (miR 26a)	Target genes: *HMGA1, HMGA2* (↑)	112

MicroRNA	Cromosome map (h)	Molecular defect	Histotype	Function	Ref.
miR-191	3p21	Overexpression	All PA	Cell proliferation	103
miR-145	5q32	Down-regulation	GH	Target genes: *c-myc, k-ras, c-fos, cyclin D2, MAPK* (↑)	106
miR-30a/b/c/d	6q13 (c); 8q24.2 (b)	Overexpression	ACTH	-	103
miR-320	8p21.3	Overexpression	GH	-	107
miR-24-1	9q22.1	Down-regulation	All PA	Predicted target genes: *VEGFR1* and several oncogenes	103
Let7-a	9q22.32	Down-regulation	All PA	Target genes: *HMGA1, HMGA2* (↑) Potential target genes: *Ras*	103, 104, 112
miR-126	9q34.3	Down-regulation	GH	Amplification of PI3K signalling; *PTTG* (↑)	106
miR-107	10q23	Overexpression	GH/ NFPA	Target gene: *AIP* (↓)	105, 111
miR-326	11q13.4	Down-regulation	GH, some PRL NFPA	Target genes: *HMGA1, HMGA2, E2F (↑)*	107
miR-141	12p13	Down-regulation	ACTH	Tumor growth and tumor local invasion	103
miR-16-1	13q14	Down-regulation	All PA	Target genes: *HMGA1, HMGA2, Bcl2* (↑)	102-104, 112
miR-15a	13q14	Down-regulation	All PA, in particular GH/PRL	Target genes: *HMGA1, HMGA2* (↑)	102, 103, 112
miR-20a	13q31.3	Overexpression	NFPA	Target gene: *Wee1*(↓)	109
miR-493	14q32.2	Overexpression	ACTH (carcinoma)	Target genes: *LGALS-3* and *RUNX2* (↓)	110
miR-381	14q32.31	Down-regulation	GH	Target gene: *PTTG* (↑)	106
miR-140	16q22.1	Overexpression	NFPA (macroadenomas)	Tumor growth	103
miR-212	17p13.3	Overexpression	All PA	Target gene: *DEDD* (↓), ↑ apoptosis	103
miR-132	17p13.3	Down-regulation	All PA	-	103
miR-152	17q21	Overexpression	All PA	Cell proliferation	103
miR-122	18q21.31	Overexpression	ACTH (carcinoma)	-	110
miR-23a	19p13.13	Overexpression	GH/PRL	-	103
miR-24-2	19p13.13	Overexpression	GH/PRL	See miR-24-1	103
		Down-regulation	ACTH/ NFPA	See miR-24-1	103
miR-155	21q21.3	Overexpression	GH/PRL/NFPA	Target gene:	109

MicroRNA	Cromosome map (h)	Molecular defect	Histotype	Function	Ref.
				Wee1 (↓)	
miR-098	Xp11.2	Down-regulation	All PA	Predicted target genes involved in cell progression, cytoskeleton and vesicle organization	103

*a transcriptional repressor of PTEN

Table 2. Differential expression of microRNAs in pituitary tumours

5. Alterations in neuropeptide signalling in pituitary tumours

Hypothalamic peptides play an essential role in normal pituitary cells and their biological effects are mediated by G-protein coupled receptors (GPCRs) [19]. In addition to their dynamic control on pituitary hormone secretion and release, they may exert trophic effects on target cells - such as GHRH and CRH on somatotrophs and corticotrophs, respectively – or limit their proliferation – such as dopamine in lactotrophs. The expression of neuropeptide receptors is generally conserved in pituitary tumours and represents the molecular basis for their pharmacological treatment with DA and SSA [2]. However, abnormal expression of these receptors may be involved in paradoxical responses or in pharmacological resistance. Neuropeptides may also be produced by the pituitary gland or ectopically by neuroendocrine tumours, and their ectopic secretion may lead to pituitary hyperplasia and/or adenoma. Finally, abnormal intracellular signalling may occur in PA, contribute to pituitary tumorigenesis and potentially influence the response to pharmacological treatment. An extensive review of such processes would be beyond the scope of this work, so we will focus on the most relevant and recent findings in this field.

5.1. Abnormalities in the cAMP-PKA pathway

The cAMP/PKA pathway is essential in pituitary cells, especially in somatotrophs and in corticotrophs. Briefly, the α-subunit of the stimulatory G protein (Gsα), encoded by the *GNAS1* gene, is required for the activation of adenyl cyclase and the generation of cAMP in somatotroph and corticotroph cells in response to GHRH and CRH, respectively, whereas the α-subunit of the inhibitory G protein (Gi) inhibits adenylate cyclase activity and decreases cAMP signalling in response to dopamine, somatostatin and their pharmacological analogues. As already reported, somatic activating mutations in the *GNAS1* gene – the *Gsp* oncogene – are frequent in somatotrophinomas whereas post-zygotic mutations are associated with the MAS syndrome. The *GNAS1* locus is under a complex imprinting control and *GNAS1*/*Gsp* mutations are exclusively found on the maternal allele. *Gsp*$^+$ somatotrophinomas were first characterized by high adenyl cyclase activity and high intracellular cAMP concentration. However, conflicting results concerning the phenotype of *Gsp*$^+$ somatotrophinomas arised from large studies comparing *Gsp*$^+$ and *Gsp*$^-$ tumours [86]. In particular, no significant differences were found concerning their hormone secretion profile and tumour aggressiveness. This could be partially explained by the development of molecular mechanisms able to counteract a sustained increase in cAMP concentration, such as an increased phosphodiesterase (PDE) activity, in particular PDE4, in *Gsp*$^+$ tumours. In addition, the *Gs* protein is instable and barely detectable in *Gsp*$^+$ tumours, whereas an overexpression of the wild-type Gsα protein can be observed in *Gsp*$^-$ tumours [86,115]. Accepting the concept that *Gsp* mutations represent an early pathogenetic event, long-standing *Gsp*$^+$ tumours may also have accumulated additional molecular abnormalities able to modify their early phenotype. However, most studies indicate that *Gsp*$^+$ somatotrophinomas are significantly smaller than their *Gsp*$^-$ counterpart and show a better response to SSA. This could be explained *in vitro* by a greater effect of cAMP decrease in the presence of high basal cAMP concentrations. The presence of a cAMP-responsive element (CRE) in the SSTR2 promoter also suggested that constitutive activation of the cAMP/PKA pathway might result in an increased sentivity to SSA, but no difference in SSTR2 expression has been found between *Gsp*$^+$ and *Gsp*$^-$ adenomas. However, considering the proliferative effects of the cAMP/PKA pathway in somatotrophs, the smaller volume of *Gsp*$^+$ tumours is intringuing and suggests that cAMP signalling is also linked to somatotroph differentiation. A few additional mutations in G proteins have been reported in PA, among which rare mutations involved in IP3/calcium signalling [86]. Additional abnormalities in cAMP signalling are represented by dysregulated protein kinase A (PKA) activity. In its inactive form, PKA is composed of two regulatory and two catalytic subunits. These latter are released when the intracellular cAMP concentration increases and bind the regulatory subunits. The inactivating mutations in the *PRKAR1A* gene encoding the type 1α regulatory subunit of PKA reported in patients affected by CNC is associated with increased cAMP signalling, probably through an altered equilibrium between regulatory and catalytic PKA subunits [57]. No somatic *PRKAR1A* mutations have been observed in PA. However, a marked reduction in PRKAR1A protein expression was reported in PA of different histotypes, due to an increase in proteasome-mediated protein degradation [116]. This was found to result in an imbalance between the R1 and R2 isoforms of the PKA regulatory subunit, which in turn was associated with an increased cell proliferation in GH_3 cells and increased Cyclin D1 expression in somatotroph PA. Following the discovery of missense and inactivating mutations in adrenal and testicular tumours, variants in the *PDE11A* gene have been reported in 17% of acromegalic patients [117]. Due their high frequency in the control population and the absence of phenotypic changes in the corresponding tumours, these variants were unlikely to be pathogenic. Accordingly, *PDE11* variants in CNC patients were not found to increase the prevalence of PA [61]. However, a single truncating mutation was observed and LOH at the corresponding locus was found in an additional tumour, with decreased PDE11A immunoreactivity in both cases, suggesting that genetic alterations in *PDE11A* may occasionally contribute to pituitary tumorigenesis [117].

5.2. Neuropeptides, neuropeptide receptors and their implications in pituitary tumour pathogenesis and treatment

Abnormal hypothalamic neuropeptide signalling has long been involved in the pathogenesis of PA. GHRH stimulates somatotroph proliferation and causes somatotroph hyperplasia in mice, with PA developing in old transgenic GHRH animals. Hypothalamic acromegaly has been exceptionally reported in patients with gangliocytomas [118] and ectopic secretion of GHRH by neuroendocrine tumours has been well characterized. In a retrospective analysis of 21 patients with ectopic acromegaly [119], most patients showed radiological evidence of pituitary enlargement, but 5 had normal pituitary imaging and 6 had suspected PA, respectively. Out of the four cases who underwent pituitary surgery, all had somatotroph hyperplasia and 2 had concomitant GH/PRL-secreting PA. Noteworthy, a MEN1 context was identified in 8/11 cases. Ectopic secretion of CRH by neuroendocrine tumours may cause ACTH-dependent hypercortisolism, but this is an exceptional condition and ectopic secretion of ACTH and other POMC-derived peptides is by far most frequent. TRH stimulates thyrotrophs and lactotrophs, mainly through the IP3/calcium pathway, and patients with long-standing, severe, primary hypothyroidism may develop pituitary thyrotroph and lactotroph hyperplasia due to an altered feedback on TRH/TSH secretion. Similar mechanisms are involved in gonadotroph hyperplasia secondary to long-standing hypogonadism (of note, pituitary hyperplasia is not a feature of menopause). However, true "feed-back" PA are rare and are likely to require additional somatic events. Abnormal/ectopic, expression of neuropeptide receptors may also occur in PA and account for some "paradoxical" responses observed *in vivo* or *in vitro* (*eg.* GH increase after TRH or GnRH stimulation in acromegalic patients) [120]. Loss of hormonal inhibition might also be involved in pituitary cell dysregulation. Dopamine maintains a tonic inhibition on PRL secretion and cell proliferation in lactotrophs through the dopaminergic receptor D2R. In prolactinomas, neovascularization by-passing the hypothalamus has been proposed to allow tumor cells to escape dopamine inhibition. D2R-deficient mice develop lactotroph hyperplasia and late-onset adenomas, especially in females [6]. However, no mutations in the *D2R* gene have been identified in human prolactinomas and most of them respond to DA in terms of prolactin normalization and tumour shrinkage. Reduced D2R expression, in particular of its short isoform, is frequently observed in resistant prolactinomas [121]. An essential role for the cytoskeleton-associated protein filamin A in D2R expression and signalling has been recently shown in MMQ cells and reduced filamin-A expression has been associated with low D2R expression and pharmacological resistance in human prolactinomas [122]. Similarly, hypothalamic somatostatin inhibits GH secretion and somatostatin receptors (SSTRs) are expressed on somatotrophinomas. Among the five SSTRs subtypes, SSTR2 and SSTR5 mediate most of the therapeutic effects of SSA in these tumours. Although there is no evidence that loss of somatostatin inhibition plays a role in pituitary tumorigenesis, abnormal somatostatin signalling may impact the outcome of pharmacological treatment [123]. Resistance to SSA in somatotrophinomas has been associated with low SSTR2 expression and a few genetic abnormalities in SSTR5, including an inactivating SSTR5 missense mutation in the third intracellular loop and LOH at the SSTR5 gene locus [117]. The truncated isoform of SSTR5, sst5TDM4, may also reduce the efficacy of SSA [124]. Finally, the pituitary gland produces neuropeptides with paracrine effects on pituitary cells (*eg.* galanin, bombesin, VIP, PACAP) [19,125]. Some of these peptides may also play a role in pituitary tumorigenesis, as suggested by animal models such as transgenic mice overexpressing galanin under the control of the GH promoter, which develop pituitary hyperplasia and adenomas [126].

6. Dysregulated cell growth and survival in pituitary tumours

Alterations in cell cycle control and imbalance between cell proliferation and apoptosis are general mechanisms in tumours. Such alterations may be driven by abnormal extracellular signalling and/or abnormal intracellular responses to extracellular signals, including constitutive activation of proliferative pathways and/or escape to normal regulatory signals.

6.1. Extracellular signalling in PA

In addition to neuropeptides, pituitary cells depend on extracellular signalling from the extracellular matrix, a variety of growth factors (GFs) and peripheral hormones secreted by target glands. Extracellular signalling molecules are involved in a complex network of paracrine and autocrine pathways, which are tightly regulated in the developing and adult pituitary [125]. Cell-to-cell signalling regulates pituitary hormone secretion, cell differentiation, growth, survival and plasticity, as well as angiogenesis. Abnormal signalling may therefore participate in pituitary tumorigenesis.

6.1.1. Growth factors and cytokines

The pituitary gland is an abundant source of GFs, in particular the FGF, EGF and VEGF families, and cytokines (the TGFβ family, interleukins and chemokines) [19,125]. Due to the abundant literature in this field, we will present an overview of the best studied GFs and related pathways in PA. FGFs play an important role in pituitary development. FGFs include >20 members and FGF signalling is mediated by 4 FGF receptors (FGFR1-4), with different isoforms (cell-bound, secreted, truncated) generated by alternative splicing. FGFs and FGFRs are involved in proliferative and anti-proliferative signals. The *heparin-binding secretory transforming (hst)* gene encoding FGF4, was first identified in prolactinomas, with strong FGF4 immunostaining being correlated with tumour invasiveness [127]. A tumour specific N-terminally truncated FGFR4 (ptdFGFR4), characterized by an exclusive intracellular localization and constitutive phosphorylation, was also identified in PA of different histotypes and proven to be tumorigenic *in vitro* and *in vivo* [128]. FGF2 has been involved in the pathogenesis of estrogen-induced experimental prolactinomas [129]. In contrast, signalling through the FGFR2 by FGF7 has anti-proliferative effects and down-regulation of FGFR2 has been reported in a subset of PA, in particular prolactinomas [130]. The TGFβ superfamily includes several members (TGFβ1-3, activin/inhibins and BMPs), which may exert either collaborative or opposing signalling on different pituitary cells and PA histotypes. TGFβ signalling is mediated by Smad proteins and generally inhibits cell proliferation. All TGFβ isoforms and their receptor TGFβ-R-II are expressed in PA, and TGFβ inhibits estrogen-induced lactotroph proliferation and PRL secretion [131]. Activin normally increases the synthesis of FSH while inhibiting that of PRL, GH and ACTH and exerts anti-proliferative effects on lactotrophs and prolactinoma cells [132]. Truncated activin receptors (Alk4) have been reported in PA, with a dominant effect opposing the antiproliferative effects of activin [133]. Inactivation of menin also blocks the anti-proliferative effects of TGFβ and activin on lactotrophs [132]. In contrast, BMP4 promotes the proliferation of GH/PRL-secreting cells and the development of prolactinomas, while inhibiting the proliferation of corticotrophs [134]. Accordingly, BMP4 is up-regulated in prolactinomas and down-regulated in corticotrophinomas [19]. Interestingly, BMP4 is down-regulated by DA in prolactinomas [108]. Other cytokines produced by the pituitary gland include interleukin 1 (IL1) 1 and TNFα, leukemia inhibitory factor (LIF), macrophage migration inhibitory factor (MIF), interferon γ, interleukins 2 (IL2) and 6 (IL6), which potential role in PA has not been extensively studied [131]. An increasing attention has been paid to IL6, which is normally produced by FCS cells but is secreted by tumour cells in PA, where it has been involved in cell proliferation, angiogenesis and oncogene-induced senescence [131]. Chemokines have also been increasingly involved in ontogenesis and cancer. The chemokine receptor CXCR4 is expressed in the normal pituitary and its ligand, the Stromal-cell Derived Factor SDF1/CXCL12, was found to increase GH/PRL secretion and cell proliferation in GH_4C_1 cells. An overexpression of CXCR4 and, to a lower extent, SDF1, has been reported in somatotrophinomas and NFPA [135]. EGF expression has been observed at all stages of pituitary development and in the adult pituitary, and the EGFR pathway contributes to pituitary physiology and tumorigenesis [136]. It is involved in the control of corticotroph and gonadotroph functions at both hypothalamic and pituitary levels and modulates hormone secretion and proliferation in GH/PRL-secreting cells. More than 60% of PA, in particular the secreting histotypes, have been shown to express EGFR by different techniques, whereas ErB2 was found in ~30% of PA, especially in NFPA [136]. Both have been positively correlated with tumour invasiveness. The EGFR pathway is of particular importance for corticotroph tumorigenesis. Overall, 75% of corticotrophinomas express EGFR [136]. The strongest positivity for EGFR and its phosphorylated form was found in corticotrophinomas and associated with p27 down-regulation [137]. Recently, nuclear localization of EGFR was observed in human and canine corticotrophinomas and associated with increased POMC transcription, whereas inhibition of EGFR tyrosine kinase activity by gefitinib decreased hormone secretion and cell proliferation *in vitro* and *in vivo* [138]. More than 50% of GH- and/or PRL-secreting PA also express EGFR [136]. However, the role of EGFR signalling in these tumours is less clearcut. EGF enhances the proliferation of lactotrophs and PRL transcription and TGFα has been involved in estrogen-related lactotroph proliferation. On the other hand, EGF is able to induce lactotroph differentiation in GH_3 cells, with a decrease in GH secretion, an increase in PRL secretion and an induction of D2R expression, with conflicting data reported on cell proliferation. Gefitinib was found to decrease cell proliferation of GH_3 cells, with a reduction in PRL and an increase in GH secretion, respectively [139]. The dual EGFR/HER2 tyrosine kinase inhibitor lapatinib showed similar or stronger effects on GH_3 cells, attenuated the effects of estrogens in estrogen-induced prolactinomas *in vivo* and suppressed PRL secretion from human prolactinomas *in vitro* [138]. Interestingly, EGFR expression was positively correlated with p27 immunostaining in somatotrophinomas [137]. The role of EGFR signalling in NFPA has not been extensively studied yet. NGF is the best characterized neurotrophin in the pituitary and NGF signalling is mediated by TrkA and $p75^{NTR}$, a member of the TNF receptor superfamily. All Trk receptors have been observed in the normal pituitary and in PA [140]. NGF plays a role in lactotroph differentiation and in the stress-related stimulation of corticotroph function, and escape to NGF control has been involved in the pathogenesis of prolactinomas. NGF induces lactotroph differentiation of GH_3 cells similarly to EGF, exerts autocrine anti-proliferative actions on prolactinoma cells and loss of NGF expression in prolactinomas has been linked to low D2R expression and pharmacological resistance [141]. The VEGF is a family of angiogenic factors composed by 6 members, including VEGFA (also known as VEGF), which effects are mediated by two tyrosine kinase receptors (VEGFR1 and KDR/Flk-1/VEGFR2). VEGF and its receptors are differentially expressed in normal pituitary cells and in PA [142]. In particular, VEGF and KDR are markedly upregulated in NFPA. Overexpression of *VEGF* and *KDR* mRNAs in PA was recently associated with extrasellar growth and a shorter recurrence-free survival, respectively [143].

6.1.2. Steroid hormones

Steroid hormones may play an important role in pituitary tumorigenesis. The best characterized model is represented by estrogen-induced lactotroph hyperplasia and prolactinomas. Estrogen-induced lactotroph hyperplasia occurs physiologically during pregnancy, but sustained estrogen exposure may lead to prolactinomas in some strains of rats. Although evidence for estrogen-induced prolactinomas in humans is very poor, prolactinoma growth and/or intra-tumoral hemorrhage may occur during pregnancy, especially in macroprolactinomas [144]. Among PA, prolactinomas express the higher concentration of ER [145] and estrogens can increase PA cell proliferation in primary culture [146]. Importantly, ERα and ERβ play distinct roles and an imbalance between these two isoforms has been reported in PA. Indeed, nuclear overexpression of ERα has been linked to tumour aggressiveness in prolactinomas and NFPA, whereas invasive NFPA were found to express lower ERβ [147]. Ablation of ERβ in mice was also associated with the development of invasive gonadotrophinomas in females [148]. Estrogens exert multiple effects on pituitary cells, especially on lactotrophs. They enhance the transcription of the *PRL* gene, as well as *PTTG* and genes encoding other growth-promoting proteins, such as *c-myc* and GFs [149]. Based on the comparison of microarray profiles obtained in human prolactinomas and in estrogen-induced rat prolactinomas, a common set of genes has been identified, supporting a major role for *E2F1*, *c-myc* and *Igf1* in their pathogenesis [92]. GFs have been involved in an interplay between FCS and lactotrophs, with the estrogen-induced increase in TGF-β3 secretion by lactotrophs being proposed to stimulate FGF release by FCS cells, which in turn stimulate latotroph proliferation. Estrogens also increase the secretion of VEGF and FGF2, thereby enhancing angiogenesis. Indeed, estrogen-induced prolactinomas are strongly vascularised, spontaneous hemorrhage may occur, and high ER concentrations were found in hemorrhagic PA [145]. In contrast, estrogens inhibit the secretion of the anti-proliferative TGFβ1 and TGFβ2 [150]. Finally, estrogens contribute to reduce the inhibitory effects of dopamine on lactotrophs, in part by favouring the expression of the long form of D2R [150]. Noteworthy, estrogens are also involved in pituitary plasticity, and a pro-apoptic role of estrogens through membrane ERs and TNF/TNFR1 has been involved in lactotroph cells renewal during the estrous cycle [151,152]. Other gonadal steroids may play a role in PA, since receptors for androgens and progesterone may also be expressed in PA and associated with the modulation of their proliferation by their relative agonists *in vitro* [145,146]. Lack of steroid feed-back on pituitary cells can also be involved in pituitary tumorigenesis, but as already mentioned, true "feed-

http://dx.doi.org/10.5772/56028

back" gonadotroph PA are very rare. The potentially aggressive Nelson's syndrome, defined by corticotrophinoma growth after bilateral surrenalectomy for Cushing's disease, provides indirect evidence that glucocorticoid excess previously contributed to control cell proliferation. However, different degrees of impaired glucocorticoid feedback are observed in Cushing's and Nelson's tumours. A glucocorticoid-receptor (GR) mutation that diminished glucocorticoid inhibition has been reported in a single Nelson's tumour, but GRs are generally overexpressed in corticotrophinomas, and at the moment the best candidates for glucocorticoid resistance are Bgr1 and HDAC2, which are involved in the GR-dependent repression of POMC and are deficient in about 50% of corticotroph PA [153]. Bgr1 is a tumour suppressor and loss of nuclear Bgr1 has been associated with loss of p27Kip1 expression [153].

6.1.3. Adhesion molecules

Adhesion molecules are important to maintain cell-to-cell contact and a normal cell morphology and tissue architecture. Similarly to other epithelial tumours, PA may develop some degree of epithelial-to-mesenchymal transition, which is associated with loss of cell adherence and tumour aggressiveness. The N- and C-cadherins are involved in pituitary development and in the organization of the adult pituitary into a functional network involving FCS cells [154]. E-cadherin has been largely recognized as a TSG in the pituitary. Reduced E-cadherin expression was first associated with an aggressive behavior in prolactinomas [155]. Subsequently, downregulation of the E-cadherin gene (*CDH1*) and decreased E-cadherin expression has been reported in different PA phenotypes. The reduced expression of E-cadherin was associated with its redistribution from the cell membrane to the nucleus in invasive tumours [156]. Similar findings were recently reported in a large series of somatotrophinomas [157]. In this latter study, pre-operative treatment with SSA was associated with increased E-cadherin expression, although its nuclear localization correlated negatively with tumour shrinkage [157]. A positive association between reduced E-cadherin expression, increased nuclear E-cadherin and tumour aggressiveness has also been reported in corticotrophinomas, with a gradual decrease from micro- to macro-adenomas and Nelson's tumours [158]. Neural adhesion molecules (NCAMs) can be modified by polysialation. Polysialated NCAMs, which are implicated in cell proliferation and migration, have been involved in pituitary tumour invasiveness [91,159].

6.2. Abnormalities in cell cycle control

The main positive regulators of the cell cycle are the cyclin dependent kinases (CDKs), which are activated by specific associations with cyclins (A, B, D, E). The progression through the different phases of the cell cycle, in particular the G_1/S and G_2/M transitions, are stimulated by cyclin/CDK complexes and suppressed by their inhibitors, CKIs. The latter are divided into the INK4 family ($p16^{Ink4a}$, $p15^{Ink4b}$, $p18^{Ink4c}$), which negatively regulates the G_1/S transition through a direct interaction with the CDK4/6 containing complexes, and the so-called "universal" Cip/Kip family ($p21^{Cip1}$, $p27^{Kip1}$, $p57^{Kip2}$), which is involved at various phases of the cell cycle by interacting with different cyclin/CDK complexes. Down-regulation of cell cycle inhibitors (*eg* CKIs, pRB) and overexpression of molecules involved in cell cycle progression (*eg*. cyclins, PTTG and HMGA proteins) are among the best characterised mechanisms of pituitary tumorigenesis [160]. The pituitary phenotype associated with genetic alterations in cell cycle regulators has been studied in several mouse models, including double mutants [160]. Some of the best characterized molecules involved in the dysregulation of cell cycle in PA are illustrated in Figure 1

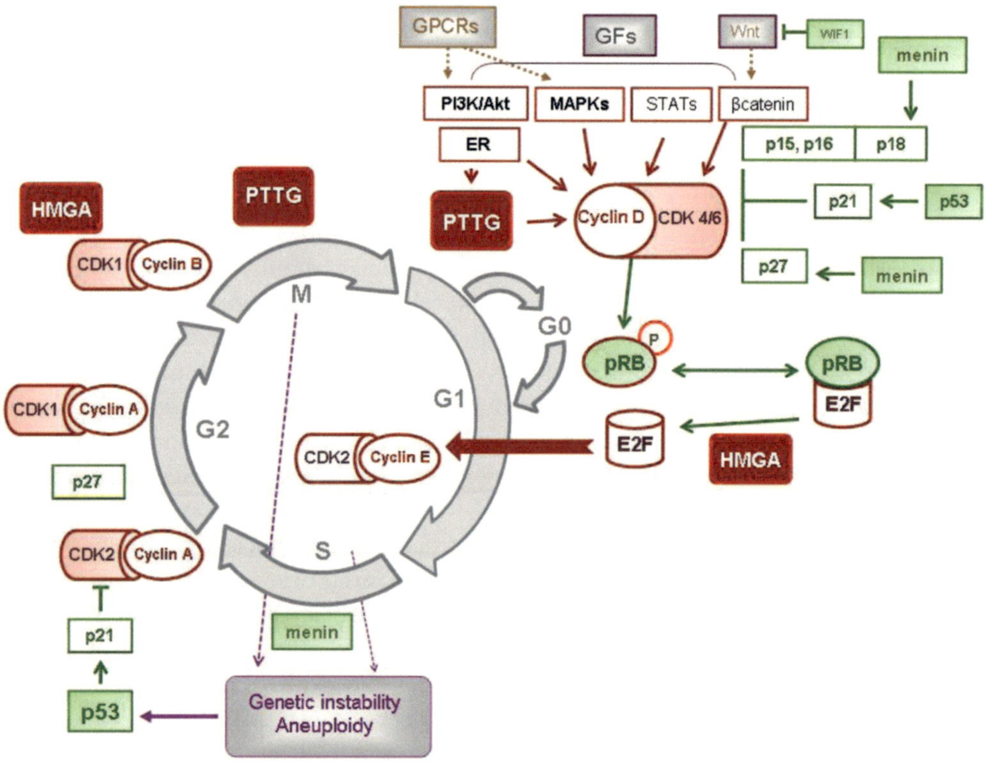

Figure 1. Cell cycle dysregulation in pituitary tumours

6.2.1. Abnormalities in cell cycle progression

Increased expression of D-type cyclins is a key event in the exit from the quiescent G_0 state under mitogenic stimulation by GFs. They activate CDK4 and CDK6, which phosphorylate pRB and therefore indirectly induce the transcription of S-phase genes by releasing TFs of the E2F family from their interaction with pRB. Transition from late G_1 to the S phase is also driven by Cyclin E/ CDK2 complexes. Overexpression of cyclins D1 and D3 has been reported in PA of different histotypes [160]. In particular, Cyclin D1 is overexpressed in ~70% of NFPA and 40% of somatotrophinomas, especially in invasive PA, with allelic imbalance suggesting gene amplification in 25% of the cases [161]. Increased GFs and Wnt/β-catenin signalling is also likely to contribute to *CCDN1/cyclinD1* expression in PA. In contrast, cyclin E overexpression has been mostly reported in corticotrophinomas, where it has recently been correlated with the loss of Bgr1 expression [162]. Overexpression of Cyclin E under the control of the POMC promoter in transgenic mice was shown to promote re-entry in the cell cycle and centrosome instability [162]. CDK4 is involved in pituitary ontogenesis. Although PA may develop in the anterior lobe of transgenic mice expressing a *CDK4* missense mutation (R24C), which inhibits its interaction with INK4 proteins, it does not appear to play a major role in human PA. The tumour suppressor function of pRB in the pituitary has long been recognized in rodents, with $pRB^{+/-}$ mice developing tumours of the intermediate lobe. In humans, loss of pRB expression in PA mainly occurs through LOH in 13q14 or promoter methylation, especially in invasive PA, though homozygous deletions in the protein-binding pocket can be found [90]. Reduced expression of the INK4 family members of CKIs - $p16^{Ink4a}$ and, to a lesser extent, $p15^{Ink4b}$, which are encoded by adjacent genes in 9p21 - has been frequently reported in PA and methylation of the $CDKN2A/p16^{Ink4a}$ gene promoter is considered as a precocious event [160]. Overall, abnormalities of the cyclinD/pRb/$p16^{Ink4a}$ pathway have been reported in 93% of NFPA and 56% of somatotrophinomas [163]. The role of $p18^{In4c}$ in pituitary tumorigenesis has been shown in mouse models. A reduced expression of $p18^{In4c}$ has been observed in a subset of PA, due to promoter methylation or, less frequently, LOH at the corresponding locus [164]. The *CDKN2C/* $p18^{In4c}$ gene is a target of menin and $p18^{In4c}$ collaborates with menin to suppress pituitary tumorigenesis. Although failure to adequately control cell cycling at G_1/S transition is considered as a mandatory step in tumorigenesis, loss of adequate control of the G_2/M transition represents an important additional event [165]. In particular, DNA damage can induce G_2 arrest as a result of the activation of ATR and ATM kinases, which activate p53-dependent and -independent intracellular cascades [165]. A reduced expression of Wee1, which induces an inhibiting phosphorylation of Cdk1 and therefore contributes to prevent G_2/M progression, has been reported in somatotrophinomas and NFPA [109]. An increased expression of Cyclin A has been reported in PA of different histotypes [160] and similar findings were reported for Cyclin B1 and B2, especially in prolactinomas [166,167]. Genes induced by p53 upon genotoxic stress include GADD45, p21 and Reprimo. GADD45γ is strongly down-regulated in most PA [168] and GADD45β has been identified as a TSG in gonadotrophinomas [169]. Reprimo has also been recently characterized as a pituitary TSG, especially in gonadotroph and somatotroph tumours [93]. Down-regulation of universal CKIs and upregulation of PTTG and HMGAs may contribute to cell cycle dysregulation at different stages.

6.2.2. The universal Cip/kip CDKI family

Both $p27^{Kip1}$ and $p21^{Cip1/Waf1}$ have been involved in pituitary tumorigenesis. The $p27^{Kip1}$ protein is normally localized in the nucleus of quiescent cells and undergoes rapid degradation upon mitogenic stimulation. Phosphorylation of $p27^{Kip1}$ is involved in its degradation through the ubiquitin/proteasome pathway. Loss of nuclear $p27^{Kip1}$ due to a reduced expression or an abnormal cytoplasmic localization has a negative prognostic value in a variety of human neoplasia. *CDKN1B/* $p27^{Kip1}$ is a haploinsufficient gene. In mice, both heterozygous and homozygous ablation of the *CDKN1B* gene induce pituitary tumours of the intermediate lobe and a collaborative effect with cyclin E up-regulation has been reported [162]. As reported hitherto, germline *CDKN1B* gene mutations are associated with MEN1-like syndromes (MEN4 in humans) [64], but this is a very rare condition. Down-regulation of $p27^{Kip1}$ has been reported in human PA, especially in corticotrophinomas and in pituitary carcinomas, due to an increased protein phosphorylation and degradation, with no significant alterations in *CDKN1B* transcripts. Of note, $p27^{Kip1}$ expression may be enhanced by other pituitary TSGs, such as E-cadherin [170] or menin [51], and by SSA in somatotrophinomas [171]. Another member of the Cip/Kip family, $p21^{Cip1/Waf1}$, is a target of p53 and induces growth arrest, essentially at the G_1/S transition but also in G_2/S. It may also be induced by oncogenes such as PTTG and Ras. The role of $p21^{Cip1/}$ in tumorigenesis is complex, since it may also have anti-apoptotic properties, depending on its subcellular localization [172]. Indeed, nuclear $p21^{Cip1}$ represses the transcriptional activity of E2F1, STAT3 and c-myc, whereas cytoplasmic $p21^{Cip1}$ binds to and inhibits pro-apoptotic molecules such as pro-caspase 3 and caspase 8 [172]. In the pituitary, the best characterized effects of $p21^{Cip1}$ are growth arrest and senescence. Using double and triple knock-out mice models for $pRb^{+/-}$, $PTTG^{-/-}$ and/or $p21^{-/-}$, p21 ablation was shown to restore tumorigenesis – induced by $pRb^{+/-}$ and abolished by $PTTG^{-/-}$ knock-out - and accelerate S-phase entry [173]. As already reported, germline *CDKN1A*/ $p21^{Cip1}$ mutations have been occasionally involved in MEN1-like syndromes [66]. Nuclear 21^{Cip1} immunostaining has been reported in secreting PA, especially somatotrophinomas [174,175]. Similar data were obtained in a recent study, which also reported a frequent cytoplasmic localization in pituitary tumours, especially NFPA and pituitary carcinomas, but not in somatotrophinomas [176].

6.2.3. PTTG

Although PTTG1 – the most abundant and widely studied member of the PTTG family, commonly referred to as PTTG - was first identified in the rat pituitary GH_4 cells, it has important oncogenic properties in a number of additional endocrine and non-endocrine neoplasia and cells overexpressing PTTG are tumorigenic *in vivo*. The biological functions of PTTG are highly complex and derive from important functional domains among which DNA-binding, SH3-binding and transactivating domains. Both nuclear and cytoplasmic localizations can be observed, nuclear shuttling being enhanced by the ubiquitous PTTG-binding protein (PBF) and by MAP kinases [177]. As a nuclear protein, PTTG has a dual role: it acts as a global TF - enhancing gene transcription either directly through binding DNA at specific promoter sites or indirectly through an interaction with other TFs - and as a securin protein - inhibiting premature separation of sister chromatids during mitosis –. PTTG functions, partners and target genes have been recently reviewed [177,178]. The securin function of PTTG is in appearent contrast with its oncogenic properties, and the multifaceted aspects of PTTG are illustrated by accumulating evidence for PTTG involvement in organ development, cell proliferation, survival and/or apoptosis, according to the experimental model and conditions. PTTG interacts with Sp1 to control progression through the G_1/S phase of the cell cycle and to suppress $p21^{Cip1}$ transcription by binding its promoter. The expression of PTTG may be increased by estrogens and GFs (EGF, FGF2), thereby creating positive feedback loops on cell proliferation [177]. PTTG expression is cell-cycle-dependent, with protein degradation occurring at anaphase and, as an estrogen inducible factor, varies according to the estrous cycle in rodents. PTTG is also involved in the control of genetic stability and angiogenesis. Detailed reviews are available on this topic [177-179]. In the normal pituitary, PTTG is expressed at low levels and is typically undetectable by IHC [177]. PTTG is necessary to pituitary development and a large body of evidence supports its dual involvement in the initiation and progression of PA [177,179]. Targeted pituitary overexpression of PTTG under the control of the α-subunit promoter in transgenic mice induced multihormonal pituitary hyperplasia with focal gonadotroph and somatotroph PA [180]. PTTG overexpression has been consistently shown to occur at both transcriptional and protein levels in PA, though conflicting data have been reported about its subcellular localization. Predominant cytoplasmic localization was first reported in PA cells [177]. Subsequently, using a monoclonal antibody, nuclear PTTG immunostaining was observed in 90% of PA of different histotypes and strongly correlated with the Ki67 labeling index ($P<0.001$), although the percentage of PTTG immunopositive nuclei was highly variable from case to case [177]. PTTG expression was also found to correlate with invasiveness in secreting PA, in particular in somatotrophinomas [177,179]. Yet, no genetic alterations have been found to explain PTTG overexpression and epigenetic changes [179] or miRs dysregulation [104] have been proposed.

6.2.4. HMGA proteins

The HMGA family of nuclear proteins - HMGA1*a*/*b*/*c* and HMGA2 - is composed of DNA-binding molecules involved in the architecture of chromatin and modulates the transcriptional activity of several TFs. They are widely expressed during embryogenesis, strongly down-regulated or silenced in normal adult tissues, and commonly re-expressed in solid tumours, including PA [181,182]. HMGAs are involved in different biological processes such as cell proliferation, cell differentiation, DNA repair [181] and interfere with the cell cycle in different ways. HMGA2 interacts with pRB and facilitates the expression of E2F1 target genes through histone modifications and acetylation of E2F1 itself, thereby promoting the G_1/S transition. HMGAs also enhance the transcription of cyclin B2, which is involved in the G_2/M transition. The critical role of HMGAs in pituitary tumorigenesis has been proven by transgenic HMGA models, which develop GH/PRL-secreting PA and additional neoplasia (eg, lipomas, fibroadenomas, T-cell lymphomas). HMGA1b and HMGA2 have been recently shown to enhance *Pit1* gene transcription and interact with the Pit1 protein [183]. Overexpression of HMGA2 was reported by IHC in 39% of human PA, in particular in FSH/LH- and ACTH-secreting PA (>60%), to a lesser extent in prolactinomas (~30%), and significantly associated with tumor invasion [184]. In contrast, HMGA2 was not detected in the normal pituitary [184]. Similarly, nuclear immunostaining for HMGA1 was observed in 62% of PA of all histotypes, with a prevalence ranging from 37% in corticotrophinomas to 100% of null cell PA, but not in the normal pituitary [185]. Overexpression of HMGA2 in prolactinomas has been explained by gene amplification and rearrangements of the HMGA2 locus in 12q14-15, with a frequent polysomy of chromosome 12, but this rarely occurs in NFPA [182,185]. Alternatively, overexpression of HMGA genes could be explained by the down-regulation of *let-7* [182] and an additional set of miRNAs [107, 112], which enforced expression was found to decrease cell proliferation in pituitary cells [107, 112].

6.3. Abnormal proliferative pathways in pituitary tumours

The Raf/MEK/ERK and PI3K/Akt/mTor pathways are typically activated by GFs but crosstalks with neuropeptide/GPCRs signalling pathways are being increasingly recognized [186]. Crosstalks between the Raf/MEK/ERK and PI3K/Akt/mTor pathways result in the modulation of ERK1/2 activity, which is involved in the regulation of cell growth and differentiation, depending on the cellular context, and represents an important proliferative pathway in cancer. Secondary activation of mTOR signalling represents an important link between cell proliferation and metabolism [187]. These pathways are essential in oncology, many drugs have been designed to target their effector molecules at different steps [188] and similar strategies may be of interest in selected PA [189,190].

6.3.1. The Ras/Raf/MEK/ERK pathway

The Ras/Raf/MEK/ERK pathway originates at the cell membrane with receptors for GFs or cytokines, which activate the GTPAse Ras protein family through the coupling complex Shc/ Grb2/SOS. The active, GTP bound, form of Ras recruits Raf proteins, which in turn activate a cascade of phosphorylations on cytoplasmic MAP kinases (MEKs and ERKs). A large number of cytoplasmic and nuclear proteins have been recognized as ERK1/2 targets, including the ribosomal S6 kinase (which in turns phosphorylates CREB), TFs (*eg.* c-myc, c-fos) and *Cyclin D1*. Activation of the Ras/Raf/MEK/ERK pathway in PA may result from increased stimulation by GFs/cytokines, overexpression or constitutive activation of their receptors, overexpression of B-Raf [191], exceptionally *H-Ras* [88] or *B-Raf* mutations [87]. Noteworthy, overexpression of B-Raf and a V600E mutation were found only in NFPA [87,191]. In an extensive western blot study, an over-phosphorylation of MEK1/2 and ERK1/2 was observed in all PA histotypes, although CyclinD1 was overexpressed in NFPA only [192]. GPCRs may activate Raf through the cAMP/PKA or the DAG/PKC pathways and therefore induce ERK1/2 phosphorylation. There is accumulating evidence that such mechanisms are relevant in different pituitary cells: ERKs have been involved in CRH-induced POMC transcription in AtT20 cells [193], gender-specific regulation of gonadotrophs by GnRH [194], GHRH induced expression of Cyclin D1 in somatotrophs [189] and the stimulation of PRL promoter activity by the *Gsp* oncogene in GH_4C_1 cells [195]. In contrast, reduced ERK1/2 activation has been involved in SSA signalling in somatotrophinomas [172].

6.3.2. The PI3K/Akt/mTOR pathway

The PI3K/AKT/mTOR pathway also initiates at the cell membrane in response to a variety of GFs and hormones, including insulin. PI3K phosphorylates phosphoinositides, resulting in the production of phosphoinositide 3-phosphate which in turn regulates the activity and intracellular localization of a number of target proteins, among which the best characterized is Akt (also known as Protein Kinase B/PKB). PI3K is negatively regulated by the tumour suppressor PTEN. The activation of Akt/PKB results in a cascade of phosphorylations, including mTOR, GSK3β, crosstalks with the Raf/MEK/ERK pathway at different levels, and has been involved in cell proliferation and motility in a number of cancers. Moreover, repression of the tumour suppressor Zac1 and activation of β-catenin through GSK3β are indirect effects of PI3K/Akt activation. The mTOR pathway is also activated by nutrients, cellular energy levels (ATP, O_2) and stress conditions; it is a major regulator of ribosomal biogenesis and protein synthesis, in particular through the activation of the ribosomal S6 kinase p70S6K and 4EBP1, which enhances the translation of *c-myc* and *Cyclin D1* mRNA [186]. Mutations and amplifications of the *PIK3CA* gene, encoding the p110 subunit of PI3K, has been reported in a large series of PA [88]. In this study, *PIK3CA* mutations were present in nearly 10% of invasive PA, whereas gene amplification, associated with protein immunostaining in a subset of cases, was found in ~30% of PA, with the highest prevalence in NFPA and no significant correlation with tumour invasiveness. Both Akt1 and Akt2 isoforms were found over-expressed and over-phosphorylated in PA, especially in NFPA, with no change in PTEN expression or sequence [196]. Increased phosphorylation of Akt, mTOR and p70S6K was reported in a genetic model of TSH-oma [197]. However, no change in mTOR and S6K expression or phosphorylation status was observed in PA [192]. Zac1, a zinc finger TF, is widely expressed in normal tissues, down-regulated in a variety of human neoplasia, and induces cell cycle arrest and apoptosis, at least in part through the induction of $p21^{Kip1}$ and $p57^{Kip2}$ [198]. It is involved in pituitary development and normally expressed by all pituitary cell types, but is strongly down-regulated in NFPA, where a complete loss of expression can be observed, especially in the null cell histotype [198]. No *Zac1* mutations have been found but epigenetic silencing is frequent and LOH at the corresponding locus (6q24-25) may occur. Interestingly, the expression of *Zac1* in somatotrophinomas is increased by SSA and correlates with the therapeutic response [198]. Data obtained in GH_3 cells indicate that this effect depends on the inhibition of PI3K/Akt signalling [198]. Zac1 appears as an essential mediator of SSA [198] and may be related to AIP [80].

6.4. Angiogenesis and hypoxia-pathways

Although angiogenesis is involved in the progression of many solid tumours, its pathogenetic role in PA is still not well defined. The normal pituitary gland is already highly vascularised and different studies on microvessel density (MVD) in PA have provided evidence for a reduced vascularity as compared to the normal tissue. On the other hand, increased vascularity can occur, as reported in estrogen-induced prolactinoma models and in some human pituitary tumours [142]. Despite conflicting results about potential factors associated with an increased vascularity (*eg.* age, male gender), most studies suggest that, in contrast to other solid tumours, there is no correlation between increased vascularity and the proliferative activity of PA [142,199]. Angiogenesis results from the balance between angiogenic and anti-angiogenic factors and requires extracellular matrix remodelling to allow the migration of endothelial cells. Among pituitary pro-angiogenic factors, VEGF and FGFs are the best characterized. Both VEGF and FGF2 are upregulated by estrogens and PTTG in PA, and correlations have been reported between the expression of PTTG and both FGF2 and VEGF-A [179].Vascular density was also associated with PTTG expression in somatotrophinomas [179]. Estrogens down-regulate thrombospondin, an anti-angiogenic factor also involved in TGFβ signalling and apoptosis [125], and thrombospondin analogues have recently proven useful in the treatment of estrogen-induced prolactinomas [200]. In contrast, with the possible exception of gonado-trophinomas, the endocrine-gland derived VEGF (EG-VEGF) was found to be down-regulated in PA [201]. Hypoxia pathways also stimulate angiogenesis, the Hypoxia-Inducible Factor (HIF)-α being the most important TF involved in the cellular response to hypoxia. Nuclear HIF-α immunostaining was reported in PA but not in the normal pituitary [202]. HIF-α protects HP75 cells from apoptosis under hypoxic conditions [203] and is stabilised by RSUME, a sumoylation factor, which is over-expressed in PA and plays an important role in VEGF-A induction under hypoxic conditions in pituitary tumour cells [204]. Angiogenesis may favour hemorrhage, and tumour apoplexy may occur, especially in pituitary macroadenomas. Hemorrhagic PA were reported to express high levels of VEGF [205, 206] and high ER concentrations [143]. Overexpression of HIF-α in MMQ cells was found to induce VEGF and the pro-apoptotic BNIP3 gene and to promote hemorrhagic transformation in MMQ cells xenografts [207]. TNFα was also found to promote VEGF and MMP-9 expression as well as tumour hemorrhage in the same model [206]. Interestingly, endoglin (CD105), a marker of endothelial proliferating cells, was found to be lower in secreting PA treated by SSA or DA than in untreated PA, indicating that inhibition of angiogenesis contributes to their therapeutic effect [208]. Anti-VEGF therapy (bevacizumab) has been proposed in experimental models of estrogen-induced [209] and dopamine-resistant [210] prolactinomas, and has been successfully used in a pituitary corticotroph carcinoma [211].

6.5. Apoptosis in pituitary tumours

As in other tissues, apoptosis is a physiological event during pituitary ontogenesis [212]. It is also believed to contribute to pituitary plasticity and may occur in PA, either spontaneously or in response to pharmacological treatment. Apoptosis is generally low in normal pituitaries and in PA, but is increased in pituitary carcinomas [213]. Apoptotic cells in PA can be detected on routine examination on the basis of their morphological changes, though they can be missed even by experienced pathologists, so that specific assays are more suitable for the definition of apoptotic indexes [214]. The ISEL and TUNEL assays, which are based on the visualization of DNA breaks, can be used on paraffin-embedded sections, but should be combined with morphological criteria to minimize artefacts [214]. Immunohistochemical detection of proteins involved in the apoptotic process such as activated caspase 3, cleaved cytokeratins or annexin-5 are also useful. As a general rule, apoptosis can be triggered by extra-cellular signalling by Fas ligand (FasL) or TNF interacting with "death receptors" or by endogenous signalling following mitochondrial or DNA damage, which is able to induce apoptosis in a p53-dependent manner. No significant relationship between p53 expression and apoptosis have been reported in PA, with the exception of nuclear p53 in corticotrophinomas [214]. An important determinant of apoptosis is the cellular expression of the Bcl2 family of proteins, which contains pro-apoptotic (*eg*. Bax, Bad) and anti-apoptotic/pro-survival (*eg*. Bcl2, Bcl-X_L) proteins, which can homo- o heterodimerize and influence cell fate. Several members of the Bcl2 family are expressed in PA, although some discrepancies have been reported about their distribution according to tumour histotype and behaviour [213-215]. Pro-apoptotic signals may be phenotype-dependent. Fas and FasL have been observed in the rat pituitary, especially in lactotrophs and somatotrophs, where they have been involved in the increased rate of apoptosis during proestrous [216], although an estrogen-dependent increase in TNFα and its receptor TNFR1 have also been implicated [151]. FasL is expressed by pituitary tumour cell lines of different lineages and Fas signalling was found to induce an arrest in cell proliferation at G_0/G_1 and apoptosis in GH_3, AtT20 and MMQ cells [217]. GH_3 cells also express TNFα and overexpression of TNFα and FasL could induce apoptosis in these cells [218]. In somatotrophs, RET heterodimerizes with its co-receptor GFRα2 and induces apoptosis *in vivo* and *in vitro* [219]. Pit-1 and p19^{ARF} (p14^{ARF} in humans) activation have been involved, leading to p53-induced apoptosis [220]. RET is a dependent receptor and both RET and its ligand GDNF are normally expressed by somatotrophs [221]. Both have also been reported in all somatotrophinomas and, to a lesser extent, in other-secreting PA [221]. Interestingly survivin, an anti-apoptotic protein of the IAP family, interacts with AIP, which enhances its stability *in vitro* and assists its mitochondrial import [222], but RET prevents survivin from binding to AIP [223]. Although ablation of RET induces somatotroph hyperplasia in mice [219], no mutation in *c-RET* has been reported in PA yet. Either, no *AIP* mutant was found to disrupt AIP-survivin interaction [223]. Studies on survivin expression in PA has lead to conflicting results [224,225]. TIM16 is a mitochondrial protein encoded by the *Magmas* gene and overexpressed in the majority of PA, in particular in corticotroph PA and cell lines, where it has been involved in cell progression and protection from apoptotic stimuli [226]. The Pituitary Tumour Apoptosis Gene (PTAG), identified by random PCR analysis of methylated genes in PA, was involved in bromocriptine-induced apoptosis in AtT20 cells [227]. Pitx2, a developmental pituitary TF involved in Wnt/β-catenin signalling, is an anti-apoptotic factor in gonadotrophs and is overexpressed in NFPA [228]. Although PTTG overexpression has been shown in different tumour cell lines to promote apoptosis, in part through p53-mediated mechanisms, it may also inhibit the transcriptional activity of p53 [177]. The potential role of PTTG in the control of apoptosis in pituitary cells remains to be further clarified. Several p53-inducible genes have been involved in cell cycle arrest and apoptosis in PA(*eg.* GADD45, Reprimo). Drug-induced apoptosis may be part of the therapeutic response to SSA and DA in PA. DA may induce apoptosis in lactotrophs through the short isoform of D2R and this effect can be sensitized by estrogens [229]. The apoptotic response to SSA has been mainly associated with SSTR2 and SSTR3, although the alternatively spliced variants of SSTR2 may have opposite effects [230].

6.6. Senescence

Senescence is an alternative tumour-suppressive cell faith to apoptosis in benign neoplasia. It is characterised by an irreversible arrest in cell proliferation and accompanied by an increase in cell cycle inhibitors such as p53, p19^{ARF}, p21^{Cip1} and p16^{Ink4a}. Because PA remain typically benign, even in the presence of invasive features, it has been proposed that a senescence buffer in PA cells exerts a protective effect against malignancy. This could in particular explain the very low prevalence of GH-secreting carcinomas and NFPA. Indeed, beta-galactosidase, a marker of senescence, was recently found overexpressed in somatotrophinomas and NFPA [176]. Interestingly, this could be explained by different molecular mechanisms. Somatotrophinomas show intranuclear p21 accumulation (possibly induced by aneuploidy and/or p53), which is able to restrain cell proliferation [176,231]. In gonadotroph PA, which express low nuclear p21^{Cip1}, high levels of clusterin have been proposed to restrain cell proliferation by triggering the CKIs p15^{Ink4b}/p16^{Ink4a}/p27^{Kip1} [232]. However, in both cases overexpression of PTTG and DNA damage are present [231,232]. Because senescence may also be activated by oncogenes, as originally described for Ras, this may apply to PTTG in pituitary tumours. Oncogene-induced senescence (OIS) is a protective mechanism against cancer which may also involve cytokines. Due to its role in pituitary development and its frequent expression in PA, IL6 is an attractive candidate for OIS in PA [131].

7. Pituitary carcinomas

Pituitary carcinomas represent about 0.2% of symptomatic primary pituitary tumours and are defined exclusively by the presence of metastases. Their prevalence may be somewhat underestimated, since metastases can be discovered post-mortem and the number of reported cases has been significantly increasing during the last 15 years [233-235]. The current interest in pituitary carcinomas certainly reflects the recent improvements in their diagnosis and therapeutic management. Their clinical characteristics have been reviewed in details elsewhere [233-236]. Briefly, most pituitary carcinomas are secreting (>80%), with malignant prolactinomas and corticotrophinomas being the most frequently encountered. They usually present as recurrent invasive macroadenomas, with an increasing degree of pharmacological resistance. Noteworthy, silent ACTH-secreting PA may become functional as malignant transformation occurs. Metastases may develop in the central nervous system (with intracranial and/or spinal localizations) or present as systemic secondary tumours, in particular in the bones, lungs or liver. Therefore, malignant transformation is a late event, which typically complicates the evolution of an aggressive PA, although exceptions have been reported. Yet, there is no specific biological marker of pituitary carcinoma and no reliable prognostic marker of potential malignant transformation in PA. The primary pituitary tumour often displays a high mitotic index and extensive p53 immunostaining, the apoptotic index is typically higher than in PA, but none of these features is invariably present and no threshold value of Ki67 or p53 immunopositivity can be defined. Several molecular abnormalities are encountered more frequently in pituitary carcinomas, such as chromosome gains, *H-Ras* mutations, overexpression of c-myc, HER2, galectin-3, loss of pRB, p27 and menin expression [233,234]. Active research is ongoing, aiming to identify molecular markers of aggressiveness and/or malignancy, which may differ according to the functional phenotype [110,237,238]. Understanding the molecular pathways of malignant transformation and progression of pituitary carcinomas should provide new tools for targeted therapies, as recently proposed for anti-VEGF or anti-EGFR therapy [138,210,211]. In addition, there is a need for reliable predictive markers of chemotherapy efficacy. Temozolomide (TMZ) has recently proven to be a very efficient tool for the treatment of pituitary carcinomas and highly aggressive PA, in particular prolactinomas [239-241]. Because changes in DNA induced by alkalylating agents may be reversed by the DNA repair enzyme O'6 methylguanine methyltransferase (MGMT), it has been proposed that, as reported in glioblastomas, MGMT status could be used as a predictive marker of TMZ efficacy in pituitary tumours. Although the first reports appeared to confirm such hypothesis [239], recent data indicate that neither MGMT immunostaining nor *MGMT* methylation status are sufficiently predictive; instead, a 3-

months clinical trial is worth regardless of MGMT status and predictive of long-term response [240,241]. In addition, the absence of correlation between MGMT gene methylation and MGMT immunostaining argues for a complex regulation of MGMT in pituitary tumours and further highlights the need for better prognostic tools [241, 242].

8. Conclusion

Pituitary tumours are very heterogeneous and their pathogenesis is multifactorial. During the last two decades, increasing knowledge about factors involved in pituitary ontogenesis, physiology and genetics have provided significant new information concerning dysregulated pathways in pituitary tumorigenesis. The rapid development of new methodological approaches allowing to explore hundreds of genes and proteins simultaneously (genomics/epigenomics/proteomics) has become an essential tool to unravel new players in pituitary tumourigenesis, although data obtained with such screening methods need to be validated on large series of pituitary tumours and integrated with functional studies. Molecular signatures of functional PA phenotypes are emerging and may provide significant information in terms of pathogenesis, prognosis and treatment. The identification of reliable markers of aggressiveness remains a priority for a better understanding and management of secreting PA resistant to conventional pharmacological treatment, NFPA and pituitary carcinomas.

Glossary

αGSU= α-glycoprotein subunit
ACP: adamantinomatous craniopharyngioma
ACTH: adrenocoticotropic hormone
AHR: aryl hydrocarbon receptor
AIP: aryl hydrocarbon receptor interacting protein
AP: anterior pituitary
BAG1: Bcl2-associated athanogene 1
Bcl2: B-cell lymphoma 2
BMP: bone morphogenetic protein
CDK: cyclin dependent kinase
CKI: cyclin dependent kinase inhibitor
CNC: Carney complex
CREB: cAMP response element-binding protein
CRH: corticotrophin-releasing hormone
GF: growth factor
GH: growth hormone
GHRH: growth-hormone-releasing hormone
GNAS1: α-subunit of the stimulatory G protein
GnRH: gonadotropin-releasing hormone
GPCR: G-protein coupled receptor
GSK-3β: glycogen synthase kinase 3β
HDAC: hystone deacetylase
HIFα: hypoxia-inducible factor α
HMGA: high mobility group AT-hook protein
IGF1: insulin-like growth factor 1
IHC: immunohystochemistry
IP3: inositol triphosphate
ISEL: immunogold electron microscopy in situ end-labeling
PAP: pituitary adenoma predisposition
PDE: phosphodiesterase
PI3K: phosphatidylinositide 3-kinases
PIK3CA: phosphatidylinositol-4,5-bisphosphate 3-kinase, catalytic subunit α
PKA: protein kinase A
PKC: protein kinase C
PKRAR1A: regulatory subunit type 1A of cAMP-dependent protein kinase
POMC: proopiomelanocortin
PPAR: peroxisome proliferator-activated receptor
PROP-1: Prophet of Pit1
PRL: prolactin

CTNNB1: cadherin-associated protein β1 (β-catenin)
D2R: D2 dopamine receptor
DA: dopamine agonist
DAPK1: death-associated protein kinase 1
EGF: epidermal growth factor
ER: estrogen receptor
Erk: extracellular-signal-regulated kinase
FasL: Fas ligand
FCS: folliculostellate cells
FGF: fibroblast growth factor
FIPA: familial isolated pituitary adenomas
FISH: Fluorescence in situ hybridization
FSH: follicle-stimulating hormone
GADD45: growth arrest and DNA damage gene
LOH: loss of heterozigosity
MAGE-A3: melanoma-associated antigen 3
MAPK: mitogen-activated protein kinase
MAS: McCune Albright syndrome
MEG3: maternally expressed gene 3
MEN1: multiple endocrine neoplasia type 1
MEN4: multiple endocrine neoplasia type 4
MGMT: methylguanine methyltransferase
miR: microRNA
MMP: matrix metalloproteinase
mTor: mammalian target of rapamycin
MVD: microvessel density
NFPA: non-functioning pituitary adenoma
PA: pituitary adenoma
PTAG: pituitary tumor derived apoptosis gene
PTTG: pituitary tumour trasforming gene
RIα: regulatory subunit type 1A
RP : Rathke's pouch
Shh: Sonic Hedgehog
SSA: somatostatin analogues
SSTR: somatostatin receptor
TGF: trasforming growth factor
TF: transcriptions factor
TNF: tumor necrosis factor
TPR: tetratricopeptide repeats
TRH: TSH-releasing hormone
TSG: tumor suppressor gene
TSH: thyroid-stimulating hormone
TUNEL: terminal deoxynucleotidyl transferase
VEGF: vascular endothelial growth factor
WHO: world health organization

Author details

Marie-Lise Jaffrain-Rea[1,2], Sandra Rotondi[1] and Edoardo Alesse[1]

1 Department of Biotechnological and Applied Clinical Sciences, University of L'Aquila, L'Aquila (AQ), Italy

2 Neuromed Institute, Pozzilli (IS), Italy

References

[1] Daly AF, Rixhon M, Adam C, Dempegioti A, Tichomirowa MA, Beckers A. High prevalence of pituitary adenomas: a cross-sectional study in the province of Liege, Belgium. The Journal of Clinical Endocrinology & Metabolism 2006;91(12) 4769-75.

[2] Arafah BM, Nasrallah MP. Pituitary tumors: pathophysiology, clinical manifestations and management. Endocrine Related Cancer 2001;8(4) 287-305.

[3] Louis DN, Ohgaki H, Wiestler OD, Cavenee WK, Burger PC, Jouvet A, Scheithauer BW, Kleihues P. The 2007 WHO classification of tumours of the central nervous system. Acta Neuropathologica 2007;114(2) 97-109.

[4] Mete O, Asa SL. Clinicopathological correlations in pituitary adenomas. Brain Pathology 2012;22(4) 443-53.

[5] Obari A, Sano T, Ohyama K, Kudo E, Qian ZR, Yoneda A, Rayhan N, Mustafizur Rahman M, Yamada S. Clinicopathological features of growth hormone-producing pituitary adenomas: difference among various types defined by cytokeratin distribution pattern including a transitional form. Endocrine Pathology 2008;19(2) 82-91.

[6] Asa SL. Transgenic and knockout mouse models clarify pituitary development, function and disease. Brain Pathology 2001;11(3) 371-84.

[7] Jaffrain-Rea ML, Di Stefano D, Minniti G, Esposito V, Bultrini A, Ferretti E, Santoro A, Faticanti Scucchi L, Gulino A, Cantore G. A critical reappraisal of MIB-1 labelling index significance in a large series of pituitary tumours: secreting versus non-secreting adenomas. Endocrine Related Cancer 2002;9(2) 103-13.

[8] De Lellis RA., Lloyd RV., Heitz PU., Eng C. World Health Organization classification of tumours: tumours of endocrine organs. Lyon: IARC press; 2004.

[9] Raverot G, Wierinckx A, Dantony E, Auger C, Chapas G, Villeneuve L, Brue T, Figarella-Branger D, Roy P, Jouanneau E, Jan M, Lachuer J, Trouillas J; HYPOPRONOS. Prognostic factors in prolactin pituitary tumors: clinical, histological, and molecular data from a series of 94 patients with a long postoperative follow-up. The Journal of Clinical Endocrinology & Metabolism 2010;95(4) 1708-16.

[10] Galland F, Lacroix L, Saulnier P, Dessen P, Meduri G, Bernier M, Gaillard S, Guibourdenche J, Fournier T, Evain-Brion D, Bidart JM, Chanson P. Differential gene expression profiles of invasive and non-invasive non-functioning pituitary adenomas based on microarray analysis. Endocrine Related Cancer 2010;17(2) 361-71.

[11] Ruebel KH, Leontovich AA, Jin L, Stilling GA, Zhang H, Qian X, Nakamura N, Scheithauer BW, Kovacs K, Lloyd RV. Patterns of gene expression in pituitary carcinomas and adenomas analyzed by high-density oligonucleotide arrays, reverse transcriptase-quantitative PCR, and protein expression. Endocrine 2006;29(3) 435-44.

[12] Clayton RN, Farrell WE. Pituitary tumour clonality revisited. Frontiers of Hormone Research 2004;32 186-204.

[13] Dworakowska D, Grossman AB. The pathophysiology of pituitary adenomas. Best Practice & Research: Clinical Endocrinology & Metabolism 2009;23(5) 525-41.

[14] Melmed S. Pathogenesis of pituitary tumors. Nature Reviews Endocrinology 2011;7(5) 257-66.

[15] Brinkmeier ML, Davis SW, Carninci P, MacDonald JW, Kawai J, Ghosh D, Hayashizaki Y, Lyons RH, Camper SA. Discovery of transcriptional regulators and signaling pathways in the developing pituitary gland by bioinformatic and genomic approaches. Genomics 2009;93(5) 449-60.

[16] Davis SW, Castinetti F, Carvalho LR, Ellsworth BS, Potok MA, Lyons RH, Brinkmeier ML, Raetzman LT, Carninci P, Mortensen AH, Hayashizaki Y, Arnhold IJ, Mendonça BB, Brue T, Camper SA. Molecular mechanisms of pituitary organogenesis: in search of novel regulatory genes. Molecular and Cellular Endocrinology 2010;323(1) 4-19.

[17] Kelberman D, Rizzoti K, Lovell-Badge R, Robinson IC, Dattani MT. Genetic regulation of pituitary gland development in human and mouse. Endocrine Reviews 2009;30(7) 790-829.

[18] De Moraes DC, Vaisman M, Conceição FL, Ortiga-Carvalho TM. Pituitary development: a complex, temporal regulated process dependent on specific transcriptional factors. Journal of Endocrinology 2012;215(2) 239-45.

[19] Perez-Castro C, Renner U, Haedo MR, Stalla GK, Arzt E. Cellular and molecular specificity of pituitary gland physiology. Physiological Reviews 2012;92(1) 1-38.

[20] Fratticci A, Grieco FA, Spilioti C, Giangaspero F, Ventura L, Esposito V, Piccirilli M, Santoro A, Gulino A, Cantore G, Alesse E, Jaffrain-Rea ML. Differential expression of neurogenins and NeuroD1 in human pituitary tumours. Journal of Endocrinology 2007;194(3) 475-84.

[21] Mantovani G, Asteria C, Pellegrini C, Bosari S, Alberti L, Bondioni S, Peverelli E, Spada A, Beck-Peccoz P. HESX1 expression in human normal pituitaries and pituitary adenomas. Molecular and Cellular Endocrinology 2006;247(1-2) 135-9.

[22] Pellegrini-Bouiller I, Manrique C, Gunz G, Grino M, Zamora AJ, Figarella-Branger D, Grisoli F, Jaquet P, Enjalbert A. Expression of the members of the Ptx family of transcription factors in human pituitary adenomas. The Journal of Clinical Endocrinology & Metabolism 1999;84(6) 2212-20.

[23] Nakamura S, Ohtsuru A, Takamura N, Kitange G, Tokunaga Y, Yasunaga A, Shibata S, Yamashita S. Prop-1 gene expression in human pituitary tumors. The Journal of Clinical Endocrinology & Metabolism 1999;84(7) 2581-4.

[24] Egashira N, Minematsu T, Miyai S, Takekoshi S, Camper SA, Osamura RY. Pituitary changes in Prop1 transgenic mice: hormone producing tumors and signet-ring type gonadotropes. Acta Histochemica and Cytochemica 2008;41(3) 47-57.

[25] Egashira N, Takekoshi S, Takei M, Teramoto A, Osamura RY. Expression of FOXL2 in human normal pituitaries and pituitary adenomas. Modern Pathology 2011;24(6) 765-73.

[26] Gueorguiev M, Grossman AB. Pituitary gland and beta-catenin signaling: from ontogeny to oncogenesis. Pituitary 2009;12(3) 245-55.

[27] Sekine S, Shibata T, Kokubu A, Morishita Y, Noguchi M, Nakanishi Y, Sakamoto M, Hirohashi S. Craniopharyngiomas of adamantinomatous type harbor beta-catenin gene mutations. American Journal of Pathology 2002;161(6) 1997-2001.

[28] Buslei R, Nolde M, Hofmann B, Meissner S, Eyupoglu IY, Siebzehnrübl F, Hahnen E, Kreutzer J, Fahlbusch R. Common mutations of beta-catenin in adamantinomatous craniopharyngiomas but not in other tumours originating from the sellar region. Acta Neuropathologica 2005;109(6) 589-97.

[29] Oikonomou E, Barreto DC, Soares B, De Marco L, Buchfelder M, Adams EF. Beta-catenin mutations in craniopharyngiomas and pituitary adenomas. Journal of Neuro-Oncology 2005;73(3) 205-9.

[30] Gaston-Massuet C, Andoniadou CL, Signore M, Jayakody SA, Charolidi N, Kyeyune R, Vernay B, Jacques TS, Taketo MM, Le Tissier P, Dattani MT, Martinez-Barbera JP. Increased Wingless (Wnt) signaling in pituitary progenitor/stem cells gives rise to pituitary tumors in mice and humans. Proceedings of the National Academy of Sciences of the United States of America 2011;108(28) 11482-7.

[31] Elston MS, Clifton-Bligh RJ. Identification of Wnt family inhibitors: a pituitary tumor directed whole genome approach. Molecular and Cellular Endocrinology 2010;326(1-2) 48-54.

[32] Wang Y, Martin JF, Bai CB. Direct and indirect requirements of Shh/Gli signaling in early pituitary development. Developmental Biology 2010;348(2) 199-209.

[33] Roessler E, Du YZ, Mullor JL, Casas E, Allen WP, Gillessen-Kaesbach G, Roeder ER, Ming JE, Ruiz i Altaba A, Muenke M. Loss-of-function mutations in the human GLI2 gene are associated with pituitary anomalies and holoprosencephaly-like features. Proceedings of the National Academy of Sciences of the United States of America 2003;100(23) 13424-9.

[34] Vila G, Papazoglou M, Stalla J, Theodoropoulou M, Stalla GK, Holsboer F, Paez-Pereda M. Sonic hedgehog regulates CRH signal transduction in the adult pituitary. FASEB Journal 2005;19(2) 281-3.

[35] Vila G, Theodoropoulou M, Stalla J, Tonn JC, Losa M, Renner U, Stalla GK, Paez-Pereda M. Expression and function of sonic hedgehog pathway components in pituitary adenomas: evidence for a direct role in hormone secretion and cell proliferation. The Journal of Clinical Endocrinology & Metabolism 2005;90(12) 6687-94.

[36] Thurston G, Kitajewski J. VEGF and Delta-Notch: interacting signalling pathways in tumour angiogenesis. British Journal of Cancer 2008;99(8) 1204-9.

[37] Raetzman LT, Ross SA, Cook S, Dunwoodie SL, Camper SA, Thomas PQ. Developmental regulation of Notch signaling genes in the embryonic pituitary: Prop1 deficiency affects Notch2 expression. Developmental Biology 2004;265(2) 329-40.

[38] Monahan P, Rybak S, Raetzman LT. The notch target gene HES1 regulates cell cycle inhibitor expression in the developing pituitary. Endocrinology 2009;150(9) 4386-94.

[39] Miao Z, Miao Y, Lin Y, Lu X. Overexpression of the Notch3 receptor in non-functioning pituitary tumours. Journal of Clinical Neuroscience 2012;19(1) 107-10.

[40] Evans CO, Moreno CS, Zhan X, McCabe MT, Vertino PM, Desiderio DM, Oyesiku NM. Molecular pathogenesis of human prolactinomas identified by gene expression profiling, RT-qPCR, and proteomic analyses. Pituitary 2008;11(3) 231-45.

[41] Jiang Z, Gui S, Zhang Y. Analysis of differential gene expression in plurihormonal pituitary adenomas using bead-based fiber-optic arrays. Journal of Neuro-Oncology 2012;108(3) 341-8.

[42] Rizzoti K. Adult pituitary progenitors/stem cells: from in vitro characterization to in vivo function. European Journal of Neuroscience 2010;32 2053–2062.

[43] Florio T. Adult pituitary stem cells: from pituitary plasticity to adenoma development. Neuroendocrinology 2011;94(4) 265-77.

[44] Hosoyama T, Nishijo K, Garcia MM, Schaffer BS, Ohshima-Hosoyama S, Prajapati SI, Davis MD, Grant WF, Scheithauer BW, Marks DL, Rubin BP, Keller C. A postnatal Pax7 progenitor gives rise to pituitary adenomas. Genes Cancer 2010;1(4) 388-402.

[45] Xu Q, Yuan X, Tunici P, Liu G, Fan X, Xu M, Hu J, Hwang JY, Farkas DL, Black KL, Yu JS. Isolation of tumour stem-like cells from benign tumours. British Journal of Cancer 2009; 101(2) 303-11.

[46] Garcia-Lavandeira M, Saez C, Diaz-Rodriguez E, Perez-Romero S, Senra A, Dieguez C, Japon MA, Alvarez CV. Craniopharyngiomas express embryonic stem cell markers (SOX2, OCT4, KLF4, and SOX9) as pituitary stem cells but do not coexpress RET/GFRA3 receptors. The Journal of Clinical Endocrinology & Metabolism 2012;97(1) E80-7.

[47] 46.Vandeva S, Jaffrain-Rea ML, Daly AF, Tichomirowa M, Zacharieva S, Beckers A. The genetics of pituitary adenomas. Best Practice & Research: Clinical Endocrinology & Metabolism 2010;24(3) 461-76.

[48] Jaffrain-Rea ML, Daly AF, Angelini M, Petriossians P, Bours V, Beckers A. Genetic susceptibility in pituitary adenomas: from pathogenesis to clinical implications. Expert Review of Endocrinology & Metabolism 2011;(2) 195-214.

[49] Agarwal SK, Ozawa A, Mateo CM, Marx SJ. The MEN1 gene and pituitary tumours. Hormone Research 2009;71 Suppl 2 131-8.

[50] Trouillas J, Labat-Moleur F, Sturm N, Kujas M, Heymann MF, Figarella-Branger D, Patey M, Mazucca M, Decullier E, Vergès B, Chabre O, Calender A, Groupe d'études des Tumeurs Endocrines. Pituitary tumors and hyperplasia in multiple endocrine neoplasia type 1 syndrome (MEN1): a case-control study in a series of 77 patients versus 2509 non-MEN1 patients. The American Journal of Surgical Pathology 2008;32(4) 534-43.

[51] Thakker RV. Multiple endocrine neoplasia type 1 (MEN1). Best Practice & Research: Clinical Endocrinology & Metabolism 2010;24(3) 355-70.

[52] Lips CJ, Dreijerink KM, Höppener JW. Variable clinical expression in patients with a germline MEN1 disease gene mutation: clues to a genotype-phenotype correlation. Clinics 2012;67 Suppl 1 49-56.

[53] Ellard S, Hattersley AT, Brewer CM, Vaidya B. Detection of a MEN1 gene mutation depends on clinical features and supports current referral criteria for diagnostic molecular genetic testing. Clinical Endocrinology 2005;62(2) 169-75.

[54] Walls GV, Lemos MC, Javid M, Bazan-Peregrino M, Jeyabalan J, Reed AA, Harding B, Tyler DJ, Stuckey DJ, Piret S, Christie PT, Ansorge O, Clarke K, Seymour L, Thakker RV. MEN1 gene replacement therapy reduces proliferation rates in a mouse model of pituitary adenomas. Cancer Research 2012;72(19) 5060-8.

[55] Dreijerink KM, Lips CJ, Timmers HT. Multiple endocrine neoplasia type 1: a chromatin writer's block. Journal of Internal Medicine 2009;266(1) 53-9.

[56] Theodoropoulou M, Cavallari I, Barzon L, D'Agostino DM, Ferro T, Arzberger T, Grübler Y, Schaaf L, Losa M, Fallo F, Ciminale V, Stalla GK, Pagotto U. Differential expression of menin in sporadic pituitary adenomas. Endocrine Related Cancer 2004;11(2) 333-44.

[57] Rothenbuhler A, Stratakis CA. Clinical and molecular genetics of Carney complex. Best Practice & Research: Clinical Endocrinology & Metabolism 2010;24(3) 389-99.

[58] Bertherat J, Horvath A, Groussin L, Grabar S, Boikos S, Cazabat L, Libe R, René-Corail F, Stergiopoulos S, Bourdeau I, Bei T, Clauser E, Calender A, Kirschner LS, Bertagna X, Carney JA, Stratakis CA. Mutations in regulatory subunit type 1A of cyclic adenosine 5'-monophosphate-dependent protein kinase (PRKAR1A): phenotype analysis in 353 patients and 80 different genotypes. The Journal of Clinical Endocrinology & Metabolism 2009;94(6) 2085-91.

[59] Yin Z, Williams-Simons L, Parlow AF, Asa S, Kirschner LS. Pituitary-specific knockout of the Carney complex gene Prkar1a leads to pituitary tumorigenesis. Molecular Endocrinology 2008;22(2) 380-7.

[60] Veugelers M, Bressan M, McDermott DA, Weremowicz S, Morton CC, Mabry CC, Lefaivre JF, Zunamon A, Destree A, Chaudron JM, Basson CT. Mutation of perinatal myosin heavy chain associated with a Carney complex variant. The New England Journal of Medicine 2004;351(5) 460-9.

[61] Libé R, Horvath A, Vezzosi D, Fratticci A, Coste J, Perlemoine K, Ragazzon B, Guillaud-Bataille M, Groussin L, Clauser E, Raffin-Sanson ML, Siegel J, Moran J, Drori-Herishanu L, Faucz FR, Lodish M, Nesterova M, Bertagna X, Bertherat J, Stratakis CA. Frequent phosphodiesterase 11A gene (PDE11A) defects in patients with Carney complex (CNC) caused by PRKAR1A mutations: PDE11A may contribute to adrenal and testicular tumors in CNC as a modifier of the phenotype. The Journal of Clinical Endocrinology & Metabolism 2011;96(1) E208-14.

[62] Dumitrescu CE, Collins MT. McCune-Albright syndrome. Orphanet Journal of Rare Diseases 2008;3 12.

[63] Lumbroso S, Paris F, Sultan C; Activating Gsalpha mutations: analysis of 113 patients with signs of McCune-Albright syndrome. A European collaborative study. The Journal of Clinical Endocrinology & Metabolism 2004;89(5) 2107-13.

[64] Pellegata NS, Quintanilla-Martinez L, Siggelkow H, Samson E, Bink K, Höfler H, Fend F, Graw J, Atkinson MJ. Germ-line mutations in p27Kip1 cause a multiple endocrine neoplasia syndrome in rats and humans. Proceedings of the National Academy of Sciences of the United States of America 2006;103(50) 19213.

[65] Pellegata NS. MENX and MEN4. Clinics (Sao Paulo) 2012;67 Suppl 1 13-8.

[66] Agarwal SK, Mateo CM, Marx SJ. Rare germline mutations in cyclin-dependent kinase inhibitor genes in multiple endocrine neoplasia type 1 and related states. The Journal of Clinical Endocrinology & Metabolism 2009;94(5) 1826-34.

[67] Ozawa A, Agarwal SK, Mateo CM, Burns AL, Rice TS, Kennedy PA, Quigley CM, Simonds WF, Weinstein LS, Chandrasekharappa SC, Collins FS, Spiegel AM, Marx SJ. The parathyroid/pituitary variant of multiple endocrine neoplasia type 1 usually has causes other than p27Kip1 mutations. The Journal of Clinical Endocrinology & Metabolism 2007;92(5) 1948-51.

[68] Xekouki P, Pacak K, Almeida M, Wassif CA, Rustin P, Nesterova M, de la Luz Sierra M, Matro J, Ball E, Azevedo M, Horvath A, Lyssikatos C, Quezado M, Patronas N, Ferrando B, Pasini B, Lytras A, Tolis G, Stratakis CA. Succinate dehydrogenase (SDH) D subunit (SDHD) inactivation in a growth-hormone-producing pituitary tumor: a new association for SDH? The Journal of Clinical Endocrinology & Metabolism 2012;97(3) E357-66.

[69] Daly AF, Jaffrain-Rea ML, Ciccarelli A, Valdes-Socin H, Rohmer V, Tamburrano G, Borson-Chazot C, Estour B, Ciccarelli E, Brue T, Ferolla P, Emy P, Colao A, De Menis E, Lecomte P, Penfornis F, Delemer B, Bertherat J, Wémeau JL, De Herder W, Archambeaud F, Stevenaert A, Calender A, Murat A, Cavagnini F, Beckers A. Clinical characterization of familial isolated pituitary adenomas. The Journal of Clinical Endocrinology & Metabolism 2006;91(9) 3316-23.

[70] Vierimaa O, Georgitsi M, Lehtonen R, Vahteristo P, Kokko A, Raitila A, Tuppurainen K, Ebeling TM, Salmela PI, Paschke R, Gündogdu S, De Menis E, Mäkinen MJ, Launonen V, Karhu A, Aaltonen LA. Pituitary adenoma predisposition caused by germline mutations in the AIP gene. Science 2006;312(5777) 1228-30.

[71] Daly AF, Vanbellinghen JF, Khoo SK, Jaffrain-Rea ML, Naves LA, Guitelman MA, Murat A, Emy P, Gimenez-Roqueplo AP, Tamburrano G, Raverot G, Barlier A, De Herder W, Penfornis A, Ciccarelli E, Estour B, Lecomte P, Gatta B, Chabre O, Sabaté MI, Bertagna X, Garcia Basavilbaso N, Stalldecker G, Colao A, Ferolla P, Wémeau JL, Caron P, Sadoul JL, Oneto A, Archambeaud F, Calender A, Sinilnikova O, Montaña-

na CF, Cavagnini F, Hana V, Solano A, Delettieres D, Luccio-Camelo DC, Basso A, Rohmer V, Brue T, Bours V, Teh BT, Beckers A. Aryl hydrocarbon receptor-interacting protein gene mutations in familial isolated pituitary adenomas: analysis in 73 families. The Journal of Clinical Endocrinology & Metabolism 2007;92(5) 1891-6.

[72] Trivellin G, Korbonits M. AIP and its interacting partners. Journal of Endocrinology 2011;210(2) 137-55.

[73] Tichomirowa MA, Barlier A, Daly AF, Jaffrain-Rea ML, Ronchi C, Yaneva M, Urban JD, Petrossians P, Elenkova A, Tabarin A, Desailloud R, Maiter D, Schürmeyer T, Cozzi R, Theodoropoulou M, Sievers C, Bernabeu I, Naves LA, Chabre O, Montañana CF, Hana V, Halaby G, Delemer B, Aizpún JI, Sonnet E, Longás AF, Hagelstein MT, Caron P, Stalla GK, Bours V, Zacharieva S, Spada A, Brue T, Beckers A. High prevalence of AIP gene mutations following focused screening in young patients with sporadic pituitary macroadenomas. European Journal of Endocrinology 2011;165(4) 509-15.

[74] Cazabat L, Bouligand J, Chanson P. AIP mutation in pituitary adenomas. New England Journal of Medicine 2011;364(20) 1974-5.

[75] Daly AF, Tichomirowa MA, Petrossians P, Heliövaara E, Jaffrain-Rea ML, BarlierA, Naves LA, Ebeling T, Karhu A, Raappana A, Cazabat L, De Menis E, Montañana CF, Raverot G, Weil RJ, Sane T, Maiter D, Neggers S, Yaneva M, Tabarin A, Verrua E, Eloranta E, Murat A, Vierimaa O, Salmela PI, Emy P, Toledo RA, Sabaté MI, Villa C, Popelier M, Salvatori R, Jennings J, Longás AF, Labarta Aizpún JI, Georgitsi M, Paschke R, Ronchi C, Valimaki M, Saloranta C, De Herder W, Cozzi R, Guitelman M, Magri F, Lagonigro MS, Halaby G, Corman V, Hagelstein MT, Vanbellinghen JF, Barra GB, Gimenez-Roqueplo AP, Cameron FJ, Borson-Chazot F, Holdaway I, Toledo SP, Stalla GK, Spada A, Zacharieva S, Bertherat J, Brue T, Bours V, Chanson P, Aaltonen LA, Beckers A. Clinical characteristics and therapeutic responses in patients with germ-line AIP mutations and pituitary adenomas: an international collaborative study. The Journal of Clinical Endocrinology & Metabolism 2010;95(11) E373-83.

[76] Raitila A, Lehtonen HJ, Arola J, Heliövaara E, Ahlsten M, Georgitsi M, Jalanko A, Paetau A, Aaltonen LA, Karhu A. Mice with inactivation of aryl hydrocarbon receptor-interacting protein (Aip) display complete penetrance of pituitary adenomas with aberrant ARNT expression. American Journal of Pathology 2010;177(4) 1969-76.

[77] Khoo SK, Pendek R, Nickolov R, Luccio-Camelo DC, Newton TL, Massie A, Petillo D, Menon J, Cameron D, Teh BT, Chan SP. Genome-wide scan identifies novel modifier loci of acromegalic phenotypes for isolated familial somatotropinoma. Endocrine Related Cancer 2009;16(3) 1057-63.

[78] Villa C, Lagonigro MS, Magri F, Koziak M, Jaffrain-Rea ML, Brauner R, Bouligand J, Junier MP, Di Rocco F, Sainte-Rose C, Beckers A, Roux FX, Daly AF, Chiovato L. Hyperplasia-adenoma sequence in pituitary tumorigenesis related to aryl hydrocarbon

receptor interacting protein gene mutation. Endocrine Related Cancer 2011;18(3) 347-56.

[79] Kasuki Jomori de Pinho L, Vieira Neto L, Armondi Wildemberg LE, Gasparetto EL, Marcondes J, de Almeida Nunes B, Takiya CM, Gadelha MR. Low aryl hydrocarbon receptor-interacting protein expression is a better marker of invasiveness in somatotropinomas than Ki-67 and p53. Neuroendocrinology 2011;94(1) 39-48.

[80] Chahal HS, Trivellin G, Leontiou CA, Alband N, Fowkes RC, Tahir A, Igreja SC, Chapple JP, Jordan S, Lupp A, Schulz S, Ansorge O, Karavitaki N, Carlsen E, Wass JA, Grossman AB, Korbonits M. Somatostatin analogs modulate AIP in somatotroph adenomas: the role of the ZAC1 pathway. The Journal of Clinical Endocrinology & Metabolism 2012;97(8) E1411-20.

[81] Kasuki L, Vieira Neto L, Wildemberg LE, Colli LM, de Castro M, Takiya CM, Gadelha MR. AIP expression in sporadic somatotropinomas is a predictor of the response to octreotide LAR therapy independent of SSTR2 expression. Endocrine Related Cancer 2012;19(3) L25-9.

[82] Finelli P, Giardino D, Rizzi N, Buiatiotis S, Virduci T, Franzin A, Losa M, Larizza L. Non-random trisomies of chromosomes 5, 8 and 12 in the prolactinoma sub-type of pituitary adenomas: conventional cytogenetics and interphase FISH study. International Journal of Cancer 2000;86(3) 344-50.

[83] Larsen JB, Schrøder HD, Sørensen AG, Bjerre P, Heim S. Simple numerical chromosome aberrations characterize pituitary adenomas. Cancer Genetics and Cytogenetics 1999;114(2) 144-9.

[84] Kontogeorgos G, Kapranos N, Tzavara I, Thalassinos N, Rologis D. Monosomy of chromosome 11 in pituitary adenoma in a patient with familial multiple endocrine neoplasia type 1. Clinical Endocrinology 2001;54(1) 117-20.

[85] Bates AS, Farrell WE, Bicknell EJ, McNicol AM, Talbot AJ, Broome JC, Perrett CW, Thakker RV, Clayton RN. Allelic deletion in pituitary adenomas reflects aggressive biological activity and has potential value as a prognostic marker. The Journal of Clinical Endocrinology & Metabolism 1997;82(3) 818-24.

[86] Lania A, Spada A. G-protein and signalling in pituitary tumours. Hormone Research 2009;71 Suppl 2 95-100.

[87] De Martino I, Fedele M, Palmieri D, Visone R, Cappabianca P, Wierinckx A, Trouillas J, Fusco A. B-RAF mutations are a rare event in pituitary adenomas. Journal of Endocrinological Investigation 2007;30(1) RC1-3.

[88] Lin Y, Jiang X, Shen Y, Li M, Ma H, Xing M, Lu Y. Frequent mutations and amplifications of the PIK3CA gene in pituitary tumors. Endocrine Related Cancer 2009;16(1) 301-10.

[89] Tanizaki Y, Jin L, Scheithauer BW, Kovacs K, Roncaroli F, Lloyd RV. P53 gene mutations in pituitary carcinomas. Endocrine Pathology 2007;18(4) 217-22.

[90] Simpson DJ, Hibberts NA, McNicol AM, Clayton RN, Farrell WE. Loss of pRb expression in pituitary adenomas is associated with methylation of the RB1 CpG island. Cancer Research 2000;60(5) 1211-6.

[91] Wierinckx A, Raverot G, Nazaret N, Jouanneau E, Auger C, Lachuer J, Trouillas J. Proliferation markers of human pituitary tumors: contribution of a genome-wide transcriptome approach. Molecular and Cellular Endocrinology 2010; 326(1-2) 30-9.

[92] Tong Y, Zheng Y, Zhou J, Oyesiku NM, Koeffler HP, Melmed S. Genomic characterization of human and rat prolactinomas. Endocrinology 2012;153(8) 3679-91.

[93] Xu M, Knox AJ, Michaelis KA, Kiseljak-Vassiliades K, Kleinschmidt-DeMasters BK, Lillehei KO, Wierman ME. Reprimo (RPRM) is a novel tumor suppressor in pituitary tumors and regulates survival, proliferation, and tumorigenicity. Endocrinology 2012;153(7) 2963-73.

[94] Jenuwein T, Allis CD. Translating the histone code. Science 2001;293(5532) 1074-80.

[95] Dudley KJ, Revill K, Clayton RN, Farrell WE. Pituitary tumours: all silent on the epigenetics front. Journal of Molecular Endocrinology 2009;42(6) 461-8.

[96] Ezzat S. Epigenetic control in pituitary tumors. Endocrine Journal 2008;55(6) 951-7.

[97] Duong CV, Emes RD, Wessely F, Yacqub-Usman K, Clayton RN, Farrell WE. Quantitative, genome-wide analysis of the DNA methylome in sporadic pituitary adenomas. Endocrine-Related Cancer 2012;19(6) 805-16.

[98] Yacqub-Usman K, Richardson A, Duong CV, Clayton RN, Farrell WE. The pituitary tumour epigenome: aberrations and prospects for targeted therapy. Nature Reviews Endocrinology 2012;8(8) 486-94.

[99] Wu X, Hua X. Menin, histone H3 methyltransferases, and regulation of cell proliferation: current knowledge and perspective. Current Molecular Medicine 2008; 8(8) 805-15.

[100] Zhang Z, Florez S, Gutierrez-Hartmann A, Martin JF, Amendt BA. MicroRNAs regulate pituitary development, and microRNA 26b specifically targets lymphoid enhancer factor 1 (Lef-1), which modulates pituitary transcription factor 1 (Pit-1) expression. The Journal of Biological Chemistry 2010;285(45) 34718-28.

[101] Yuen T, Ruf F, Chu T, Sealfon SC. Microtranscriptome regulation by gonadotropin-releasing hormone. Molecular and Cellular Endocrinology 2009;302(1) 12-7.

[102] Bottoni A, Piccin D, Tagliati F, Luchin A, Zatelli MC, degli Uberti EC. miR-15a and miR-16-1 down-regulation in pituitary adenomas. Journal of Cellular Physiology 2005;204(1) 280-5.

[103] Bottoni A, Zatelli MC, Ferracin M, Tagliati F, Piccin D, Vignali C, Calin GA, Negrini M, Croce CM, Degli Uberti EC. Identification of differentially expressed microRNAs by microarray: a possible role for microRNA genes in pituitary adenomas. Journal of Cellular Physiology 2007;210(2) 370-7.

[104] Sivapragasam M, Rotondo F, Lloyd RV, Scheithauer BW, Cusimano M, Syro LV, Kovacs K. MicroRNAs in the human pituitary. Endocrine Pathology 2011;22(3) 134-43.

[105] Trivellin G, Butz H, Delhove J, Igreja S, Chahal HS, Zivkovic V, McKay T, Patócs A, Grossman AB, Korbonits M. MicroRNA miR-107 is overexpressed in pituitary adenomas and inhibits the expression of aryl hydrocarbon receptor-interacting protein in vitro. American Journal of Physiology – Endocrinology and Metabolism 2012;303(6) E708-19.

[106] Mao ZG, He DS, Zhou J, Yao B, Xiao WW, Chen CH, Zhu YH, Wang HJ. Differential expression of microRNAs in GH-secreting pituitary adenomas. Diagnostic Pathology 2010;5 79.

[107] D'Angelo D, Palmieri D, Mussnich P, Roche M, Wierinckx A, Raverot G, Fedele M, Croce CM, Trouillas J, Fusco A. Altered microRNA expression profile in human pituitary GH adenomas: down-regulation of miRNA targeting HMGA1, HMGA2, and E2F1. The Journal of Clinical Endocrinology & Metabolism 2012;97(7) E1128-38.

[108] Wang C, Su Z, Sanai N, Xue X, Lu L, Chen Y, Wu J, Zheng W, Zhuge Q, Wu ZB. microRNA expression profile and differentially-expressed genes in prolactinomas following bromocriptine treatment. Oncology Reports 2012;27(5) 1312-20.

[109] Butz H, Likó I, Czirják S, Igaz P, Khan MM, Zivkovic V, Bálint K, Korbonits M, Rácz K, Patócs A. Down-regulation of Wee1 kinase by a specific subset of microRNA in human sporadic pituitary adenomas. The Journal of Clinical Endocrinology & Metabolism 2010;95(10) E181-91.

[110] Stilling G, Sun Z, Zhang S, Jin L, Righi A, Kovācs G, Korbonits M, Scheithauer BW, Kovacs K, Lloyd RV. MicroRNA expression in ACTH-producing pituitary tumors: up-regulation of microRNA-122 and -493 in pituitary carcinomas. Endocrine 2010;38(1) 67-75.

[111] Palumbo T, Faucz FR, Azevedo M, Xekouki P, Iliopoulos D, Stratakis CA. Functional screen analysis reveals miR-26b and miR-128 as central regulators of pituitary somatomammotrophic tumor growth through activation of the PTEN-AKT pathway. Oncogene 2012 [Epub ahead of print].

[112] Palmieri D, D'Angelo D, Valentino T, De Martino I, Ferraro A, Wierinckx A, Fedele M, Trouillas J, Fusco A. Downregulation of HMGA-targeting microRNAs has a critical role in human pituitary tumorigenesis. Oncogene 2012;31(34) 3857-65.

[113] Zhou Y, Zhang X, Klibanski A. MEG3 noncoding RNA: a tumor suppressor. Journal of Molecular Endocrinology 2012; 48(3) R45-53.

[114] Cheunsuchon P, Zhou Y, Zhang X, Lee H, Chen W, Nakayama Y, Rice KA, Tessa Hedley-Whyte E, Swearingen B, Klibanski A. Silencing of the imprinted DLK1-MEG3 locus in human clinically nonfunctioning pituitary adenomas. American Journal of Pathology 2011;179(4) 2120-30.

[115] Pertuit M, Barlier A, Enjalbert A, Gérard C. Signalling pathway alterations in pituitary adenomas: involvement of Gsalpha, cAMP and mitogen-activated protein kinases. Journal of Neuroendocrinology 2009;21(11) 869-77.

[116] Lania AG, Mantovani G, Ferrero S, Pellegrini C, Bondioni S, Peverelli E, Braidotti P, Locatelli M, Zavanone ML, Ferrante E, Bosari S, Beck-Peccoz P, Spada A. Proliferation of transformed somatotroph cells related to low or absent expression of protein kinase a regulatory subunit 1A protein. Cancer Research 2004;64(24) 9193-8.

[117] Peverelli E, Ermetici F, Filopanti M, Elli FM, Ronchi CL, Mantovani G, Ferrero S, Bosari S, Beck-Peccoz P, Lania A, Spada A. Analysis of genetic variants of phosphodiesterase 11A in acromegalic patients. European Journal of Endocrinology 2009;161(5) 687-94.

[118] Asa SL, Scheithauer BW, Bilbao JM, Horvath E, Ryan N, Kovacs K, Randall RV, Laws ER Jr, Singer W, Linfoot JA, Thorner MO, Vale W. A case for hypothalamic acromegaly: a clinicopathological study of six patients with hypothalamic gangliocytomas producing growth hormone-releasing factor. The Journal of Clinical Endocrinology & Metabolism 1984;58 796-803.

[119] Garby L, Caron P, Claustrat F, Chanson P, Tabarin A, Rohmer V, Arnault G, Bonnet F, Chabre O, Christin-Maitre S, du-Boullay H, Murat A, Nakib I, Sadoul JL, Sassolas G, Claustrat B, Raverot G, Borson-Chazot F; GTE Group. Clinical characteristics and outcome of acromegaly induced by ectopic secretion of growth hormone-releasing hormone (GHRH): a French nationwide series of 21 cases. The Journal of Clinical Endocrinology & Metabolism 2012;97(6) 2093-104.

[120] Senovilla L, Núñez L, de Campos JM, de Luis DA, Romero E, Sánchez A, García-Sancho J, Villalobos C. Multifunctional cells in human pituitary adenomas: implications for paradoxical secretion and tumorigenesis. The Journal of Clinical Endocrinology & Metabolism 2004;89(9) 4545-52.

[121] Molitch ME. Pharmacologic resistance in prolactinoma patients. Pituitary 2005;8(1) 43-52.

[122] Peverelli E, Mantovani G, Vitali E, Elli FM, Olgiati L, Ferrero S, Laws ER, Della Mina P, Villa A, Beck-Peccoz P, Spada A, Lania AG. Filamin-A is essential for dopamine D2 receptor expression and signaling in tumorous lactotrophs. The Journal of Clinical Endocrinology & Metabolism 2012;97(3) 967-77.

[123] Lania A, Mantovani G, Spada A. Genetic abnormalities of somatostatin receptors in pituitary tumors. Molecular and Cellular Endocrinology 2008;286(1-2) 180-6.

[124] Durán-Prado M, Saveanu A, Luque RM, Gahete MD, Gracia-Navarro F, Jaquet P, Dufour H, Malagón MM, Culler MD, Barlier A, Castaño JP. A potential inhibitory role for the new truncated variant of somatostatin receptor 5, sst5TMD4, in pituitary adenomas poorly responsive to somatostatin analogs. The Journal of Clinical Endocrinology & Metabolism 2010;95(5) 2497-502.

[125] Denef C. Paracrinicity: the story of 30 years of cellular pituitary crosstalk. Journal of Neuroendocrinology 2008;20(1) 1-70.

[126] Perumal P, Vrontakis ME. Transgenic mice over-expressing galanin exhibit pituitary adenomas and increased secretion of galanin, prolactin and growth hormone. Journal of Endocrinology 2003;179(2) 145-54.

[127] Shimon I, Hinton DR, Weiss MH, Melmed S. Prolactinomas express human heparin-binding secretory transforming gene (hst) protein product: marker of tumour invasiveness. Clinical Endocrinology 1998;48(1) 23-9.

[128] Ezzat S, Zheng L, Zhu XF, Wu GE, Asa SL. Targeted expression of a human pituitary tumor-derived isoform of FGF receptor-4 recapitulates pituitary tumorigenesis. The Journal of Clinical Investigation 2002;109(1) 69-78.

[129] Mukdsi JH, De Paul AL, Petiti JP, Gutiérrez S, Aoki A, Torres AI. Pattern of FGF-2 isoform expression correlated with its biological action in experimental prolactinomas. Acta Neuropathologica 2006;112(4) 491-501.

[130] Zhu X, Lee K, Asa SL, Ezzat S. Epigenetic silencing through DNA and histone methylation of fibroblast growth factor receptor 2 in neoplastic pituitary cells. Amercian Journal of Pathology 2007;170(5) 1618-28.

[131] Haedo MR, Gerez J, Fuertes M, Giacomini D, Páez-Pereda M, Labeur M, Renner U, Stalla GK, Arzt E. Regulation of pituitary function by cytokines. Hormone Research 2009;72(5) 266-74.

[132] Lebrun JJ. Activin, TGF-beta and menin in pituitary tumorigenesis. Advances in Experimental Medicine and Biology 2009;668 69-78.

[133] Danila DC, Zhang X, Zhou Y, Haidar JN, Klibanski A. Overexpression of wild-type activin receptor alk4-1 restores activin antiproliferative effects in human pituitary tumor cells. The Journal of Clinical Endocrinology & Metabolism 2002;87(10) 4741-6.

[134] Giacomini D, Acuña M, Gerez J, Nagashima AC, Silberstein S, Páez-Pereda M, Labeur M, Theodoropoulou M, Renner U, Stalla GK, Arzt E. Pituitary action of cytokines: focus on BMP-4 and gp130 family. Neuroendocrinology 2007;85(2) 94-100.

[135] Barbieri F, Bajetto A, Stumm R, Pattarozzi A, Porcile C, Zona G, Dorcaratto A, Ravetti JL, Minuto F, Spaziante R, Schettini G, Ferone D, Florio T. Overexpression of stromal cell-derived factor 1 and its receptor CXCR4 induces autocrine/paracrine cell proliferation in human pituitary adenomas. Clinical Cancer Research 2008;14(16) 5022-32.

[136] Cooper O, Vlotides G, Fukuoka H, Greene MI, Melmed S. Expression and function of ErbB receptors and ligands in the pituitary. Endocrine Related Cancer 2011;18(6) R197-211.

[137] Theodoropoulou M, Arzberger T, Gruebler Y, Jaffrain-Rea ML, Schlegel J, Schaaf L, Petrangeli E, Losa M, Stalla GK, Pagotto U. Expression of epidermal growth factor receptor in neoplastic pituitary cells: evidence for a role in corticotropinoma cells. Journal of Endocrinology 2004;183(2) 385-94.

[138] Fukuoka H, Cooper O, Ben-Shlomo A, Mamelak A, Ren SG, Bruyette D, Melmed S. EGFR as a therapeutic target for human, canine, and mouse ACTH-secreting pituitary adenomas. The Journal of Clinical Endocrinology 2011;121(12) 4712-21.

[139] Vlotides G, Siegel E, Donangelo I, Gutman S, Ren SG, Melmed S. Rat prolactinoma cell growth regulation by epidermal growth factor receptor ligands. Cancer Research 2008;68(15) 6377-86.

[140] Assimakopoulou M, Zolota V, Chondrogianni C, Gatzounis G, Varakis J. p75 and TrkC neurotrophin receptors demonstrate a different immunoreactivity profile in comparison to TrkA and TrkB receptors in human normal pituitary gland and adenomas. Neuroendocrinology 2008;88(2) 127-34.

[141] Missale C. Nerve growth factor, D2 receptor isoforms, and pituitary tumors. Endocrine 2012;42(3) 466-7.

[142] Lloyd RV, Vidal S, Horvath E, Kovacs K, Scheithauer B. Angiogenesis in normal and neoplastic pituitary tissues. Microscopy Research and Technique 2003;60(2) 244-50.

[143] Sánchez-Ortiga R, Sánchez-Tejada L, Moreno-Perez O, Riesgo P, Niveiro M, Picó Alfonso AM. Over-expression of vascular endothelial growth factor in pituitary adenomas is associated with extrasellar growth and recurrence. Pituitary 2012 [Epub ahead of print].

[144] Molitch ME. Prolactinoma in pregnancy. Best Practice & Research Clinical Endocrinology & Metabolism 2011;25(6) 885-96.

[145] Jaffrain-Rea ML, Petrangeli E, Ortolani F, Fraioli B, Lise A, Esposito V, Spagnoli LG, Tamburrano G, Frati L, Gulino A. Cellular receptors for sex steroids in human pituitary adenomas. Journal of Endocrinology 1996; 151(2) 175-84.

[146] Caronti B, Palladini G, Bevilacqua MG, Petrangeli E, Fraioli B, Cantore G, Tamburrano G, Carapella CM, Jaffrain-Rea ML. Effects of 17 beta-estradiol, progesterone and tamoxifen on in vitro proliferation of human pituitary adenomas: correlation with specific cellular receptors. Tumour Biology 1993;14(1) 59-68.

[147] Zhou W, Song Y, Xu H, Zhou K, Zhang W, Chen J, Qin M, Yi H, Gustafsson JA, Yang H, Fan X. In nonfunctional pituitary adenomas, estrogen receptors and slug contribute to development of invasiveness. The Journal of Clinical Endocrinology & Metabolism 2011;96(8) E1237-45.

[148] Fan X, Gabbi C, Kim HJ, Cheng G, Andersson LC, Warner M, Gustafsson JA. Gonadotropin-positive pituitary tumors accompanied by ovarian tumors in aging female ERbeta-/- mice. Proceedings of the National Academy of Sciences of the United States of America 2010;107(14) 6453-8.

[149] Heaney AP, Fernando M, Melmed S. Functional role of estrogen in pituitary tumor pathogenesis. The Journal of Clinical Investigation 2002;109(2) 277-83.

[150] Sarkar DK. Genesis of prolactinomas: studies using estrogen-treated animals. Frontiers of Hormone Research 2006;35 32-49.

[151] Zaldivar V, Magri ML, Zárate S, Jaita G, Eijo G, Radl D, Ferraris J, Pisera D, Seilicovich A. Estradiol increases the expression of TNF-α and TNF receptor 1 in lactotropes. Neuroendocrinology 2011;93(2) 106-13.

[152] Zárate S, Jaita G, Ferraris J, Eijo G, Magri ML, Pisera D, Seilicovich A. Estrogens induce expression of membrane-associated estrogen receptor α isoforms in lactotropes. PLoS One 2012;7(7) E41299.

[153] Dworakowska D, Grossman AB. The molecular pathogenesis of corticotroph tumours. European Journal of Clinical Investigation 2012;42(6) 665-76.

[154] Chauvet N, El-Yandouzi T, Mathieu MN, Schlernitzauer A, Galibert E, Lafont C, Le Tissier P, Robinson IC, Mollard P, Coutry N. Characterization of adherens junction protein expression and localization in pituitary cell networks. Journal of Endocrinology 2009;202(3) 375-87.

[155] Qian ZR, Li CC, Yamasaki H, Mizusawa N, Yoshimoto K, Yamada S, Tashiro T, Horiguchi H, Wakatsuki S, Hirokawa M, Sano T. Role of E-cadherin, alpha-, beta-, and gamma-catenins, and p120 (cell adhesion molecules) in prolactinoma behavior. Modern Pathology 2002;15(12) 1357-65.

[156] Elston MS, Gill AJ, Conaglen JV, Clarkson A, Cook RJ, Little NS, Robinson BG, Clifton-Bligh RJ, McDonald KL. Nuclear accumulation of e-cadherin correlates with loss of cytoplasmic membrane staining and invasion in pituitary adenomas. The Journal of Clinical Endocrinology & Metabolism 2009;94(4) 1436-42.

[157] Fougner SL, Lekva T, Borota OC, Hald JK, Bollerslev J, Berg JP. The expression of E-cadherin in somatotroph pituitary adenomas is related to tumor size, invasiveness, and somatostatin analog response. The Journal of Clinical Endocrinology & Metabolism 2010;95(5) 2334-42.

[158] Evang JA, Berg JP, Casar-Borota O, Lekva T, Kringen MK, Ramm-Pettersen J, Bollerslev J. Reduced levels of E-cadherin correlate with progression of corticotroph pituitary tumours. Clinical Endocrinology 2011;75(6) 811-8.

[159] Trouillas J, Daniel L, Guigard MP, Tong S, Gouvernet J, Jouanneau E, Jan M, Perrin G, Fischer G, Tabarin A, Rougon G, Figarella-Branger D. Polysialylated neural cell

adhesion molecules expressed in human pituitary tumors and related to extrasellar invasion. Journal of Neurosurgery 2003; 98(5) 1084-93.

[160] Quereda V, Malumbres M. Cell cycle control of pituitary development and disease. Journal of Molecular Endocrinology 2009;42(2) 75-86.

[161] Hibberts NA, Simpson DJ, Bicknell JE, Broome JC, Hoban PR, Clayton RN, Farrell WE. Analysis of cyclin D1 (CCND1) allelic imbalance and overexpression in sporadic human pituitary tumors. Clinical Cancer Research 1999;5(8) 2133-9.

[162] Roussel-Gervais A, Bilodeau S, Vallette S, Berthelet F, Lacroix A, Figarella-Branger D, Brue T, Drouin J. Cooperation between cyclin E and p27(Kip1) in pituitary tumorigenesis. Molecular Endocrinology 2010;24(9) 1835-45.

[163] Simpson DJ, Frost SJ, Bicknell JE, Broome JC, McNicol AM, Clayton RN, Farrell WE. Aberrant expression of G(1)/S regulators is a frequent event in sporadic pituitary adenomas. Carcinogenesis 2001;22(8) 1149-54.

[164] Kirsch M, Mörz M, Pinzer T, Schackert HK, Schackert G. Frequent loss of the CDKN2C (p18INK4c) gene product in pituitary adenomas. Genes Chromosomes Cancer. 2009;48(2) 143-54.

[165] Foijer F, te Riele H. Check, double check: the G2 barrier to cancer. Cell Cycle 2006;5(8) 831-6.

[166] Wierinckx A, Auger C, Devauchelle P, Reynaud A, Chevallier P, Jan M, Perrin G, Fèvre-Montange M, Rey C, Figarella-Branger D, Raverot G, Belin MF, Lachuer J, Trouillas J. A diagnostic marker set for invasion, proliferation, and aggressiveness of prolactin pituitary tumors. Endocrine Related Cancer 2007;14(3) 887-900.

[167] De Martino I, Visone R, Wierinckx A, Palmieri D, Ferraro A, Cappabianca P, Chiappetta G, Forzati F, Lombardi G, Colao A, Trouillas J, Fedele M, Fusco A. HMGA proteins up-regulate CCNB2 gene in mouse and human pituitary adenomas. Cancer Research 2009;69(5) 1844-50.

[168] Zhang X, Sun H, Danila DC, Johnson SR, Zhou Y, Swearingen B, Klibanski A. Loss of expression of GADD45 gamma, a growth inhibitory gene, in human pituitary adenomas: implications for tumorigenesis. The Journal of Clinical Endocrinology & Metabolism 2002;87(3) 1262-7.

[169] Michaelis KA, Knox AJ, Xu M, Kiseljak-Vassiliades K, Edwards MG, Geraci M, Kleinschmidt-DeMasters BK, Lillehei KO, Wierman ME. Identification of growth arrest and DNA-damage-inducible gene beta (GADD45beta) as a novel tumor suppressor in pituitary gonadotrope tumors. Endocrinology 2011;152(10) 3603-13.

[170] St Croix B, Sheehan C, Rak JW, Flørenes VA, Slingerland JM, Kerbel RS. E-Cadherin-dependent growth suppression is mediated by the cyclin-dependent kinase inhibitor p27(KIP1). Journal of Cellular Biology 1998;142(2) 557-71.

[171] Hubina E, Nanzer AM, Hanson MR, Ciccarelli E, Losa M, Gaia D, Papotti M, Terreni MR, Khalaf S, Jordan S, Czirják S, Hanzély Z, Nagy GM, Góth MI, Grossman AB, Korbonits M. Somatostatin analogues stimulate p27 expression and inhibit the MAP kinase pathway in pituitary tumours. European Journal of Endocrinology 2006;155(2) 371-9.

[172] Abbass T, Dutta A. p21 in cancer: intricate networks and multiple activities. Nature Review in Cancer 2009; 9(6) 400-14.

[173] Chesnokova V, Zonis S, Kovacs K, Ben-Shlomo A, Wawrowsky K, Bannykh S, Melmed S. p21(Cip1) restrains pituitary tumor growth. Proceedings of the National Academy of Sciences of the United States of America 2008;105(45) 17498-503.

[174] Hiyama H, Kubo O, Kawamata T, Ishizaki R, Hori T. Expression of cyclin kinase inhibitor p21/WAF1 protein in pituitary adenomas: correlations with endocrine activity, but not cell proliferation. Acta Neurochirurgica 2002;144(5) 481-8.

[175] Neto AG, McCutcheon IE, Vang R, Spencer ML, Zhang W, Fuller GN. Elevated expression of p21 (WAF1/Cip1) in hormonally active pituitary adenomas. Annals of Diagnostic Pathology 2005;9(1) 6-10.

[176] Alexandraki KI, Munayem Khan M, Chahal HS, Dalantaeva NS, Trivellin G, Berney DM, Caron P, Popovic V, Pfeifer M, Jordan S, Korbonits M, Grossman AB. Oncogene-induced senescence in pituitary adenomas and carcinomas. Hormones 2012;11(3) 297-307.

[177] Vlotides G, Eigler T, Melmed S. Pituitary tumor-transforming gene: physiology and implications for tumorigenesis. Endocrine Reviews 2007;28(2) 165-86.

[178] Tong Y, Eigler T. Transcriptional targets for pituitary tumor-transforming gene-1. Journal of Molecular Endocrinology 2009;43(5) 179-85.

[179] Salehi F, Kovacs K, Scheithauer BW, Lloyd RV, Cusimano M. Pituitary tumor-transforming gene in endocrine and other neoplasms: a review and update. Endocrine Related Cancer 2008;15(3) 721-43.

[180] Abbud RA, Takumi I, Barker EM, Ren SG, Chen DY, Wawrowsky K, Melmed S. Early multipotential pituitary focal hyperplasia in the alpha-subunit of glycoprotein hormone-driven pituitary tumor-transforming gene transgenic mice. Molecular Endocrinology 2005;19(5) 1383-91.

[181] Cleynen I, Van de Ven WJ. The HMGA proteins: a myriad of functions (Review). International Journal of Oncology 2008;32(2) 289-305.

[182] Fedele M, Fusco A. Role of the high mobility group A proteins in the regulation of pituitary cell cycle. Journal of Molecular Endocrinology 2010;44(6) 309-18.

[183] Palmieri D, Valentino T, De Martino I, Esposito F, Cappabianca P, Wierinckx A, Vitiello M, Lombardi G, Colao A, Trouillas J, Pierantoni GM, Fusco A, Fedele M. PIT1

upregulation by HMGA proteins has a role in pituitary tumorigenesis. Endocrine Related Cancer 2012;19(2) 123-35.

[184] Qian ZR, Asa SL, Siomi H, Siomi MC, Yoshimoto K, Yamada S, Wang EL, Rahman MM, Inoue H, Itakura M, Kudo E, Sano T. Overexpression of HMGA2 relates to reduction of the let-7 and its relationship to clinicopathological features in pituitary adenomas. Modern Pathology 2009;22(3) 431-41.

[185] Wang EL, Qian ZR, Rahman MM, Yoshimoto K, Yamada S, Kudo E, Sano T. Increased expression of HMGA1 correlates with tumour invasiveness and proliferation in human pituitary adenomas. Histopathology 2010;56(4) 501-9.

[186] May LT, Hill SJ. ERK phosphorylation: spatial and temporal regulation by G protein-coupled receptors. The International Journal of Biochemistry & Cell Biology 2008;40(10) 2013-7.

[187] Pópulo H, Lopes JM, Soares P. The mTOR Signalling Pathway in Human Cancer. International Journal of Molecular Sciences 2012;13(2) 1886-918.

[188] McCubrey JA, Steelman LS, Franklin RA, Abrams SL, Chappell WH, Wong EW, Lehmann BD, Terrian DM, Basecke J, Stivala F, Libra M, Evangelisti C, Martelli AM. Targeting the RAF/MEK/ERK, PI3K/AKT and p53 pathways in hematopoietic drug resistance. Advances in Enzyme Regulation 2007;47 64-103.

[189] Suojun Z, Feng W, Dongsheng G, Ting L. Targeting Raf/MEK/ERK pathway in pituitary adenomas. European Journal of Cancer 2012;48(3) 389-95.

[190] Cakir M, Grossman AB. Targeting MAPK (Ras/ERK) and PI3K/Akt pathways in pituitary tumorigenesis. Expert Opinion on Therapeutic Targets 2009;13(9) 1121-34.

[191] Ewing I, Pedder-Smith S, Franchi G, Ruscica M, Emery M, Vax V, Garcia E, Czirják S, Hanzély Z, Kola B, Korbonits M, Grossman AB. A mutation and expression analysis of the oncogene BRAF in pituitary adenomas. Clinical Endocrinology 2007;66(3) 348-52.

[192] Dworakowska D, Wlodek E, Leontiou CA, Igreja S, Cakir M, Teng M, Prodromou N, Góth MI, Grozinsky-Glasberg S, Gueorguiev M, Kola B, Korbonits M, Grossman AB. Activation of RAF/MEK/ERK and PI3K/AKT/mTOR pathways in pituitary adenomas and their effects on downstream effectors. Endocrine Related Cancer 2009;16(4) 1329-38.

[193] Kovalovsky D, Refojo D, Liberman AC, Hochbaum D, Pereda MP, Coso OA, Stalla GK, Holsboer F, Arzt E. Activation and induction of NUR77/NURR1 in corticotrophs by CRH/cAMP: involvement of calcium, protein kinase A, and MAPK pathways. Molecular Endocrinology 2002;16(7) 1638-51.

[194] Bliss SP, Navratil AM, Xie J, Roberson MS. GnRH signaling, the gonadotrope and endocrine control of fertility. Frontiers in Neuroendocrinology 2010;31(3) 322-40.

[195] Pertuit M, Romano D, Zeiller C, Barlier A, Enjalbert A, Gerard C. The gsp oncogene disrupts Ras/ERK-dependent prolactin gene regulation in gsp inducible somatotroph cell line. Endocrinology 2011;152(4) 1234-43.

[196] Musat M, Korbonits M, Kola B, Borboli N, Hanson MR, Nanzer AM, Grigson J, Jordan S, Morris DG, Gueorguiev M, Coculescu M, Basu S, Grossman AB. Enhanced protein kinase B/Akt signalling in pituitary tumours. Endocrine Related Cancer 2005;12(2) 423-33.

[197] Lu C, Willingham MC, Furuya F, Cheng SY. Activation of phosphatidylinositol 3-kinase signaling promotes aberrant pituitary growth in a mouse model of thyroid-stimulating hormone-secreting pituitary tumors. Endocrinology 2008;149(7) 3339-45.

[198] Theodoropoulou M, Stalla GK, Spengler D. ZAC1 target genes and pituitary tumorigenesis. Molecular and Cellular Endocrinology 2010;326(1-2) 60-5.

[199] Pizarro CB, Oliveira MC, Pereira-Lima JF, Leães CG, Kramer CK, Schuch T, Barbosa-Coutinho LM, Ferreira NP. Evaluation of angiogenesis in 77 pituitary adenomas using endoglin as a marker. Neuropathology 2009;29(1) 40-4.

[200] Recouvreux MV, Camilletti MA, Rifkin DB, Becu-Villalobos D, Díaz-Torga G. Thrombospondin-1 (TSP-1) analogs ABT-510 and ABT-898 inhibit prolactinoma growth and recover active pituitary transforming growth factor-β1 (TGF-β1). Endocrinology 2012;153(8) 3861-71.

[201] Raica M, Coculescu M, Cimpean AM, Ribatti D. Endocrine gland derived-VEGF is down-regulated in human pituitary adenoma. Anticancer Research 2010;30(10) 3981-6.

[202] Vidal S, Horvath E, Kovacs K, Kuroki T, Lloyd RV, Scheithauer BW. Expression of hypoxia-inducible factor-1alpha (HIF-1alpha) in pituitary tumours. Histology and Histopathology 2003;18(3) 679-86.

[203] Yoshida D, Kim K, Noha M, Teramoto A. Anti-apoptotic action by hypoxia inducible factor 1-alpha in human pituitary adenoma cell line, HP-75 in hypoxic condition. Journal of Neuro-oncology 2006;78(3) 217-25.

[204] Shan B, Gerez J, Haedo M, Fuertes M, Theodoropoulou M, Buchfelder M, Losa M, Stalla GK, Arzt E, Renner U. RSUME is implicated in HIF-1-induced VEGF-A production in pituitary tumour cells. Endocrine Related Cancer 2012;19(1) 13-27.

[205] Jin Kim Y, Hyun Kim C, Hwan Cheong J, Min Kim J. Relationship between expression of vascular endothelial growth factor and intratumoral hemorrhage in human pituitary adenomas. Tumori 2011;97(5) 639-46.

[206] Xiao Z, Liu Q, Mao F, Wu J, Lei T. TNF-α-induced VEGF and MMP-9 expression promotes hemorrhagic transformation in pituitary adenomas. International Journal of Molecular Sciences 2011;12(6) 4165-79.

[207] Xiao Z, Liu Q, Zhao B, Wu J, Lei T. Hypoxia induces hemorrhagic transformation in pituitary adenomas via the HIF-1α signaling pathway. Oncology Reports 2011;26(6) 1457-64.

[208] Rotondo F, Sharma S, Scheithauer BW, Horvath E, Syro LV, Cusimano M, Nassiri F, Yousef GM, Kovacs K. Endoglin and CD-34 immunoreactivity in the assessment of microvessel density in normal pituitary and adenoma subtypes. Neoplasma 2010;57(6) 590-3.

[209] Miyajima K, Takekoshi S, Itoh J, Kakimoto K, Miyakoshi T, Osamura RY. Inhibitory effects of anti-VEGF antibody on the growth and angiogenesis of estrogen-induced pituitary prolactinoma in Fischer 344 Rats: animal model of VEGF-targeted therapy for human endocrine tumors. Acta Histochemica Cytochemica 2010;43(2) 33-44.

[210] Luque GM, Perez-Millán MI, Ornstein AM, Cristina C, Becu-Villalobos D. Inhibitory effects of antivascular endothelial growth factor strategies in experimental dopamine-resistant prolactinomas. Journal of Pharmacology and Experimental Therapeutics 2011;337(3) 766-74.

[211] Ortiz LD, Syro LV, Scheithauer BW, Ersen A, Uribe H, Fadul CE, Rotondo F, Horvath E, Kovacs K. Anti-VEGF therapy in pituitary carcinoma. Pituitary. 2012;15(3) 445-9.

[212] Saraga-Babic M, Bazina M, Vukojevic K, Bocina I, Stefanovic V. Involvement of pro-apoptotic and anti-apoptotic factors in the early development of the human pituitary gland. Histology and Histopathology 2008;23(10) 1259-68.

[213] Kulig E, Jin L, Qian X, Horvath E, Kovacs K, Stefaneanu L, Scheithauer BW, Lloyd RV. Apoptosis in nontumorous and neoplastic human pituitaries: expression of the Bcl-2 family of proteins. American Journal of Pathology 1999;154(3) 767-74.

[214] Kapranos N, Kontogeorgos G, Horvath E, Kovacs K. Morphology, molecular regulation and significance of apoptosis in pituitary adenomas. Frontiers of Hormone Research 2004;32 217-34.

[215] Sambaziotis D, Kapranos N, Kontogeorgos G. Correlation of bcl-2 and bax with apoptosis in human pituitary adenomas. Pituitary 2003;6(3) 127-33.

[216] Jaita G, Zárate S, Ferrari L, Radl D, Ferraris J, Eijo G, Zaldivar V, Pisera D, Seilicovich A. Gonadal steroids modulate Fas-induced apoptosis of lactotropes and somatotropes. Endocrine 2011;39(1) 21-7.

[217] Chen L, Zhuang G, Li W, Liu Y, Zhang J, Tian X. RGD-FasL induces apoptosis of pituitary adenoma cells. Cellular & Molecular Immunology 2008;5(1) 61-8.

[218] Candolfi M, Jaita G, Pisera D, Ferrari L, Barcia C, Liu C, Yu J, Liu G, Castro MG, Seilicovich A. Adenoviral vectors encoding tumor necrosis factor-alpha and FasL induce apoptosis of normal and tumoral anterior pituitary cells. Journal of Endocrinology 2006;189(3) 681-90.

[219] Cañibano C, Rodriguez NL, Saez C, Tovar S, Garcia-Lavandeira M, Borrello MG, Vidal A, Costantini F, Japon M, Dieguez C, Alvarez CV. The dependence receptor Ret induces apoptosis in somatotrophs through a Pit-1/p53 pathway, preventing tumor growth. EMBO Journal 2007;26(8) 2015-28.

[220] Diaz-Rodriguez E, García-Lavandeira M, Perez-Romero S, Senra A, Cañibano C, Palmero I, Borrello MG, Dieguez C, Alvarez CV. Direct promoter induction of p19Arf by Pit-1 explains the dependence receptor RET/Pit-1/p53-induced apoptosis in the pituitary somatotroph cells. Oncogene 2012;31(23) 2824-35.

[221] Japón MA, Urbano AG, Sáez C, Segura DI, Cerro AL, Diéguez C, Alvarez CV. Glial-derived neurotropic factor and RET gene expression in normal human anterior pituitary cell types and in pituitary tumors. The Journal of Clinical Endocrinology & Metabolism 2002;87(4) 1879-84.

[222] Kang BH, Xia F, Pop R, Dohi T, Socolovsky M, Altieri DC. Developmental control of apoptosis by the immunophilin aryl hydrocarbon receptor-interacting protein(AIP) involves mitochondrial import of the survivin protein. The Journal of Biological Chemistry 2011;286(19) 16758-67.

[223] Vargiolu M, Fusco D, Kurelac I, Dirnberger D, Baumeister R, Morra I, Melcarne A, Rimondini R, Romeo G, Bonora E. The tyrosine kinase receptor RET interacts in vivo with aryl hydrocarbon receptor-interacting protein to alter survivin availability. The Journal of Clinical Endocrinology & Metabolism 2009;94(7) 2571-8.

[224] Wasko R, Waligorska-Stachura J, Jankowska A, Warchol JB, Liebert W, Sowinski J. Coexpression of survivin and PCNA in pituitary tumors and normal pituitary. Neuro Endocrinology Letters 2009;30(4) 477-81.

[225] Formosa R, Gruppetta M, Falzon S, Santillo G, DeGaetano J, Xuereb-Anastasi A, Vassallo J. Expression and clinical significance of Wnt players and survivin in pituitary tumours. Endocrine Pathology 2012;23(2) 123-31.

[226] Tagliati F, Gentilin E, Buratto M, Molè D, degli Uberti EC, Zatelli MC. Magmas, a gene newly identified as overexpressed in human and mouse ACTH-secreting pituitary adenomas, protects pituitary cells from apoptotic stimuli. Endocrinology 2010;151(10) 4635-42.

[227] Bahar A, Simpson DJ, Cutty SJ, Bicknell JE, Hoban PR, Holley S, Mourtada-Maarabouni M, Williams GT, Clayton RN, Farrell WE. Isolation and characterization of a novel pituitary tumor apoptosis gene. Molecular Endocrinology 2004;18(7) 1827-39.

[228] Acunzo J, Roche C, Defilles C, Thirion S, Quentien MH, Figarella-Branger D, Graillon T, Dufour H, Brue T, Pellegrini I, Enjalbert A, Barlier A. Inactivation of PITX2 transcription factor induced apoptosis of gonadotroph tumoral cells. Endocrinology 2011;152(10) 3884-92.

[229] Radl DB, Ferraris J, Boti V, Seilicovich A, Sarkar DK, Pisera D. Dopamine-induced apoptosis of lactotropes is mediated by the short isoform of D2 receptor. PLoS One 2011;6(3) e18097.

[230] Grozinsky-Glasberg S, Shimon I, Korbonits M, Grossman AB. Somatostatin analogues in the control of neuroendocrine tumours: efficacy and mechanisms. Endocrine Related Cancer 2008;15(3) 701-20.

[231] 223. Chesnokova V, Melmed S. Pituitary senescence: the evolving role of Pttg. Molecular and Cellular Endocrinology 2010;326(1-2) 55-9.

[232] Chesnokova V, Zonis S, Zhou C, Ben-Shlomo A, Wawrowsky K, Toledano Y, Tong Y, Kovacs K, Scheithauer B, Melmed S. Lineage-specific restraint of pituitary gonadotroph cell adenoma growth. PLoS One 2011;6(3) e17924.

[233] Ragel BT, Couldwell WT. Pituitary carcinoma: a review of the literature. Neurosurgical Focus 2004;16(4) E7.

[234] Kaltsas GA, Nomikos P, Kontogeorgos G, Buchfelder M, Grossman AB. Clinical review: Diagnosis and management of pituitary carcinomas. The Journal of Clinical Endocrinology & Metabolism 2005;90(5) 3089-99.

[235] Colao A, Ochoa AS, Auriemma RS, Faggiano A, Pivonello R, Lombardi G. Pituitary carcinomas. Frontiers of Hormone Research 2010;38 94-108.

[236] van der Klaauw AA, Kienitz T, Strasburger CJ, Smit JW, Romijn JA. Malignant pituitary corticotroph adenomas: report of two cases and a comprehensive review of the literature. Pituitary 2009;12(1) 57-69.

[237] Ruebel KH, Leontovich AA, Jin L, Stilling GA, Zhang H, Qian X, Nakamura N, Scheithauer BW, Kovacs K, Lloyd RV. Patterns of gene expression in pituitary carcinomas and adenomas analyzed by high-density oligonucleotide arrays, reverse transcriptase-quantitative PCR, and protein expression. Endocrine 2006;29(3) 435-44.

[238] Sav A, Rotondo F, Syro LV, Scheithauer BW, Kovacs K. Biomarkers of pituitary neoplasms. Anticancer Research 2012;32(11) 4639-54.

[239] Syro LV, Ortiz LD, Scheithauer BW, Lloyd R, Lau Q, Gonzalez R, Uribe H, Cusimano M, Kovacs K, Horvath E. Treatment of pituitary neoplasms with temozolomide: a review. Cancer 2011;117(3) 454-62.

[240] Raverot G, Sturm N, de Fraipont F, Muller M, Salenave S, Caron P, Chabre O, Chanson P, Cortet-Rudelli C, Assaker R, Dufour H, Gaillard S, François P, Jouanneau E, Passagia JG, Bernier M, Cornélius A, Figarella-Branger D, Trouillas J, Borson-Chazot F, Brue T. Temozolomide treatment in aggressive pituitary tumors and pituitary carcinomas: a French multicenter experience. The Journal of Clinical Endocrinology & Metabolism 2010;95(10) 4592-9.

[241] Raverot G, Castinetti F, Jouanneau E, Morange I, Figarella-Branger D, Dufour H, Trouillas J, Brue T. Pituitary carcinomas and aggressive pituitary tumours: merits and pitfalls of temozolomide treatment. Clinical Endocrinology 2012;76(6) 769-75.

[242] Salehi F, Scheithauer BW, Kros JM, Lau Q, Fealey M, Erickson D, Kovacs K, Horvath E, Lloyd RV. MGMT promoter methylation and immunoexpression in aggressive pituitary adenomas and carcinomas. Journal of Neuro-oncology 2011;104(3) 647-57.

Chapter 3

Aging and Subclinical Thyroid Dysfunction

Corrêa V. M. da Costa and D. Rosenthal

Additional information is available at the end of the chapter

http://dx.doi.org/10.5772/55194

1. Introduction

1.1. Endocrinology of aging

Aging is inevitable. Although it has been intensively studied and discussed, its cause(s) are still in the realm of hypotheses. Two main theories hold the center of the stage at the moment: 1) aging occurs in accordance with genetic pre- programmed events or 2) it is not genetically programmed but results from an accumulation of random events [1, 2]. Either way, changes in cellular/molecular function are common denominators to be found in all processes that characterize biological aging, but these changes occur with different timing and specificity among different cells, tissues or organs [3]. This chapter will briefly review some important aspects of current knowledge about aging process and its impact on thyroidal function.

The endocrine system is as affected by aging as are other systems. Yet, again, not all of its components are affected at the same time or in the same way. During aging, physiologic functions decline gradually, cellular protein synthesis is diminished as well as immune function. There is also an increase in fat mass, a loss of muscle mass and strength, and a decrease in bone mineral density that contribute to declining health status.

Two important clinical changes occur in endocrine activity during aging, involving pancreas and thyroid gland. About 40% of individuals between the ages of 65 and 74 years and 50% of those older than 80 years have impaired glucose tolerance or diabetes mellitus, and in almost 50% of elderly adults with diabetes the disease is undiagnosed [4]. Pancreatic secretion, insulin receptor and insulin signaling pathways changes associated with aging are critical components of the endocrinology of aging. In addition to relatively decreased insulin secretion by the beta cells, peripheral insulin resistance related to poor diet, physical inactivity, increased abdominal fat mass, and decreased lean body mass contribute to the deterioration of glucose metabolism

[4]. Other hormonal systems exhibit lowered circulating hormone concentrations during normal aging, and these changes have been considered mainly physiologic. The decrease in human gonadic function with consequent decline in circulating estrogen and testosterone, and increase in serum gonadotropins (FSH and LH), is a classic example. A decrease in growth hormone (GH) and insulin-like growth factor-I (IGF-I) are most probably due do a decline in hypothalamic growth hormone releasing hormone (GHRH), and also a part of the aging process in mammals [4, 5]. The aged adrenal cortex is affected in its capacity to produce dehydroepiandrosterone (DHEA). In contrast the glucocorticoids produced in the adrenal cortex fasciculate layer tend to be more responsive to stimuli, have a slightly delayed clearance rate, and are less entrained to the circadian phase in aged subjects than in young ones. Although not all authors agree [6], most report that healthy elder subjects have higher cortisol levels presumably in response to increased corticotrophin (ACTH) secretion [7, 8]. It is difficult to evaluate - in humans - if this discordance is gender-related. An increased hypothalamus-pituitary-adrenal activity is also seen in aged rats, more due to an increase in hypothalamic vasopressin (AVP) synthesis and secretion than to increases in corticotrophin releasing hormone (CRH), and may be related to a decrease in glucocorticoid receptor activity both at the hypothalamus/pituitary and at peripheral tissues [9, 10].

2. Problem statement

2.1. Aging and thyroid dysfunction

Age-related thyroid dysfunction is common. Lowered plasma thyroxine (T4) and increased thyrotropin concentrations occur in 5% to 10% of elderly women [11]. Autoimmunity or an age-associated disease frequently are the primarily cause of these abnormalities rather than a natural consequence of the aging process. Several immunological abnormalities have been described in aging process. A well-recognized age-associated immune abnormality is the general production of both organ- and nonorgan-specific autoantibodies. Aging is frequently associated with the appearance of thyroid autoantibodies, but the biological and clinical significance of this is still unknown. Some data have shown that these thyroid autoantibodies are rare in healthy centenarians and in other highly selected aged populations, whereas they are frequently observed in unselected or hospitalized elderly patients, thus suggesting that these autoantibodies are not the consequence of the aging process itself, but rather are related to age-associated disease [12].

Thyroid autoimmunity and subclinical hypothyroidism have also been implicated in the pathogenesis of other age-associated disorders like coronary heart disease [13]. A major, unresolved issue is whether, and to what extent, the complex physiological changes seen in the hypothalamus-pituitary-thyroid axis contribute to the pathogenesis of age-associated diseases such as atherosclerosis, coronary heart disease and neurological disorders [11].

With improvements in biochemical testing and increasing numbers of relatively asymptomatic individuals being subjected to blood testing, subclinical hypothyroidism and subclinical hyperthyroidism have become the most frequent thyroid disease. The clinical complications and functional consequences and effects on quality of life have been extensively addressed as well as the therapeutic options, however because of the lack of large randomized clinical trials, the evidence for choosing one treatment over another is minimal [14].

Normal aging is accompanied by a slight decrease in pituitary thyrotropin (TSH) release and especially by decreased peripheral metabolism of T4, which results in a gradual age-dependent decline in serum triiodothyronine (T3) concentrations without changes in T4 levels [11]. This slight decrease in plasma T3 concentrations occurs largely within the broad normal range of the healthy elderly population and has not been clearly related to functional changes during the aging process. The deleterious effects of overt thyroid dysfunction in elderly individuals are clearly recognized, but the clinical relevance of mild forms of hypothyroidism and hyperthyroidism are a matter of debate. The prevalence of thyroid disease increases with age and all forms of thyroid disease are encountered. However, the clinical manifestations are different from those encountered in younger patients. In the elderly, autoimmune hypothyroidism is particularly prevalent. Hyperthyroidism is mainly characterized by cardiovascular symptoms and is frequently due to toxic nodular goiters. Thyroid carcinoma is also more aggressive [15].

Molecular biology studies have considerably broadened our knowledge of thyroid tumorigenesis. Follicular cell proliferation is mainly regulated by TSH but also is controlled by extracellular growth factors that essentially modify intra- cellular signaling pathways after binding to membrane receptors. It is known that "in *vitro*" TSH stimulates cell cycle progression and proliferation in cooperation with insulin or IGF-I in various thyrocyte culture systems, including rat thyroid cell lines (FRTL-5, WRT and PCCl-3), and in primary cultures of rat, dog, sheep and human thyroid cells [16]. Park *et al.* demonstrated that the TSH proliferative effect is, at least in part, mediated by an increase in expression of an adaptor molecule of the IGF-I receptor (p66Shc) [17]. These data suggest that the synergistic proliferative effect of TSH and insulin/IGF-I on the thyroid gland may also occur "in *vivo*".

Tumor growth occurs when the normal equilibrium of regulatory pathways is disrupted, either through enhancement of stimulatory pathways or deficient inhibitory pathways [18]. Epidemiological studies show that cancer is primarily a disease of the aged. Cancer rates increase dramatically in humans beginning in the sixth and seventh decades of life. Although the complex relationship between cancer and aging has long been recognized, a clear understanding of the mechanisms underlying this relationship has remained elusive. Recently, Hinkal and Donehower reviewing this issue focused on a decline in function of tumor-suppressing genes like p53 during aging, associated with the development of tumors in many different tissues in mice. Among the hundreds of tumor-suppressing genes now identified, p53 may be the most important. The p53 gene is mutated in over half of all human cancers, and it has been estimated that more than 80% of human cancers have dysfunctional p53 signaling [19]. In fact, decreased expression of tumor- suppressing genes, may be associated with higher cancer incidence in aged subjects, but one can not discard higher function of genes involved in cellular proliferation probably also present in aged subjects.

Ras proteins are involved in the transduction of growth factor signals by surface receptors, and are key components of downstream signaling through several pathways. Ras activation of the Raf serine/threonine kinases, and activation of the ERK mitogen-activated protein kinases (MAPKs) is an important signaling pathway for many Ras effects [20]. Thyroidal proliferation can be induced by growth factors, and it is known that oncogenic mutations of Ras-family genes play an important role in malignant transformation and tumor progression in the follicular epithelium of the thyroid gland. In fact, De Vita *et al.* showed in FRTL5 thyroid cells that the overexpression of mutated RAS gene inhibits the expression of thyroid differentiation markers in a dose-dependent way [63]. Overexpression of three different Ras isoforms (H-, K- and N-Ras) exert similar effects on the thyroid phenotype: loss of thyroid differentiation, with decrease in thyroidal differentiation markers proteins as thyroglobulin, thyroperoxidase, Na+/I- symporter, TSH receptor, thyroid oxidase and thyroid specific combination of transcription factors, Titf 1, Foxe 2 and Pax 8 [21].

Ras proteins comprise a group of 20- to 25-KDa proteins that are involved in transduction of signals elicited by activated surface receptors, acting as molecular switches in many processes governing cellular growth and differentiation. The Ras-pERK pathway can also be modulated by thyroid hormones. In the hypothyroid rat there is a clear positive modulation of Ras, but this does not affect pERK, which shows a slight decrease. In contrast, thyroidal pERK increases in T4-induced hyperthyroidism, but there are no changes in RAS expression [22].

Effects of aging on Ras expression are still very much unexplored. In rat thyroids from both genders aging duplicated Ras expression, but its signal transduction by pERK was decreased, suggesting a failure in this pathway [23]. These results could be involved in the impaired thyroidal function observed in old rats. Ras activation of Raf serine/threonine kinases, and activation of the ERK mitogenactivated protein kinases is an important signaling pathway for many Ras effects, the others being the activation of phosphatidylinositol-3 kinase or the Ral-small GTPases. As far as we know, an increase in the protooncogene Ras expression in the thyroid from aged rats has not been detected previously. Further studies are required to elucidate the pathways involved in this increases in Ras expression during the aging process, and to correlate them with the known morphologic and functional changes that affect the aging thyroid gland.

2.2. Aging and hypothalamus-pituitary-thyroid axis

The effect of aging on the hypothalamus-pituitary-thyroid function is still a subject of controversies. The hypothalamus-pituitary-thyroid axis undergoes a significant number of complex physiological alterations associated with aging. However, direct age-related changes need to be distinguished from indirect alterations caused by simultaneous thyroid or non- thyroidal illness, or other physiological or pathophysiological states whose incidence increases with age. Several changes formerly believed to be a direct result of the aging process have subsequently been shown to be due to the increased prevalence of subclinical thyroid disease and/or the result of non-thyroidal illness. This makes interpretation of thyroid function tests difficult in the elderly [11].

Pituitary thyrotropin (TSH) stimulates all steps of thyroid hormones biosynthesis and is the major regulator of the thyroid gland morphology and function. TSH production and secretion are stimulated by the hypothalamic thyrotropin-releasing hormone (TRH) and suppressed by thyroid hormones, in a classic negative feedback control system.

In a revision of several population studies Surks and Hollowell report that the TSH distribution of aged humans - without thyroid disease - progressively shift to higher concentrations, suggesting that the prevalence of subclinical hypothyroidism could have been overestimated in many other studies [24]. The main point that is being discussed for some time by endocrinologists is whether the increase in the serum immunoreactive TSH of aged subjects, and related changes in thyroid function, are a "physiologic" consequence of aging on the hypothalamus-pituitary-thyroid axis or if they reflect alterations induced by acute or chronic non-thyroid illnesses and/or use of drugs, both more frequent in the elder population [25, 26].

In fact there are strong evidences pointing to a decrease hypothalamus-pituitary-thyroid axis activity with aging, be it in humans [27, 28] or in rats [29, 30, 31]. Thyroid hormone production and metabolism are altered by aging. Serum T4 and T3 are significantly reduced in old male rats, but the serum T3 seems to be less affected in elder female rat [30, 31, 32]. Decreases in serum T3, associated or not with lower T4, are present in aged humans [26], however it should be emphasized that although significantly decreased the thyroid hormone and TSH concentrations mostly remain within the range considered as normal.

The decrease in T3 levels, and in the metabolism of T4 in elder subjects has been attributed to a diminished 5'- deiodinase type I (D1) activity. In fact, we and others have found lower hepatic and thyroid D1 activity in aging rats, but males seem to be more affected than females [30, 33, 34]. The resulting lower serum T3/T4 ratio can also be attributed, at least in part, to a preferential release of T3 by the thyroid of the aged rat, both basal and after TSH stimulation [35]. The effect of aging on pituitary deiodinases type 1 and type 2 (D1, D2) is still awaiting further confirmatory studies. Donda and Lemarchand-Beraud found an increase of D1 and deiodinase type 2 (D2) activities in the pituitary of old male rats, while we found both pituitary deiodinase activities to be decreased in the old female rat [36]. No further information seems to be available, although suggestions of a "partial central hypothyroidism" and less efficient response of the hypothalamic-pituitary axis to lower circulating thyroid hormones are found often enough [32].

Hypothalamic TRH content is reduced in aged rats [32, 35] and thyrotroph response to TRH is mostly reported as decreased, both in rats [29, 32, 36] and [37, 38] in humans. Non-stimulated

TSH concentration has also been reported as relatively diminished by aging in a large population of older persons without hyperthyroidism, and in aging patients with resistance to thyroid hormone (and their non-affected relatives) [27].

In fact, Carlé *et al.* detected four-fold higher average serum TSH in younger (0-20 years) than in the older (80+ years) patients with untreated primary, spontaneous autoimmune hypothyroidism, while there was no age-dependent variation in serum T4. The well-known inverse linear correlation between T4 and log TSH was maintained in both groups, but the serum TSH/T4 ratio was lower in the elder patients than in the young ones. Thus, for the same degree of thyroid failure, the serum TSH is lower among the elderly. Since serum T4 is the parameter best associated with the degree of tissue hypothyroidism, a lower TSH at diagnosis/follow-up of elder patients may suggest that their degree of hypothyroidism is less severe than it really is. Furthermore, and of interest for the clinical endocrinologist, a longer time may be needed after thyroid hormone withdrawal before elder patients with thyroid cancer reach sufficiently high TSH values to allow an effective radioiodine treatment [28].

The increase of pituitary thyrotroph hormonal secretion, when stimulated by the low levels of thyroid hormones, is also significantly impaired in the old rat, even when the thyroid hormones levels are dramatically reduced by MMI treatment [31]. "Normal" circulating levels of TSH are frequently seen in aged rats, in spite of their low serum thyroid hormone levels [30, 31, 36]. This may be attributed to the secretion of a TSH with increased sialylation and diminished biological activity [39] as reported in some types of central hypothyroidism [40] and/or to a diminished response of the thyroid to TSH (less TSH receptors or defective transduction of its signal). A diminished effect of a less biologically active TSH can explain the low thyroid hormone concentration of the aged rat, that could be in part mediated by a decrease in the TPO and Tg expression as found by us in the thyroid gland of aged male (but not female) rat [30].

Thus, at the moment, we must consider that the hypothalamus-pituitary-thyroid axis is affected at all three levels by normal aging, and a reduced responsiveness of target cells/tissues to the effects of thyroid hormones levels rounds-off the picture of a mild state of "total" hypothyroidism that occurs during the aging process, and that may vary according to gender and species evaluated.

Aging also affect thyroid morphology, Messina *et al.* reported a reduction of the hypothalamus-pituitary-thyroid axis activity, with anatomical (weight) and physiological (uptake of iodine and hormone synthesis) age-related adaptations, that result in a reduction of thyroid function [41]. Nevertheless, the authors consider this state as different from hypothyroidism since the thyroid hormones tend to remain within the range considered as normal. In F344 rats, the follicular area and the area of the follicular lumen increased and the height of follicular epithelial cells decreased at 20.5 months, indicating low thyrocyte activity; concomitantly serum T3, T4 and TSH concentrations also decreased with age, confirming that in F344 male rats the aged thyroid shows structural and functional changes [42].

Figure 1 summarizes our current knowledge on aging process and its impact on thyroidal function and regulation.

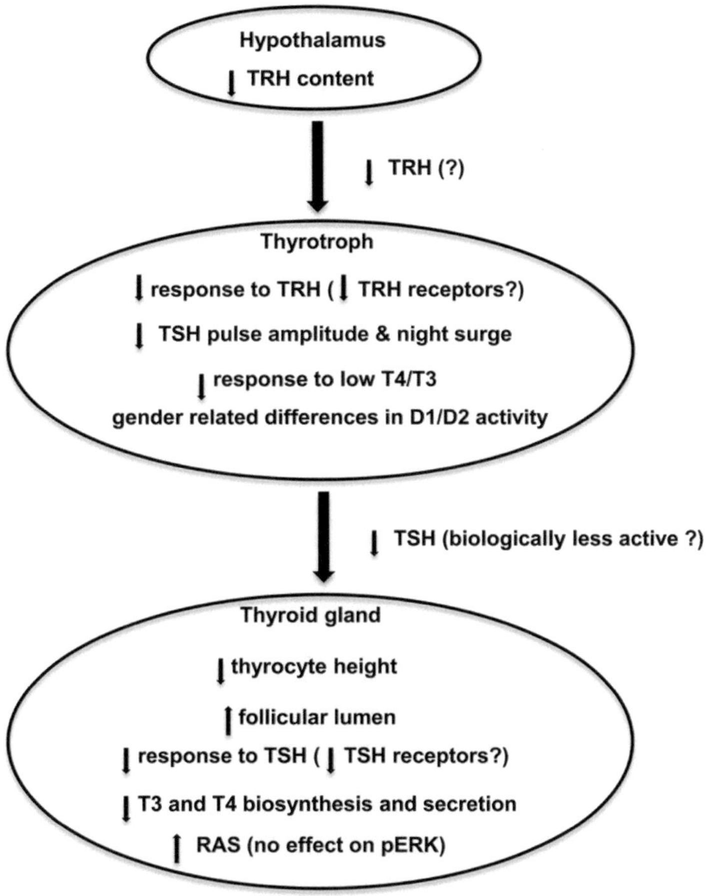

Figure 1. A schematic view of aging effects on thyroid regulation and function.

2.3. Subclinical hypothyroidism

The term "subclinical hypothyroidism" was first introduced in the early 1970s coincident with the introduction of serum TSH measurements. Subclinical hypothyroidism is defined biochemically as a high serum TSH concentration and normal serum free T4 and T3 concentrations. Some investigators also consider patients who have normal basal serum TSH and supranormal serum TSH responses to thyrotropin-releasing hormone (TRH) to have subclinical hypothyroidism. By definitions, patients with subclinical hypothyroidism cannot be identified on the basis of symptoms and signs [43].

Subclinical hypothyroidism is present in about 4% to 8.5% of adults in the United States who are without known thyroid disease [44]. Subtle thyroid dysfunction often affects the oldest-old fraction of the elderly population (i.e., those >85 years). In 85-year-old healthy individuals, hypothyroidism was in the subsequent 4 years associated with lower all-cause and cardiovascular mortality rates compared with euthyroid individuals [45]. In a group of 400 men with a mean age of 78 years, Van den Beld and colleagues [46] showed that low serum levels of free T4 and T3 (with normal reverse T3 [rT3]) concentrations were associated with better physical performance and 4-year survival, whereas subjects with low serum levels of T3 and high rT3 concentrations did not show a survival advantage and had lower levels of physical activity. These two studies support the concept that some degree of physiologically decreased thyroid activity at the tissue level may have favorable effects in the oldest-old subjects, but caution should be exercised when interpreting the predictive value of thyroid dysfunction in the elderly, which may produce contradictory results if not considered in the appropriate context [15].

Subclinical hypothyroidism has been associated with heart failure [48] and with increased odds of metabolic syndrome [49], but the significance of increased serum TSH in elder subjects is still *sub judice*. Thus, treatment of subclinical hypothyroidism to prevent heart failure and cardiovascular disease in older people should be better evaluated in large randomized clinical trials.

Thyroid hormones have an important role in many organic functions and their deficiency causes a wide spectrum of clinical presentations and symptoms. Neuromuscular manifestations are well established in overt hypothyroidism and impaired muscle function is frequently observed. Thyroid hormone deficiency may also interfere substantially with various aspects of physical, mental and social well-being. The evidence for improvement of psychiatric symptoms with hormonal treatment of hypothyroidism, and the use of T3 to potentiate the response to treatment of depressive disorders suggest a direct relationship between thyroid hormones and psychiatric symptoms. Neurobiological evidence seems to corroborate the hypothesis of an organic basis of the effects of thyroid hormone on the brain and on psychiatric symptoms. There is some evidence that subclinical hypothyroidism may also be responsible for findings classically described in hypothyroidism. Symptoms and signs of hypothyroidism have been frequently found in subclinical hypothyroidism patients, as reported by many authors. In fact, Reuters et al described an improvement in some physical aspects of quality of life after L-T4 treatment in patients with subclinical hypothyroidism [50].

The frequency of subclinical hypothyroidism, varies from 6.5 to 15% in elder subjects [51, 52] Subclinical hypothyroidism has been associated with clustering of cardiovascular risk factors, such as hypertension, diabetes mellitus, dyslipidaemia and hyperuricaemia [53], as well as with the development of insulin resistance, which is evident both in vivo and in vitro studies. The latter may be attributed to decreased insulin-stimulated rates of glucose transport in cells, due to impaired translocation of GLUT4 glucose transporters on the plasma membrane [54].

Multiple studies, with conflicting results, have examined the association of subclinical hypothyroidism with cardiovascular risk and mortality. A recent reanalysis of the Whickham Survey suggested a clear association of subclinical hypothyroidism with ischemic heart disease and mortality [55]. However, a meta-analysis of 15 observational studies indicated that increased cardiovascular risk is evident only in younger individuals with subclinical hypothyroidism [56]. In patients with type 2 diabetes mellitus, subclinical hypothyroidism has been found to be associated with reduced all-cause mortality [57]. Furthermore, age-related subtle thyroid hypofunction has been related to longevity [58]. Part of the heterogeneity in these studies may be related to differences in participants' age, sex or TSH level. In a recent meta-analysis combining data on 55,287 participants from 11 prospective studies, subclinical hypothyroidism was associated with an increased risk of coronary heart disease and mortality in patients with TSH levels higher than 10 IU/L, these associations did not differ in age, sex or ethnicity [51].

Treatment of subclinical hypothyroidism remains controversial [52, 53, 59]. Although there are no randomized controlled trials documenting decreased cardiovascular morbidity or mortality, some studies have suggested that treatment of subclinical hypothyroidism may result in improvement of cardiovascular risk factors, such as insulin sensitivity, glucose metabolism, soluble intercellular adhesion molecule-1 [60], endothelial progenitor cell levels [61], abnormalities in high-density lipoprotein metabolism [62], and common carotid intima-media thickness [63]. According to the American Association of Clinical Endocrinologists, treatment is indicated in patients with TSH levels above 10 IU/ml or in patients with TSH levels between 5 and 10 IU/ml along with goiter or positive anti-thyroid peroxidase antibodies, since these patients have increased rates of progression to overt hypothyroidism. However, it should be kept in mind that TSH levels are sometimes transiently elevated, due to recovery from non-thyroidal illness or medication use. As a result, it has been recommended that TSH measurement should be repeated after 6–8 weeks in order to confirm the diagnosis of subclinical hypothyroidism, prior to any consideration of initiating therapy [52].

The prevalence of thyroid disease increases with age but very often presents different clinical manifestations from those found in younger patients. Autoimmune hypothyroidism is particularly prevalent in the elderly, and may be one of the factors that underlies an increased serum TSH reported by various studies in this population [64]. Hyperthyroidism is less common in among older subject, is frequently due to toxic nodular goiters, is mainly characterized by cardiovascular symptoms, and its manifestations are generally milder than in the younger patients. The associated decrease in TSH may also be less marked than that found in Graves' disease. Thus, the question of whether changes in circulating TSH levels in the elderly indicate a "physiologic adaptation" or are a reflection of associated health disturbances is still pertinent and awaiting further evaluation.

3. Conclusion

The effect of aging on the hypothalamus-pituitary-thyroid function is still a subject of controversies. Normal aging is accompanied by a slight decrease in pituitary thyrotropin release and especially by decreased peripheral degradation of T4, which results in a gradual age-dependent decline in serum triiodothyronine concentrations without changes in T4 levels. This slight decrease in plasma T3 concentrations occurs largely within the broad normal range of the healthy elderly population and has not been clearly related to functional changes during the aging process.

The frequency of subclinical hypothyroidism, varies from 6.5 to 15% in older subjects and treatment of subclinical hypothyroidism remains controversial. However, it should be kept in mind that TSH levels are sometimes transiently elevated, due to recovery from nonthyroidal illness or medication use.

Author details

Corrêa V. M. da Costa* and D. Rosenthal

*Address all correspondence to: vmccosta@biof.ufrj.br

Laboratório de Fisiologia Endócrina Doris Rosenthal, Instituto de Biofísica Carlos Chagas Filho, Universidade Federal do Rio de Janeiro, Rio de Janeiro, Brazil

References

[1] Austad SN. Is aging programmed? Aging cell, 2004;3: 249-251.

[2] Hayflick L. Biological aging is no longer an unsolved problem. Ann NY Acad Sci 2007; 1100:1-13.

[3] Chahal HS, Drake WM. The endocrine system and ageing. J Pathol 2007;211: 173-180.

[4] Peters AL, Davidson MB. Aging and diabetes. In: Alberti KGMM, Zimmet P, Defrozo RA, Keen H, eds. International Textbook of Diabetes Mellitus. Chichester, UK: John Wiley & Sons; 1997:1151.

[5] Frutos MG, Cacicedo L, Fernández C, Vicent D, Velasco B, Zapatero H, Sánchez-Franco F. Insights into a role of GH secretagogues in reversing the age-related decline in the GH/IGF-I axis. Am J Physiol Endocrinol Metab 2007;293: E1140-E1152.

[6] Baranowska B, Wolinska-Witort E, Bik W, Baranowska-Bik A, Martynska L, Chmielowsa M. Evaluation of neuroendocrine status in longevity. Neurobiol Aging 2007;28: 774-783.

[7] Ferrari M, Mantero F. Male aging and hormones: the adrenal cortex. J Endocrinol Invest 2005;28 (11 Suppl): 92-95.

[8] Giordano R, Bo A, Pellegrino M, Vezzari M, Baldi M, Picu A, Balbo M, Bonelli L, Migliaretti G, Ghigo E, Arvat E. Hypothalamus-pituitary-adrenal hyperactivity in human aging is partially refractory to stimulation by mineralocorticoid receptor blockade. J Clin Endocrinol Metab 2005;90: 5656-5662.

[9] Keck ME, Hatzinger M, Wotjak CT, Landgraf R, Holsboer F, Neumann ID. Aging alters intrahypothalamic release patterns of vasopressin and oxitocin in rats. Eur J Neurosci 2000;12: 1487-1494.

[10] Hatzinger M, Wotjak CT, Naruo T, Simchen R, Keck ME, Landgraf R, Holsboer F, Neumann ID. Endogenous vasopressin contributes to hypothalamic- pituitary-adrenocortical alterations in aged rats. J Endocrinol 2000;164: 197-205.

[11] Mariotti S, Franceschi C, Cossarizza A, Pinchera A. The aging thyroid. Endocr Rev. 1995;16:686.

[12] Pinchera A, Mariotti S, Barbesino G, Bechi R, Sansoni P, Fagiolo U, Cossarizza A, Franceschi C. Thyroid autoimmunity and ageing. Horm Res 1995;43(1-3):64-68.

[13] Mariotti S. Mild hypothyroidism and ischemic heart disease: is age the answer? J Clin Endocrinol Metab. 2008;93:2969.

[14] Goichot B, Pearce SH. Subclinical thyroid disease: Time to enter the age of evidence-based medicine. Thyroid 2012;22:765-768.

[15] Chiovato L, Mariotti S, Pinchera A. Thyroid diseases in the elderly. *Baillie`res Clin Endocrinol Metab*1997;11(2):251–270.

[16] Kimura T, van Keymeulen A, Goldstein J, Fusco A, Dumont JE, Roger PP. Regulation of thyroid cell proliferation by TSH and others factors: A critical evaluation of *in vitro* models. Endocr Rev, 2001; 22: 631-656.

[17] Park YJ, Kim TY, Lee SH, Kim H, Shong M, Yoon YK, Cho BY, Park DJ. p66Shc expression in proliferating thyroid cells is regulated by thyrotropin receptor signaling. Endocrinology, 2005;146: 2473-2480.

[18] Schlumberger M, Pacini F. Oncogenes and tumor suppressor genes In: Schlumberger & Pacini, (ed.), Nucle´on, France, 1999; 61-81.

[19] Hinkal G, Donehower LA. Decline and fall of the tumor suppressor. Proc Natl Acad Sci USA, 2007; 104: 18347-18348.

[20] Shields JM, Pruit K, McFall A, Shaub A, Der CJ. Understanding Ras: 'it ain't over 'til it's over'. Trends Cell Biol, 2000;10: 147-154.

[21] De Vita G, Bauer L, Corre◎a da Costa VM, De Felice M, Baratta MG, De Menna M, DiLauro R. Dose-dependent inhibition of thyroid differentiation by ras oncogenes. Mol Endocrinol, 2005; 19: 76-89.

[22] Leal ALRC, Pantaleão TU, Moreira DG, Marassi MP, Pereira VS, Rosenthal D, Corrêa da Costa VM. Hypothyroidism and hyperthyroidism modulates Ras-MAPK intracellular pathway in murine thyroids. Endocrine, 2007; 31: 174-178.

[23] Moreira DG. [Effects of aging on regulation and function of the murine thyroid gland] (portuguese). PhD Thesis, Federal University of Rio de Janeiro; 2007.

[24] Surks MI, Hollowell JG. Age-specific distribution of serum thyrotropin and antithyroid antibodies in U.S. population: Implica- tions for the prevalence of subclinical hypothyroidism. J Clin Endocrinol Metab 92: 4575-4582 (2007).

[25] Maiti BR, Sarkar S, Sarkar R, Sengupta SC, Pradhan D, Chatterjee A. Inhibtions of thyroidal and extra-thyroidal T3, T4 and thyroperoxidase profiles with elevation of basal TSH following lithium treatment in adult and aged rats. Acta Endocrinologica, 2010;2:171-184.

[26] Mitrou P, Raptis SA, Dimitriadis G. Thyroid disease in older people. Maturitas 2011;70:5-9.

[27] Weiss RE, Refetoff. Resistance to thyroid hormone. Rev Endocr Metab Disord, 2000; 1: 97-108.

[28] Carlé A, Laurberg P, Pedersen IB, Perrild H, Ovesen L, Rasmussen LB, Jorgensen T, Knudsen N. Age modifies the pituitary TSH response to thyroid failure. Thyroid, 2007;17: 139-144.

[29] Cizza G, Brady LS, Calogero AE, Bagdy G, Lynn AB, Kling MA, Blackman MR, Chrousos GP, Gold PW. Central hypothyroidism is associated with advanced age in male Fisher 344/N rats: *in vivo* and *in vitro* studies. Endocrinology, 1992; 131: 2672-2680.

[30] Corre◎a da Costa VM, Moreira DG, Rosenthal D. Thyroid function and age: gender related differences. J Endocrinol, 2001;171: 193-198.

[31] Moreira DG, Marassi MP, Corre◎a da Costa VM, Carvalho DP, Rosenthal D. Effects of ageing and pharmacological hypothyroid- ism on pituitary-thyroidal axis of Dutch-Miranda and Wistar rats. Exp Gerontol, 2005;40: 330-334.

[32] Greeley GH Jr, Lipton MA, Kizer JS. Serum thyroxine, triiodothyronine and TSH levels and TSH release after TRH in aging male and female rats. Endocr Res, 1982;9: 169-177.

[33] Corrêa da Costa VM, Rosenthal D. Effect of aging on thyroidal and pituitary T4-5′-deiodinase activity in female rats. Life Sci, 1996;18: 1515-1520.

[34] Donda A, Lemarchand-Beraud T. Aging alters the activity of 5′-deiodinase in the adenohypophysis, thyroid gland, and liver of the male rat. Endocrinology, 1989; 124: 1305-1309.

[35] Pekary AE, Hershman JM, Sugawara M, Gieschen KI, Sogol PB, Reed AW, Pardridge WM, Walfish PG, Preferential release of triiodothyronine: and intrathyroidal adaptation to reduced serum thyroxine in aging rats. J Gerontol, 1983;18: 653-659.

[36] Donda A, Reymond MJ, Lemarchand-Beraud T. Influence of age on the control of thyrotropin secretion be thyrotropin-releasing hormone in the male rat. Neuroendocrinology, 1989;49: 389-394.

[37] Monzani F, Del Guerra P, Caraccio N, Del Corso L, Casolaro A, Mariotti S, Pentimone F. Age-related modifications in the regulation of the hypothalamic-pituitary-thyroid axis. Horm Res, 1986;46: 107-112.

[38] Chakraborti S, Chakraborti T, Mandal M, Das S, Batabyal SK. Hypothalamic-pituitary-thyroid axis status during development of aging process. Clin Chim Acta, 1999;288: 137-145.

[39] Oliveira JH, Barbosa ER, Kasamatsu T, Abucham J. Evidence for thyroid hormone as positive regulator of serum thyrotropin bioactivity. J Clin Endocrinol Metab, 2007;92: 3108-3113.

[40] Oliveira JH, Persani L, Beck-Pecoz P, Abucham J. Investigating the paradox of hypothyroidism and increased serum thyrotropin (TSH) levels in Sheehan's syndrome: characterization of TSH carbohydrate content and bioactivity. J Clin Endocrinol Metab, 2001;86: 1694-1699.

[41] Messina G, Viceconti N, Triti B. Variations in anatomy and physiology of the thyroid gland in old age. Recenti Prog Med 1997;88: 281-286.

[42] Takaoka M, Teranishi M, Furukawa T, Manabe S, Goto N. Age-related changes in thyroid lesions and function in F344/DuCrj rats. Exp Anim 1995; 44: 57-62.

[43] Ross DS, Subclinical hypothyroidism. In: Braverman & Utiger (ed) Werner & Ingbar's The Thyroid: A Fundamental and Clinical Text. Lippincott Williams & Wilkins, 2005; p1070-1078.

[44] Surks MI, Ortiz E, Daniels GH, Sawin CT, Col NF, Cobin RH, Franklyn JA, Hershman JM, Burman KD, Denke MA, Gorman C, Cooper RS, Weissman NJ. Subclinical thyroid disease: scientific review and guidelines for diagnosis and management. JAMA. 2004;291:228.

[45] Gussekloo J, van Exel E, de Craen AJ, Meinders AE, Frölich M, Westendorp RG. Thyroid status, disability and cognitive function, and survival in old age. JAMA. 2004;292:2591. 16.

[46] van den Beld AW, Visser TJ, Feelders RA, Grobbee DE, Lamberts SW. Thyroid hormone concentrations, disease, physical function, and mortality in elderly men. J Clin Endocrinol Metab. 2005;90:6403.

[47] Mariotti S. Thyroid function and aging: do serum 3,5,3′-triiodothyronine and thyroid-stimulating hormone concentrations give the Janus response? J Clin Endocrinol Metab. 2005;90:6735.

[48] Nanchen D, Gussekloo J, Westendorp RGJ, Stott DJ, Jukerna JW, Trompet S, Ford I, Welsh P, Sattar N, Macfarlane PW, Mooijaart SP, Rodondi N, de Craen AJ; Subclinical thyroid dysfunction and the risk of heart failure in older persons at high cardiovascular risk. J Clin Endocrinol Metab, 2012;97(3):852-861.

[49] Waring AC, Rodondi N, Harrison S, Kanaya AM, Simonsick EM, Miljkovic I Satterfield S, Newman AB, Bauer DC. Thyroid function and prevalent and incident metabolic syndrome in older adults: the health, ageing and body composition study. Clinical Endocrinology, 2012;76:911-918.

[50] Reuters, VS, Almeida CP, Teixeira PFS, Vigário PS, Ferreira MM, Castro CLN, Brasil, MA, Costa AJL, Buescu A, Vaisman M Effects of subclinical hypothyroidism treatment on psychiatric symptoms, muscular complaints, and quality of life. Arquivos Brasileiros de Endocrinologia e Metabologia 2012;56:128-136.

[51] Rodondi N, den Elzen WPJ, Bauer DC, Cappola AR, Razvi S, Walsh JP, Asvold BO, Iervasi G, Imaizumi M, Collet TH, Bremner A, Maisonneuve P, Sgarbi JA, Khaw KT, Vanderpump MP, Newman AB, Cornuz J, Franklyn JA, Westendorp RG, Vittinghoff E, Gussekloo J Subclinical hypothyroidism and the risk of coronary heart disease and mortality. JAMA 2010;304:1365–74.

[52] Klubo-Gwiezdzinska J, Wartofsky L. Thyrotropin blood levels, subclinical hypothyroidism, and the elderly patient. Arch Intern Med 2009;169(21):1949–51.

[53] Ceresini G, Morganti S, Maggio M, Usberti E, Fiorino I, Artoni A, Teresi G, Belli S, Ridolfi V, Valenti G, Ceda GP. Subclinical thyroid disease in elderly subjects. Acta Biomed 2010;81(Suppl. 1):31–6.

[54] Maratou E, Hadjidakis D, Kollias A, Tsegka K, Peppa M, Alevizaki M, Mitrou P, Lambadiari V, Boutati E, Nikzas D, Tountas N, Economopoulos T, Raptis SA, Dimitriadis G. Studies of insulin resistance in patients with clinical and subclinical hypothyroidism. Eur J Endocrinol 2009;160(5):785–90.

[55] Razvi S, Jola U, Weaver JU, Vanderpump MP, Pearce SHS. The incidence of ischemic heart disease and mortality in people with subclinical hypothyroidism: reanalysis of the Whickham survey cohort. J Clin Endocrinol Metab 2010;95:1734–40.

[56] Razvi S, Shakoor A, Vanderpump M, Weaver JU, Pearce SHS. The influence of age on the relationship between subclinical hypothyroidism and ischemic heart disease: a metaanalysis. J Clin Endocrinol Metab 2008;93:2998–3007.

[57] Ssthyapalan T, Manuchehri AM, Rigby AS, Atkin SL. Subclinical hypothyroidism is associated with reduced all-cause mortality in patients with type 2 diabetes. Diabetes Care. 2010 Mar;33(3):e37.

[58] Consonello A, Montesanto A, Berardelli M, De Rango F, Dato S, Mari V, Mazzei B, Lattanzio F, Passarino G.. A cross-section analysis of FT3 age-related changes in a group of old and oldest-old subjects, including centenarians' relatives, shows that a down-regulated thyroid function has a familial component and is related to longevity. Age Ageing 2010;39:723–7.

[59] Vilar HC, Saconato H, Valente O, Atallah AN. Thyroid hormone replacement for subclinical hypothyroidism. Cochrane Database Syst Rev 2007;18(3):CD003419.

[60] Kowalska I, Borawski J, Nikolajuk A, Budlewski T, Ooziomek E, Górska M, Straczkowski M. Insulin sensitivity, plasma adiponectin and sICAM concentrations in patients with subclinical hypothyroidism: response to levothyroxine therapy. Endocrine 2011, 40(1):95-101

[61] Shakoor SK, Aldibbiat A, Ingoe LE, Shakoor SK, Aldibbiat A, Ingoe LE. Endothelial progenitor cells in subclinical hypothyroidism: the effect of thyroid hormone replacement therapy. J Clin Endocrinol Metab 2010;95(1):319–22.

[62] Sigal GA, Medeiros-Neto G, Vinagre JC, Diament J, Maranhao RC. Lipid metabolism in subclinical hypothyroidism: plasma kinetics of triglyceride-rich lipoproteins and lipid transfers to high-density lipoprotein before and after levothyroxine treatment. Thyroid 2011; 21(4):347-53

[63] Kim SK, Kim SH, Park KS, Park SW, Cho YW. Regression of the increased common carotid artery-intima media thickness in subclinical hypothyroidism after thyroid hormone replacement. Endocr J, 2009;56(6):753–8.

[64] Chahal HS, Drake WM. The endocrine system and ageing. J Patholol, 2007;211:173-180.

Chapter 4

Detection of Iodine Deficiency Disorders (Goiter and Hypothyroidism) in School-Children Living in Endemic Mountainous Regions, After the Implementation of Universal Salt Iodization

Imre Zoltán Kun, Zsuzsanna Szántó, József Balázs, Anisie Năsălean and Camelia Gliga

Additional information is available at the end of the chapter

http://dx.doi.org/10.5772/54188

1. Introduction

1.1. Physiological aspects

Iodine and thyroid hormones are indispensable for somatic growth and development of several organs and systems in the fetus and infant. Their most important action is on the development of central nervous system in the critical period of life: from the fetal life up to the third year of age (Dobbing & Sands, 1973; Delong, 1989; Delange, 2000; Koibuchi & Chin, 2000). Thyroid hormone primary is involved in myelination and neuronal-glial cell differentiation (Bernal, 2005), brain maturation, and is crucial in the development and maintenance of normal physiological processes (Joffe & Sokolov, 1994, Neale et al., 2007).

1.2. Etiology and pathophysiology of Iodine Deficiency Disorders (IDD)

Insufficient dietary iodine intake is the most important etiological factor of disorders caused by iodine deficiency, but goitrogens (perchlorates, thiocyanates), physiological periods with high requirement of iodine (puberty, pregnancy, lactating period), increased urinary iodine excretion (nephrosis syndrome), high thyroxine binding globuline level (hyperestrogenism, oral contraceptives), lack of selenium, latent thyroid enzyme defects and autoimmune thyroid processes may contribute as well (Brook et al., 2008; Delange & Dunn, 2005).

Insufficient iodine intake leads to reduced thyroid hormone production, and all the consequences of iodine deficiency.

Iodine deficiency occuring during the critical period of life induces the most damaging complications: irreversible mental retardation and cretenism (Hetzel, 1983; Stanbury, 1994; Delange, 2001; Boyages, 1994, Bleichrodt, 1994). In severely endemic areas, cretenism may affect up to 5-15% of the population, being the most common cause of mental retardation (Glinoer, 2001, Morreale de Escobar et al., 2004; Pearce, 2009). However, milder brain impairments appear most frequently, such as poor school performance, reduced intellectual ability, impaired work capacity (Stanbury, 1994), apathy, lassitude, diminished mental capacity, verbal and hearing impairments.

In children iodine deficiency causes goiter and reduced growth velocity as well. During time diffuse goiters can transform into uni- or multinodular goiters. These nodules can become autonomous, inducing hyperthyroidism, especially after administration of iodine.

1.3. Clinical aspects – High-risk populational groups

Iodine deficiency induces a large spectrum of organic and functional consequences grouped under the general heading of iodine deficiency disorders (IDD) (Hetzel, 1983). IDD reflect this public health problem more relevantly than the term „goiter". This group of disturbances is characterised by all of the ill-effects of iodine deficiency specific to different physiological stages (fetus, newborn, infant, schoolchild, adolescent, adult, especially pregnant woman) (Hetzel, 1983; Stanbury, et al., 1998; Lauberg et al., 2000; de Benoist et al., 2004; Delange & Dunn, 2005), that can be prevented by adequate intake of iodine.

The population groups being at the highest risk to develop IDD and severe consequences are fetuses, children under 2 years of age, pregnant and lactating women. The most devastating outcome of IDD is increased perinatal mortality and mental retardation. In infants iodine deficiency is the most frequent cause of preventable mental damage worldwide (de Benoist et al., 2004).

In school-age children and adolescents the main clinical manifestations are diffuse endemic goiter, subclinical thyroid dysfunctions (mainly hypothyroidism and rarely hyperthyroidism), and impaired mental function, retarded physical development as the impact of iodine deficiency on the central nervous system. The iodine-deficient thyroid gland in children is highly susceptible to nuclear radiation (Hetzel, 1983; Stanbury et al., 1998; Lauberg et al., 2000; de Benoist et al., 2004; Delange & Dunn, 2005, Zimmermann, 2009, Andersson et al., 2007).

In moderate iodine-deficient regions hypothyroidism may appear in children (Brook et al., 2008), at the same time delayed neurodevelopment with defective neuromotor and cognitive ability were also met (Vermiglio et al., 1990; Bleichrodt & Born, 1994; Pop et al., 2003).

Clinically euthyroid school-children in iodine-deficient regions have subtle or overt neuropsychointellectual deficits compared to iodine-sufficient children in the same ethnic, demographic, nutritional and socioeconomic system (Vermiglio et al., 1990; Fenzi et al., 1990). The intelligence quotient may be reduced with about 10-15% in children living in mild, moderate iodine deficient areas (Bleichrodt & Born, 1994).

The attention deficit and hyperactivity disorders (AD-HD) appear significantly more frequently in mild-moderate iodine-deficient geographical areas than in iodine-replete regions (Vermiglio et al., 2004). AD-HD was often observed in developed European countries known currently with mild-moderate iodine deficiency (Vermiglio et al., 2004).

1.4. Epidemiology

Several regions worldwide are believed to be iodine deficient of different degree, but the true extent is not fully known. 50% of the world population was estimated to live in countries with iodine deficiency. IDD represented a major public health problem in the whole world at the end of the 20th and the beginning of the 21th century. In 1999 IDD did affect 2.225 billion people (38.4% of the world population) in 130 countries. About 700 million people (12.6% of the population) had goiter (WHO et al., 1999). In 1994, 43 million individuals were estimated to be mentally handicapped as a consequence of iodine deficiency.

Europe is considered a mild to moderate iodine-deficient continent. Endemic goiter was often reported in Europe, especially in mountainous areas. The reevaluation of iodine status in the late 1980's indicated that most European countries were still iodine deficient (Gutekunst & Scriba, 1989). Thus, programs for the elimination of iodine deficiency were initiated in several regions. In 1997 a study involving 26 European countries showed mild to severe iodine deficiency in many regions, and a dramatic return of the deficiency within 5 to 7 years after the interruption of iodized salt program (Delange et al., 1998). In 1999 the World Health Organization (WHO), the United Nations Children's Fund (UNICEF) and the International Council for the Control of Iodine Deficiency Disorders (ICCIDD) reported that 18 countries in Western and Central Europe, including Romania and 14 countries in Eastern Europe were still affected by iodine deficiency; then Denmark, France and Ireland were added to them. About 275 million people (31.6% of the population) were affected by IDD, and 130 million had goiter (15%) (WHO et al., 1999).

Romania was considered an European endemic region at the end of the 20th century, where goiter frequency was very variable in different areas. The highest frequency was reported in hilly-mountainous regions, such as Maramureş (mountainous northern zone) the Carpathian Mountains, as well as the Transylvanian Basin (located at the center of the country). In 1993 the incidence of goiter was 1.19-26.45% in school-age children. In 1994-1995 the Thyromobil project realized in Braşov and Timişoara districts detected goiter by ultrasound in 13.5% of boys and in 10.1% of girls with age between 6-12 years. The incidence of goiter assessed by physical examination was 2.9-36.3% in 16 counties (Simescu & Ionescu, 1998). In conclusion, at the end of the 20th century iodine deficiency disorders remained a serious public health problem in our contry.

During 2002-2004 the evaluation of iodine status in the whole territory of Romania has shown that 80% of the counties (especially rural regions) were moderately iodine deficient areas, the prevalence of endemic goiter was 0-40% and urinary iodine excretion

(UIE) was reduced in 2/3 of studied individuals, detecting very low levels in pregnant women (Goldner, 2005).

Mureş County is a 6,700 square km large hilly-mountainous region in Transylvanian Basin, located in the center of Romania, populated with about 600,000 inhabitants. Similar investigations were performed here in 1950's (Cornea, 1957), which were continued until the '80 years, some of the results being published (Vasilescu et al., 1986, Hetzel et al., 1987). After that IDD survey by modern methods (UIE and thyroid ultrasound volumetry) were recommended. In 1998-1999 school-children from localities near the superior and middle hydrographical basin of the river Mureş, including Târgu Mureş (the capital city of Mureş County) were screened. The results showed mild iodine deficiency in most rural localities, moderate iodine deficiency in some villages, and normal iodine state in Târgu Mureş (Balázs et al., 1998, 2000/a,2000/b). Our survey targeting neonatal and maternal screening, performed during 2001-2006, investigated the impact of universal salt iodization on the iodine status of these high-risk populations, and it showed that Mureş County is a moderately mild iodine-deficient area (Kun et al., 2003, Kun, 2006, Kun et al., 2007, Szántó et al., 2007).

1.5. Official strategies to eliminate iodine deficiency disorders worldwide

In 1990 the heads of States and Governments and other senior officials on the occasion of the World Summit for Children assumed a solemn obligation to eliminate the iodine deficiency disorders. In 2002 an international agreement for the long-term elimination of IDD until 2005 was accepted at the special Session of UNO dedicated to childhood health. The World Health Organization criteria to eliminate IDD through universal iodization of alimentary salt were the use of iodized salt at least in 90% of households, adequate iodine-concentration of salt (20-40mg/kg), and the implementation in practice of these measurements at least within two years. Reviewing the IDD status in Europe, a marked improvement in the status of iodine nutrition was observed, especially in the central parts of the continent (Delange, 2002; Vitti et al., 2003, Gerasimov, 2002).

1.6. National strategy on the elimination of IDD in Romania

The legislative measures for the elimination of endemic goiter were controlled for decades by the 637/1955 and the 1056/1962 Governmental Decisions, which ordered among others the distribution of potassium iodide (KI) tablets in school-age children. Thus, legislation on salt iodization did exist, but being not enforced it could not eradicate goiter. So, several Romanian counties, especially hilly-mountainous and rural regions remained iodine deficient according to the above presented data. In 1995 a new governmental order (No. 779/1995) proposed to review the prevention measures of IDD. In 1997 the 21 National Program of the Romanian Ministry of Health intentioned to reduce the frequency of IDD with at least 10% during the following 5 years. Romania has been taken part at the European strategy to eliminate iodine deficiency in Europe on the basis of the WHO criteria from 2002. Extended surveys were performed in Braşov County, Banat (in the central and the western region of the country, respectively, both being parts of the Thyromobil project), Moldova (the eastern territory) and Dobrogea (south-eastern region), as well as Bucharest, the capital of the country (Simescu, 1999). The nationwide surveys conducted in 2002 have shown that non-iodized salt was still present in Romanian households: 31% of the households in urban and 37% in rural localities (Government of Romania, 2005).

In the frame of the general strategy the following measurements were taken: a governmental decision (No. 586/5 June 2002) was adopted regarding universal salt iodization (mean KIO_3 content of salt 34±8.5mg/kg – i.e. 25.5-42.5mg/kg, higher than previously); the use of iodized alimentary salt has become mandatory since 2003, and the compulsory iodization of salt used in baking industry was decided in 2004. In addition, the National Committee for universal salt iodization and IDD elimination (with multisectorial participation) was founded in 2004; in the same year the National Strategy on the elimination of IDD during 2004-2012 was elaborated and adopted by governmental decision (Government of Romania, 2005). In 2005 the National Strategy on the elimination of IDD was founded in the Institute of Public Health Bucureşti. Consequently, the use of iodized salt in households increased to 96% in 2004 (compared to 53% in 2002) according to data furnished by the Institute of Mother and Child's Protection, but on the other hand iodine content of alimentary salt proved to be insufficient (63%). Therefore, iodine supplementation was necessary, and 10% of school-children received iodine tablets, prescribed by general practitioners. Consequently the iodine-supplementation of school-children and pregnant women has improved considerably after the first 2 years of obligatory use of iodized alimentary salt, the urinary iodine excretion (UIE) becoming almost normal. With all the efforts IDD was still persisting in 2005, requiring enforced monitoring system of iodized salt production and consumption, strengthen the health promotion network etc. (Goldner, 2005).

1.7. Indicators to assess baseline IDD status and to monitor and evaluate the IDD control programs

Individual evaluation of IDD is based on clinical exam (physical examination to determine thyroid size and signs of thyroid dysfunctions, inclusion the case into populational group at risk for IDD, psychoneurosomatic assessment of children and adolescents), as well as laboratory and imagistical findings (UIE, TSH, FT_4, FT_3, radioiodine uptake, thyroid ultrasound and scintigraphy, fine-needle aspiration biopsy of thyroid nodules).

The epidemiological evaluation of a geoclimatic area includes the determination of iodine content of the water and soil, and the assessment of different types of IDD in the population by indicators of iodine status at baseline and during the salt iodization program (impact indicators: median UIE, goiter frequency and high TSH levels) and by indicators evaluating the degree of successfullness and sustainability of the salt iodization programs (sustainability indicators).

Indicators used to assess the iodine status of school-age children are median UIE, the prevalence of goiter determined by inspection/palpation or ultrasound, and the level of thyroglobulin (Tg).

Urinary iodine excretion (UIE) is a sensitive tool to indicate the present iodine status, being useful to evaluate the recent changes of iodine intake in the target population (Gorstein, 2001).

Median UIE (μg/L)	Iodine deficiency	Iodine intake
< 20	severe	insufficient
20-49	moderate	insufficient
50-99	mild	insufficient

Table 1. The degree of iodine deficiency in school-age children based on the median UIE, according to WHO classification (WHO et al., 2001).

The **frequency of goiter** (total goiter prevalence – TGP) reflects the population's history of iodine nutrition but not its present iodine status, because thyroid size becomes normal for months or years after the correction of iodine deficiency. This indicator is useful to assess the severity of IDD at baseline and the long-term impact of control programs (de Benoist et al., 2004), but it is of limited usefulness in assessing the impact of programs once salt iodization has commenced (WHO et al., 2001).

Indicator	The degree of iodine deficiency		
	mild	moderate	severe
Prevalence of goiter assessed by inspection and palpation [%]	5-19.9	20-29.9	≥30
Frequency of thyroid volume >97th percentile by ultrasound* [%]	5-19.9	20-29.9	≥30
Mean serum Tg level [ng/mL]	10-19.9	20-39.9	≥40

*corresponding to the upper normal limit of thyroid volume

Table 2. The degree of iodine deficiency in school-age children based on goiter prevalence, according to WHO classification (WHO et al., 1994, 2001).

The screening of thyroid volume assessed by inspection and palpation may furnish subjective bias in as much as 30-40% of the cases (Delange, 1994; Gutekunst & Teichert, 1993; WHO et al., 1994; Vitti et al., 1994), being imprecise mostly for small goiters. Therefore, thyroid ultrasound (US) is a far better method to detect goiter in population, especially in children (Gutekunst & Teichert, 1993). It determines more accurately and objectively the thyroid size, but there is no agreement on reference values. The upper normal limit of thyroid volume in children living in normal iodine-supply regions was elaborated (Delange et al., 1997). In the following years the reevaluation of previous measurements and the standardization of values in iodine-deficient regions were suggested, because the values provided on the basis of data collected in Europe (Delange et al., 1997) were overestimated by 30% (Zimmermann et al., 2001). Reliable new values have been provided in iodine-sufficient school-children (Zimmermann et al., 2004).

A geographical region is defined as iodine-deficient if the median UIE is below 100μg/L or the prevalence of goiter is higher than 5% among school-age children (aged 6 to 12 years) (WHO et al., 2001).

The **serum TSH level** as an indicator of iodine status is particularly used in neonatal screening programs. A region is considered iodine-deficient if the frequency of serum TSH>5mIU/L is higher than 3% (WHO et al., 1994; 2001). In school-children the level of TSH measured together with free-thyroxine (FT_4) determines the thyroid dysfunction (subclinical or overt hypothyroidism) which has appeared in the context of iodine deficiency.

The major goal of IDD elimination programs is to ensure the sustained elimination of iodine deficiency. The sustainability is evaluated by median UIE, besides other sustainability indicators (the proportion of households consuming adequately iodized salt, and programmatic indicators, such as the effectiveness of public health authorities and salt industry to monitor and control the whole procession). Sustained elimination of iodine deficiency is ensured if the proportion of target population with UIE<100μg/L is under 50%, and of those with UIE<50μg/L is below 20% (WHO et al., 2001).

1.8. Iodine requirement, IDD prophylaxis in school-age children

The human body needs very small amount of iodine (in average 200μg/day), but the intake should be continuous. The recommended daily iodine intake varies by references. In 2001 the WHO/UNICEF/ICCIDD recommended 120μg/day iodine for school-children (6 to 12 years) and 150 μg for individuals above 12 years, but with these amounts the recommended UIE of 100-200μg/L was not obtained, reaching only 55-80μg/L. In addition to table salt, iodization of animal food and bottled table water can contribute to iodine intake (Andersson et al., 2007; Szybinski, 2011).

1.9. Current iodine status worldwide

Iodine deficiency continues to be a major public health problem in many parts of the world. World statistics show that 1.6 billion people are at risk of being affected by the reduced iodine in their diet, 50 million children are suffering of IDD and every year 100.000 children are born with cretenism worldwide. In 2002 a number of 14 countries of Western and Central Europe have reached a normal status of iodine nutrition, 3 countries were close to iodine sufficiency, but 13 countries, including Romania did remain with persisting IDD (Delange, 2002).

The WHO/UNICEF/ICCIDD report published in 2007 stated that 70% of the world population had access to iodized salt (Andersson et al., 2007), although only 41 countries worldwide can be classified as consuming adequate iodine. Using the median UIE of <100μg/L as the current indicator for insufficient iodine intake, 2 billion people remain at risk for iodine deficiency (Andersson et al., 2007). The recent WHO/ICCIDD study on IDD carried out in 2011 showed that national surveys covered 114 countries, and since 2007 new data have been obtained from 74 countries. From these data it emerged that populations of 37 countries were still classified as iodine deficient, of which 9 had moderate and 28 mild deficiency. IDD in population show a declining tendency, from 54% in 2003 to 47% in 2007 and 37% in 2011. Corresponding results for school-age children were 36.5%, 31.5% and 30.5%, respectively. However, only 32% of these studies were carried out in known iodine deficient areas. In the European Union only 44% of population live in iodine sufficient areas (Andersson, 2011). The experience accumulated thus far has shown that the prevention and control of iodine deficiency requires monitoring to be sustainable.

Endemic cretinism as the most severe complication of IDD was practically eradicated as late as the second half of the 20th century by prophylactic programs conducted worldwide, but serious consequences of IDD are persisting and currently iodine deficiency still remained a major populational health problem.

The iodine status of Mureş County has not been evaluated since 2000. Similarly, the impact of universal salt iodization program initiated in 2003 was not studied in Mureş County. In 2006 we proposed to evaluate the outcome of universal salt iodization in school-age children from iodine-deficient regions of Mureş County, after the legislative changes targeting the improvement of iodine status in Romania were initiated.

2. Objectives

Our primary objective was to evaluate the impact of universal salt iodization (with increased KIO_3-content) at school-age children living in formerly iodine-deficient areas from Mures County (mainly from rural mountainous regions). Secondly, we proposed to assess the frequency and grade of endemic goiter, as well as of thyroid dysfunctions in children from these well known iodine-deficient regions. Additionaly, we intended to diagnose other etiological factors of goiter and hypothyroidism, such as juvenile chronic autoimmune thyroiditis (Hashimoto's disease).

3. Material and methods

Material. The target population was school-age children, having 8-14 years of age of both sexes, living in mountainous rural localities of Mureş County known as iodine deficient regions in 1999-2000, before the implementation of universal salt iodization.

In October 2006 the team of endocrinologists from Endocrinology Clinic Târgu Mureş investigated 135 school-children (Vth-VIIIth classes) from three villages known as endemic areas in Gurghiu Valley: 55 children from Caşva, 30 from Glăjărie and 50 from Ibăneşti. The total population of these three localities is estimated by the censuses of population and housing realized in Romania in 2002: Caşva had 569, Glăjărie 1797 and Ibăneşti 2377 inhabitants.

The endocrinologists arrived to schools located in the mentioned geographical areas, and the children of classes between Vth-VIIIth were examined at the school's health room. This screening activity was previously planed, thus the children were told not to eat on the morning of investigations.

Locality	Mean age (years)	No. boys	No. girls	Total number
Caşva	11.51±1.89	34	21	55
Glăjărie	11.80±1.32	20	10	30
Ibăneşti	12.80±1.23	24	26	50
Total	12.05±1.64	78 (57.7%)	57 (42.3%)	135

Table 3. Mean age and gender distribution of school-children living in the studied mountainous villages of Mureş County

Methods. Data recording was completed with initials, age, gender, hight, weight, physical examination, laboratory and imagistic information for every child. In all cases physical examination and thyroid ultrasonography were performed, then urine and blood samples were collected in order to measure UIE, the level of TSH (thyrotropin), free-thyroxine (FT_4) and anti-thyroid peroxidase antibodies (TPO-Ab).

Samples of drinking water and alimentary salt accesible in the local food marts in every locality were collected in order to measure their iodine content.

Firstly family and personal history were taken, than physical examination and thyroid ultrasonography were performed.

Family history of thyroid dysfunctions, goiter, or any known thyroid disease of parents and other relatives was clarified. In the case of 82 children we could take a valuable familial anamnesis. Personal history of thyroid disease also was registered.

Physical examination consisted of general examination of organs and segments of the body, focusing on the possible signs and symptoms of thyroid disorders.

Anthropometric parameters were determined. *Hight* and *weight* were measured and compared to the standard, being calculated the height-SDS and weight-SDS. Normal height and weight charts of Prader for both sexes from Switzerland reported in 1989 were used, as these are accepted for children living in Romania and similar charts adapted for the Romanian population are not available.

We distributed the casuistry in cohorts with/without hypothyroidism, with/without iodine deficiency, and the mean height and weight of the group was calculated, as well as the data between groups were compared by statistical means.

Local examination of the anterior and lateral cervical regions including the regional lymph nodes represents an important part of the investigation. Inspection and palpation of thyroid gland provided information about the size, consistency and surface of the thyroid, as well as the existence of palpable thyroid nodules and cervical lymph node enlargement. Goiter was clinically defined according to the WHO criteria in 1960 for the classification of thyroid size (Perez et al., 1960). Goiter was diagnosed if its size was grade 1a (palpable thyroid lobes larger than the terminal phalanges of the subject's thumbs), grade 1b (visible with the extended neck), grade 2 (visible with the head in normal position, but the goiter does not extends beyond the medial edge of the sternocleidomastoidian muscles) or grade 3 (visible at a distance and it extends beyond the previous limits) (Perez et al., 1960). Nodules in the thyroid that is otherwise not enlarged fall into grade 1 category (Delange & Dunn, 2005). The inspection and palpation of the anterior and lateral cervical regions were effectuated at all school-age children included in our study.

Thyroid ultrasound (US) was performed in all cases by a portable instrument (Sono Ace 600 – SA-600) using a 7.5-MHz linear transducer. The volume of thyroid lobes was measured and the total thyroid volume was calculated. The structure of thyroid tissue and the presence/absence of thyroid nodules were also investigated.

The volume of each thyroid lobe was calculated by the formula: V = lenght × width × depth × 0.479 (all values expressed in cm), than they were added together to obtain the total volume of the gland. The isthmus was ignored unless a nodule was present. In our study the volume of lobes was calculated automatically by the computer of the US equipment.

We evaluated our data according to values of ultrasound provided by the Thyromobil project performed in Europe (Delange et al., 1997 – Table 4.) and to data furnished by Zimmermann et al. (Zimmermann et al., 2004 – Table 5.) for all children with age between 6-12 years. The thyroid volume measured in 13-14 years-old adolescents was compared to values provided by Delange et al., 1997.

The measured thyroid volumes were also adjusted to the body surface area (BSA) and the obtained data were evaluated according to the upper normal limits (Table 5).

Body surface area was calculated using a variant of Dubois formula:

BSA (m^2) = 0.007184 x Height(cm)$^{0.725}$ x Weight(kg)$^{0.425}$.

After evaluation of thyroid volume for every children, the frequency and the grade of goiter was determined in the cohort.

	Upper normal limit of thyroid volume (mL)									
Age (years)	6	7	8	9	10	11	12	13	14	15
Boys	5.4	5.7	6.1	6.8	7.8	9.0	10.4	12.0	13.9	16.0
Girls	5.0	5.9	6.9	8.0	9.2	10.4	11.7	13.1	14.6	16.1
BSA (kg/m²)	0.8	0.9	1.0	1.1	1.2	1.3	1.4	1.5	1.6	1.7
Boys	4.7	5.3	6.0	7.0	8.0	9.3	10.7	12.2	14.0	15.8
Girls	4.8	5.9	7.1	8.3	9.5	10.7	11.9	13.1	14.3	15.6

Table 4. Age- and BSA-adjusted upper normal limit of thyroid volume measured by ultrasound for children living in iodine-sufficent areas (Delange et al., 1997).

	Median P97 of thyroid volume (mL)									
Age (years)	6	7	8	9	10	11	12	13	14	15
Boys	2.91	3.29	3.71	4.19	4.73	5.34	6.03	-	-	-
Girls	2.84	3.26	3.76	4.32	4.98	5.73	6.59	-	-	-
BSA (kg/m²)	0.8	0.9	1.0	1.1	1.2	1.3	1.4	1.5	1.6	1.7
Boys	2.95	3.32	3.73	4.2	4.73	5.32	5.98	6.73	7.57	-
Girls	2.91	3.32	3.79	4.32	4.92	5.61	6.40	7.29	8.32	-

Table 5. Age- and BSA-ajusted median values (97th percentile – P97) for thyroid volume measured by ultrasound for children living in iodine-sufficent areas (Zimmermann et al., 2004).

The standards of normal thyroid volume according to age and BSA are very different in the references, so at last we evaluated our results on the basis of the values obtained in the region surrounding Iaşi, (in Moldova, eastern part of Romania) provided by the team of endocrinologists from Iaşi (Vulpoi et al., 2002; Zbranca et al., 2008).

Intellectual capacity of 59 children was evaluated by school performances provided by the school's teaching and medical stuff. School performance spectrum was distributed into four subgroups: very good, good, mediocre and low capacity.

In order to measure **urinary iodine excretion** (UIE), the 24-hours urine was collected, than the whole urine quantity was mixed and a 50mL sample was retained and transported to the laboratory. Urinary iodine concentration was determined with the colorimetric procedure based on the Sandell-Kolthoff reaction, using ammonium persulfate (WHO et al., 2001; Dunn et al., 1993).

After obtaining absolute urinary iodine levels for individuals, mean and median UIE values were calculated for our studied groups.

Urinary iodine excretion measurement expressed in μg/L refers to the median value of the UIE calculated for the target population. We estimated the impact of universal salt iodization to eliminate iodine deficiency at school-age children by the interpretation of UIE based on WHO criteria (Table 1).

The assessment of **thyroid function** was also performed. Serum TSH, FT_4 and TPO-Ab levels were determined from 5 mL total blood collected by venipuncture into heparinized tubes.

Serum TSH and free-T_4 levels were measured from venous blood in the morning in all children included in the study. Third generation ECLIA (electrochemiluminescence immunoassay) was applied at the Central Laboratory of Emergency Clinical Hospital Mureş County. Normal range for TSH was considered between 0.27-4.2mIU/L and for FT_4 between 0.932-1.71ng/dL. We evaluated the presence and the severity of hypothyroidism, being diagnosed overt primary hypothyroidism in case of high TSH with reduced FT_4, and subclinical form if TSH was increased and FT_4 normal or at the lower normal limit.

The level of **anti-thyroid peroxidase antibodies** (TPO-Ab) was measured in every schoolchildren. Values under 50IU/mL were considered normal. TPO-Ab above 50IU/mL indicates the presence of juvenile form of Hashimoto's thyroiditis.

Iodine content of drinking water in each village in question was measured. Water samples were collected from the main fountains used by the majority of inhabitants in every localities, and from the water supply network in the school, respectively. These samples were processed by the Laboratory Unit Mureş of the Romanian Academic Research Institute. The iodine-concentration of water under 50μg/L was considered low.

Iodine content of alimentary salt available in the local food marts was also determined. According to the legislative measures the iodine content of the salt must be between 25.5-42.5mg/kg of potassium iodate (KIO_3).

The collected data were systematised and statistically processed. The parameters between groups were compared statistically with T-Student test and Chi-square-test. Homologue parameters between the groups were considered statistically different, if P-value<0.05.

4. Results

Anthropometric parameters of the 135 school-age children living in the three studied mountainous villages (Caşva, Glăjărie, Ibăneşti,) show similar distribution (Table 6.). From the whole cohort 6 children had height below --2SD (mean -2.27±0.24).

Family history was positive for thyroid disturbances (including goiter) in 11 children from the 82 cases with precise data (13.4%). A proportion of 54.5% of children (6/11) with positive family history presented goiter and/or hypothyroidism vs. 32.4% (23/71) of individuals without family history for thyroid condition. The difference between the groups was not significant (P-value: 0.18, OR: 2.50, 95%CI: 0.69-9.07).

Parameter	Studied villages from Mureş County			whole cohort
	Caşva	Glăjărie	Ibăneşti	
Mean W-SDS [SD]	+0.13±1.06	+0.32±1.18	-0.11±1.20	+0.08±1.15
Minimum W-SDS [SD]	-2.26	-2.58	-2.88	-2.88
Median W-SDS [SD]	-0.06	+0.34	+0.005	+0.18
Maximum W-SDS [SD]	+3.18	+2.44	+2.79	+3.18
Mean H-SDS [SD]	-0.10±0.98	+0.07±1.10	+0.02±1.05	-0.01±1.03
Minimum H-SDS [SD]	-2.28	-2.72	-2.30	-2.72
Median H-SDS [SD]	-0.04	+0.005	+0.18	0.00
Maximum H-SDS [SD]	+2.33	+2.20	+2.43	+2.43

W- and H-SDS: weight and height standard deviation score

Table 6. Anthropometric parameters of school-age children living in mountainous villages from Mureş County

Physical examination of the anterior and lateral cervical regions has shown a 51.1% owerall goiter frequency. In all cases diffuse goiter was palpable. In more than half of the cases only small goiter (grade Ia) was present, and goiter grade II was met very rarely (6.7% of all children).

Locality	Number of cases	Thyroid size on physical examination				Owerall goiter frequency
		Grade 0	Grade Ia	Grade Ib	Grade II	
Caşva	55	56.4% (31/55)	27.3% (15/55)	10.9% (6/55)	5.4% (3/55)	43.6% (24/55)
Glăjărie	30	53.3% (16/30)	26.7% (8/30)	16.7% (5/30)	3.3% (1/30)	46.7% (14/30)
Ibăneşti	50	36% (18/50)	30% (15/50)	22% (11/50)	10% (5/50)	62% (31/50)
Total	135	48.1%	28.1%	16.3%	6.7%	51.1%

Table 7. The distribution of thyroid size according to WHO classification

Thyroid volume assessment by ultrasound Thyroid ultrasound was performed in every child enrolled in our study in 2006, the data regarding thyroid volume were calculated in function to age and BSA (Tables 8. and 9.).

Age [years]	Subjects [number]	Thyroid volume [mL]			
		Min.	Max.	Median	Mean
8	5	2.77	5.23	3.16	3.67±1.04
9	7	3.18	4.87	3.67	3.82±0.63
10	10	4.11	10.24	5.29	5.82±1.77
11	24	3.62	8.37	6.36	6.01±1.61
12	26	2.65	21	5.71	6.46±3.42
13	33	4.45	16.04	7.86	8.42±3.09
14	30	3.61	13.18	7.73	8.17±2.47

Table 8. Age-related minimum, maximum, median, and mean thyroid volume measured by ultrasound in the investigated school-children

BSA [m^2]	Subjects [number]	Thyroid volume [mL]			
		Min.	Max.	Median	Mean
0.8	1				2.77
0.9	1				7.15
1.0	11	2.95	9.03	4.66	4.70±1.64
1.1	17	3.18	6.80	4.87	4.78±1.01
1.2	24	2.65	9.02	5.34	5.78±1.89
1.3	18	3.15	11.78	6.71	7.29±2.38
1.4	30	3.62	14.80	6.78	7.06±2.83
1.5	19	5.60	14.55	7.61	8.86±2.69
1.6	5	6.62	9.41	7.85	7.93±1.01
1.7	9	7.17	21.00	10.73	11.80±4.39

Table 9. BSA-related minimum, maximum, median, and mean thyroid volume measured by ultrasound in the investigated school-children

The thyroid volume of every child was compared to data furnished by Delange et al. in 1997 and Zimmermann et al. in 2004 (see Tables 4. and 5.), then the frequency of goiter in the studied villages from Mureş County was determined.

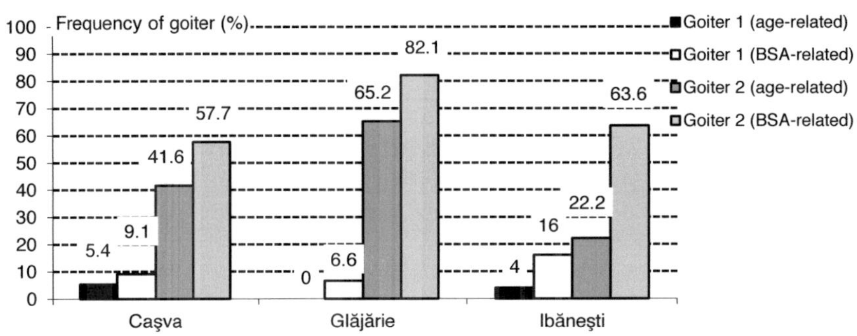

Figure 1. The frequency of goiter in school-children living in mountainous villages from Mureş County, Romania. Goiter 1 – the results evaluated according to Delange et al. 1997; Goiter 2 – the results were classified corresponding to data of Zimmermann et al. 2004.

Figure 1. shows a very variable goiter frequency according to the used standards, being situated between 5.4-57.7% in Caşva, between 0-82.1% in Glăjărie and between 4-63.6% in Ibăneşti. Evaluation of our results based on the normal values provided by Iaşi County, a formerly iodine-deficient Romanian region (Zbranca et al., 2008), shows that goiter was detected in 9 (16.3%) children living in Caşva, in 4 (13.3%) school-children from Glăjărie, and in 14 (28%) subjects from Ibăneşti.

The frequency of goiter in the whole investigated group was 20% (27 children from the total number of 135 cases), compared to standards provided by Vulpoi et al., 2002, Zbranca et al., 2008. All cases of goiter were diffuse.

The frequency of goiter assessed by physical examination and ultrasound were compared, and distributed regarding to gender. The overall goiter frequency provided by ultrasound was significantly higher in girls than in boys (28% vs. 14.1%). Thyroid enlargement was almost similar in both sexes in the subgroup from Caşva, twice and more than three times higher in girls from Glăjărie and Ibăneşti, respectively, although stratified data according to localities show non-significant differences between the subgroups (Table 10).

Locality	Frequency of goiter assessed by physical examination		Frequency of goiter assessed by ultrasound	
	Girls	Boys	Girls	Boys
Caşva	47.6% (10/21)	41.1% (14/34)	14.2% (3/21)	17.6% (6/34)
	Not significant (NS)		Not significant (NS)	
Glăjărie	50% (5/10)	45% (9/20)	20% (2/10)	10% (2/20)
	NS		NS	
Ibăneşti	73% (19/26)	50% (12/24)	42.3% (11/26)	12.5% (3/24)
	NS		NS	
Total	59.6% (34/57)	44.8% (35/78)	28% (16/57)	14.1% (11/78)
	P:0.11, RR:1.32, 95%CI:0.959-1.841		**P:0.052, RR:1.99, 95%CI:1.001-3.959**	

Table 10. Gender distribution of frequency of goiter assessed by physical examination and thyroid ultrasound

We divided the cohort in two groups according to age: one group with children between 6-12 years (72 cases) and the other with subjects between 12-14 years (63 cases). The frequency of goiter assessed by physical examination in the first group was 40.2% (29/72) with no difference between sexes (48.2% in girls and 41.8% in boys), and 58.7% (37/63) in the second group with difference almost significant between sexes (71.4% in girls and 48.5% in boys, P: 0.078, OR: 2.64, 95%CI: 0.9221-7.599).

Urinary iodine excretion measurement

In 2006, at about 2-2.5 years after the implementation in practice of universal salt iodization the mean UIE of the 135 children living in the three mentioned villages from Gurghiu Valley was 85.37±60.05μg/L. The median UIE of 74.88μg/L indicates globally a mild iodine deficiency, but stratified data show large interindividual variations within children.

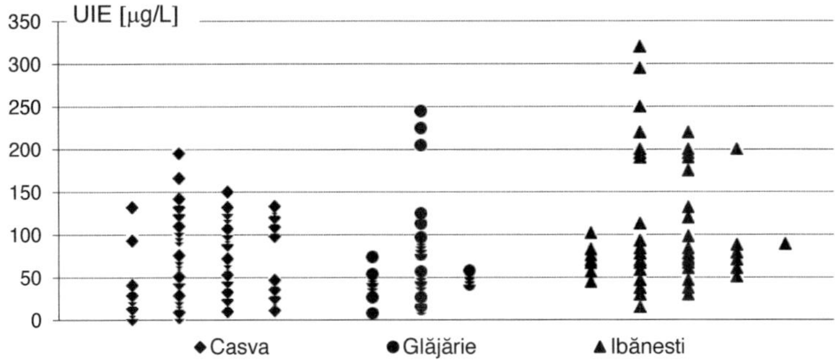

Figure 2. Distribution of individual values of UIE in school-children living in the three studied villages from Mureş County in 2006

UIE below normal range was detected in 68.1% of the cohort. The proportion of UIE <50μg/L reached 30.3%, and that of UIE <100μg/L was 68.1%, which are above the maximal values (20% for UIE <50μg/L and 50% for UIE <100μg/L) of adequate iodine-supply conditions. A large part of the group (60.9%) had mildly or moderately low UIE.

Indicators of iodine status	Data from the studied villages			Whole cohort
	Caşva	Glăjărie	Ibăneşti	
Mean UIE [μg/L]	72.91	75.42	117.84	85.37
Median UIE [μg/L]	67.00	53.50	81.00	74.88
Mean UIE ± SD [μg/L]	72.91±48.63	75.42±60.30	117.84±91.95	85.37±60.05
Frequency of cases with UIE<100μg/L [%]	67.3 (37/55 cases)	76.6 (23/30 cases)	64 (32/50 cases)	68.1 (92/135)
Frequency of cases with UIE<50μg/L [%]	40 (22/55 cases)	36.6 (11/30 cases)	16 (8/50 cases)	30.3 (41/135)
Frequency of goiter assessed by US [%]	16.3 (9/55 cases)	13.3 (4/30 cases)	28 (14/50 cases)	20 (27/135)

Table 11. The indicators of iodine status and of universal salt iodization program sustainability in school-children from mountainous villages in 2006

Thyroid function. In the whole group mean TSH level was 2.32±1.04mIU/L and mean FT_4 concentration 1.07±0.12ng/dL. These values are situated in the normal range, but individual hormonal results showed primary hypothyroidism in 24 (17,7%) children. Fifteen of them had mild overt hypothyroidism and 9 subclinical form, the mean TSH being 5.28±0.73mIU/L (normal: 0.27-4.2) and mean FT_4 0.86±0.05ng/dL (normal: 0.932-1.70).

In Caşva the mean TSH was normal (2.34±1.00mIU/L). Nine (16.3%) children had primary hypothyroidism. In Glăjărie the mean TSH and FT_4 were also normal (2.12±0.93mIU/L and 1.08±0.13, respectively), and 5 school-children (16.6%) were detected with hypothyroidism

(4 mild overt and 1 subclinical form). In Ibăneşti 10 subjects (20%) were diagnosed with thyroid insufficiency (6 mild overt and 4 subclinical).

We did not detect any case of hyperthyroidism.

TPO-Ab was negative (<50IU/mL) in all 135 cases, which means that juvenile chronic autoimmune thyroiditis was not met in this cohort, and hypothyroidism was not caused by this thyroid disease, rather it was induced by iodine deficiency.

We did not found considerable or significant differences of somatic development in children with or without iodine-deficiency, with or without hypothyroidism.

Intellectual performances of 59 children were recorded, and than we distributed them into two groups: one (1. subgroup) with children having mediocre and low learning capacity (32 cases), and the other (2. subgroup) consisting of individuals with good or very good performances (27 cases). The goiter frequency based on ultrasound was 22.5% in the first, and 17.8% in the second group (P-value >0.05). We compared the mean UIE, TSH and FT_4 between the subgroups of children with different school performances, but we did not found significant differences, excepting a tendency of reducing school performances with the gradually increasing values of TSH and decreasing levels of FT_4 (Figure 3.).

Our results recorded in 2006 show that the **water sample** from Caşva contains 3.8μg/L iodine, and the iodized alimentary salt 16.02mg/kg (which was lower than the ordered concentration of 34±8.5mg/kg). In Glăjărie the iodine content of the water from the central fountain was 1.0μg/L, from the parish yard 1.9μg/L, in the running water from the school 0.45μg/L and from the medical unit 4.2 μg/L. The iodine content of water from Ibăneşti was 0.6μg/L and of the iodized alimentary salt 51.64mg/kg (which was higher than the allowed upper normal concentration).

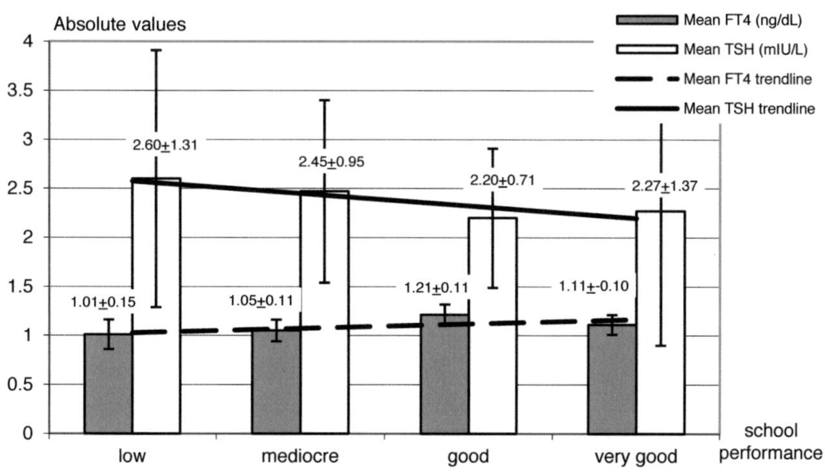

Figure 3. The mean TSH and FT_4 levels in subgroups of children distributed according to school performances

5. Discussion

In 2003 the Romanian governmental decision regarding universal salt iodization was implemented into practice, and in 2006, after about 2.5-3 years, we evaluated the impact of this program in regions of Mureş County known as moderate or mild iodine deficient.

In order to evaluate the impact of universal salt iodization program in Romania in the context of national strategy on the elimination of iodine deficiency disorders from 2003, we compared our results reflecting iodine status in localities from Mureş County after the implementation of this program with those before it. Thus, we compared the indicators of iodine status in Mureş County reported in 1998-1999 by Balázs et al. (1998; 2000/a; 2000/b), before the governmental measures, with the same indicators measured by us in 2006. The mentioned data in 1998/99 were obtained in the superior and middle hydrographic basin of the Mureş river, investigating a group of 508 school-children living in areas surrounding locality Deda (situated in a mountainous region in Mureş County). From the 508 school-age children 26.97% (137 cases) were living in urban and 73.03% (371) in rural localities.

Physical examination of thyroid gland by palpation and inspection was performed in both studies (in 1998/99 and in that presented now). Thyroid size determined by local physical examination was evaluated according to WHO criteria (0, Ia, Ib, II, III subgroups) in the mentioned former studies. According to the Bourdoux classification the volume of thyroid gland was enlarged by palpation in 45.27% of children: grade Ia goiter observed in 29.92% (152 cases), grade Ib in 14.17% (72), and grade II in 1.18% (6 children). Those studies highlighted the high frequency of low grade goiter in rural localities in comparison with a lower frequency observed in urban regions (Balázs et al., 1998).

In the present work physical examination shows an owerall goiter frequency of 51.9%, prevailing small goiters (grade Ia) in all studied villages (more than half of goiters), large goiters being very rare (grade II only in 6.7% of all cohort). Comparing the data of the two series we could not found any improvement in the overall frequency of goiter (45.28% in 1999 vs. 51.1% in 2006), but we must take into account, that in the previous study children came from several localities (including Târgu Mureş, the capital city of Mureş County) with different iodine status (mild or moderate iodine deficient, as well as with normal iodine supply). A considerable number of the enrolled children were from Târgu Mureş, a city which proved to be without iodine deficiency. In the present work we focused on mountainous villages, known before as iodine deficient regions, some of them (Caşva and Glăjărie) known partly isolated in socioeconomical and geographical point of view.

In our study physical examination of thyroid gland shows variable goiter frequency in the three localities: it is the highest in Ibăneşti (62.0%) vs. the other two localities (46.7% in Glăjărie and 43.6% in Caşva). This result is not in concordance with the fact that Ibăneşti is the largest among the three localities, with better socioeconomical status and lesser isolated. An explanation might reside in the differences in age, gender and pubertal stage of the children. In Ibăneşti the mean chronological age of school-age children enrolled in the study is higher (12.05 years vs. 11.51 and 11.80 years in the other two localities), and the distribution between sexes is almost 1:1 (differing evidently from boys:girls-ratio of 2:1 in Glăjărie and 3:2 in Caşva). Taking into account that the girls from Ibăneşti were older, between 12-14-years, the pubertal stage was higher in this group. Balázs et al. (1998) have reported the increased incidence of grade Ib and II goiter in children with pubertal onset compared to those being in prepubertal stage, as pubertal onset is an important facilitating factor for goiter development. This is in concordance with our data, too, related to gender. The overall goiter frequency provided by ultrasound was significantly higher in girls than in boys (28% vs. 14.1%): although goiter appeared almost with the same frequency in both sexes from Caşva (14.2% in girls and 17.6% in boys), but it was more than 3-times more frequent in girls than in boys living in Ibăneşti (42.3% vs. 12.5%). Euthyroid pubertal goiter is especially frequent in adolescents, because iodine metabolism is accelerated during this period of life (Delange & Ermans, 1967).

Than we compared our data obtained in 2006 to the results recorded during April-June 1999 at school-age children living in Deda, a mountainous rural locality, presumed as iodine deficient area. In that study 36.22% of the children had goiter, mainly of small size, without considerable differences between the sexes (Balázs et al., 2000/a) – the goiter being assessed by inspection/palpation. This result is similar to that in the present study (40.2% in children with age between 6-12 years), without any significant differences between the groups. It must be emphasized, that the lack of gender differences may be attributed to inspection/palpation method for the diagnosis of goiter. Taking into account the subjectivity and bias of physical examination of thyroid gland, especially in young children, as this method of evaluation estimates goiter presence with an error as much as 30-40%, our interpretation was based mainly on thyroid ultrasound.

The objective determination of thyroid volume by ultrasound provided the exact size of the thyroid, however it was difficult to chose the adequate standards for the normal thyroid volume fitting to the goiter estimation in our region. The references published during the last 2-3 decades provide very variable standards for the upper normal limit of thyroid ultrasound volumetry adjusted for age, gender and BSA.

We evaluated firstly the age- and BSA-adjusted goiter frequency compared to the reference values provided by the Thyromobile survey accross Europe (Delange et al., 1997), and thereafter we reevaluated the results according to parameters published by Zimmermann (2004), but we obtained very different results (Figure 1.). After all we chose the standards provided by a team of endocrinologists from Iaşi performed on a cohort living in a formerly iodine deficient Romanian region (Vulpoi et al., 2002; Zbranca et al., 2008). Thus, goiter frequency in our cohort assessed by ultrasound was 20%, with a considerable difference between the sexes (28% in girls and 14.1% in boys).

In the study of Balázs et al. (2000/a) thyroid ultrasonography was also performed in 83 children living in Târgu Mureş. The mean thyroid volume determined by ultrasound among these children was 5.22±1.51cm^3, adjusted to a mean body surface area of 1.23±0.14 m^2. Goiter evaluated by ultrasound was detected in 33.73% of the children, mainly small goiters (grade Ia), predominantly in girls (about 2/3 in girls and 1/3 in boys).

The 20% of goiter frequency (diagnosed by ultrasound) detected in school-age children by us, reflects a mild/moderate iodine deficiency in the studied three mountainous villages from Mureş County in 2006. The stratified results of each locality showed that Caşva and Glăjărie were mildy iodine deficient areas (reflected by 16.3 and 13.3% goiter, respectively), and Ibăneşti moderately iodine deficient (with 28% goiter).

So, we observed a significant reduction of goiter frequency after the measures taken in the frame of universal salt iodization, compared to the results obtained by Balázs et al. in 1998/99 (the overall goiter frequency 20% in 2006 vs. 33.73% in 1999 – P-value: 0.025, RR: 1.687, 95%CI: 1.073-2.652). As thyroid enlargement reflects the former iodine status, i.e. the history of iodine nutrition for the previous several months/1-2 years, this means a significant improvement of iodine status in the studied regions, reflecting the beneficial outcome of universal salt iodization.

Urinary iodine excretion reflects the present iodine status of a geographical region. Determination of UIE with Sandell-Kolthoff reaction, using ammonium persulfate was the laboratory method used in the both series of study (realized in 1998/99 and in 2006) performed in Mureş County, so the absolute values could be compared.

In 1998/99 the majority of rural localities situated on the superior and middle hydrographical basin of the river Mureş were mildly iodine-deficient areas, the rest being moderately deficient. The mean UIE was 100.22μg/L, but with a high interindividual variation: SD ± 73.37 (Balázs et al., 1998). The mountainous rural region of Deda was considered moderately iodine deficient in 1998, the normal UIE being detected only in 6.9% of cases, and the mean UIE being 59.95±30.22μg/L. Although in Târgu Mureş the mean UIE was within the normal range (130.05±75.45μg/L), normal individual UIE levels >100μg/L were observed only in 56.79% of the children (Balázs et al., 1998; 2000/a; 2000/b).

In 2006, at about 2-2.5 years after the implementation in practice of universal salt iodization the mean urinary iodine excretion measured in the 135 school-age children living in the three mentioned villages from Gurghiu Valley was 85.37±60.05μg/L. Median value of 74.88μg/L indicates an overall mild iodine deficiency. In order to compare this result with that from 1999, the median UIE in 1999 was calculated based on the mean UIE in 1999 (59.95±30.22μg/L) using the formula recommended by WHO (median UIE = 1.128 + 0.864 × mean UIE – WHO et al., 2001). Thus, the estimated median UIE was 52.29μg/L before the universal salt iodization program.

The median UIE compared to the previous studies shows also a considerable improvement in the iodine status of rural regions from Mureş County, being in concordance with the significant reduction of goiter frequency discussed previously. So, we observed better median UIE in Ibăneşti (81.00μg/L), in contrast with Glăjărie, known as the most isolated and with less socioeconomical background (having the lowest median UIE: 53.50μg/L).

In the studies performed before universal salt Iodization highly variable interindividual UIE concentrations were observed, although the mean value indicated only a mild iodine deficiency. Normal UIE was found only in 6.9% of school-age children, which means a frequency of cases with UIE<100μg/L of 93.1%. In 2006 a large proportion (68.1%) of studied school-children had still mildly or moderately low UIE. Similarly to the studies performed in 1998/99, the results of the present work show large interindividual variations of UIE (SD: ±60.05μg/L).

Values below normal range (UIE <100μg/L) were detected in 68.1% of our cohort, which is improved compared to data obtained in 1998/1999. Indead, the proportion of cases with normal UIE has increased significantly in 2006 compared to that determined in 1998/1999 (31.9% vs. 6.9%, P-value<0.0001, RR: 1.268, 95%CI: 1.183-1.581). However, this increase has not attained yet the most important criteria of normal iodine-supply conditions, i.e. the maximal value of 50% UIE <100μg/L (the 68.1% is still above of this limit with 18.1%); similarly, in our present study the proportion of UIE <50μg/L is 30.3%, for normal iodine-supply it must be ≤20%. These results show that the universal salt iodization program could not be ensured at an optimal level, being not sustained continuously.

The iodine status of the studied localities from Mureş County in 2006 was evaluated by the following indicators: median UIE for the current iodine status, frequency of goiter assessed by ultrasound for the history of iodine nutrition of the previous months-years, and the frequency of UIE concentrations below 100μg/L and below 50μg/L for the sustainability of universal salt iodization program (Table 12.).

Interpretation of indicators	Data from every studied villages			Whole cohort
	Caşva	Glăjărie	Ibăneşti	
Current iodine status in 2006 (by median UIE)	mild iodine deficiency	mild iodine deficiency	mild iodine deficiency	mild iodine deficiency
Former iodine status (before 2006) (by frequency of goiter)	mild iodine deficiency	mild iodine deficiency	moderate iodine deficiency	mild/moderate iodine deficiency
Sustained elimination of iodine deficiency (by % cases with UIE<100μg/L and UIE<50μg/L)	not ensured	not ensured	not ensured	not ensured

Table 12. The interpretation of indicators showing the iodine status among school-children in the three mountainous villages in 2006

During 2006 the frequency of goiter in school-age children was 20% which is improved to that observed in 1998/99 (33.73%), but it has not reached normal levels yet, being situated at the borderline between mild and moderate iodine deficiency (5-19.9% and 20-29.9%, respectively). Our results show an improved iodine status in 2006: the mean UIE rose to 85.37±60.05μg/L, median UIE to 74.88μg/L, and 30.8% of children had normal urinary iodine excretion. Analysing separately the groups in every village, the mean UIE are different in some degree: 72.91±48.63μg/L in Caşva, 75.42±60.30μg/L in Glăjărie and 117.84±91.95 μg/L in Ibăneşti. Median UIE has improved compared to the situation in 1998/99, but it remained at subnormal levels, indicating a mild iodine deficiency in all three villages. The indicators for the estimation of sustained elimination of iodine deficiency were at subnormal levels. Studies performed during 2002-2004 reported an improvement of overall median UIE in school-age Romanian children from 70 (in urban) and 60µg/L (in rural areas) in 2002 to 105 and 100µg/L, respectively, until 2004. At the Second National Conference for the elimination of IDD held at Bucharest in 2005, the Mother and Child Care Institute "Alfred Rusescu" reported that in children of 6-7-years of age the overall iodine status tended to normalize, the median UIE reaching 100µg/L (Stănescu, 2005). Although the median UIE became almost normal (105 in urban and 100µg/L in rural localities), a large interindividual variation were found, reflected by the SD of ±60µg/L (Stănescu, 2005). Important differences between iodine status of rural and urban environment were observed. Mild iodine deficiency was recorded in 33.5% of the population, 11% presented moderate and 2.4% severe forms (Stănescu, 2005), although 96.3% of the housholds used iodized salt. These results could derive from the facts that more than half of the families used salt with inadequate iodine content (under 15mg iodine/kg salt), 3/4 of the families consumed iodized salt but in an inadequate manner (adding salt before and during cooking) which reduces the content of iodine; the frequency of iodized salt consumption is higher in families with the higher educational level of the mother.

In conclusion, on the basis of the indicators for iodine status the mountainous villages located in Mureş Conty, known as mild/moderate iodine deficient regions in 1999, remained in the same iodine deficiency category during 2006, however the absolute values of indicators were considerably, some even significantly improved. The indicators situated before at the lower limit of mild/moderate iodine deficiency interval, after-wise were shifted to the middle zone and upper limit of this range. The universal salt iodization had a beneficial impact on iodine deficient rural regions, as expected, but its sustainability must be maintained, i.e. the effectiveness of public health authorities and salt industry to monitor and control the whole procession must be consolidated. The elimination strategy of IDD in mountainous rural areas remains a very important public health program, as the iodine content of water and soil is very low here. Water samples taken from the main water-provision points from every village showed that the iodine content of drinking water was very low in every locality, as expected in mountainous rural regions. Thus general measures to increase the iodine content of the water should be applied. The iodine content of the running water measured in 1998/99 and 2006 was very variable (the mean value being X=10.15µg/L, SD±9.85 – Balázs et al., 1998), but in all cases the iodine concentration was much more under the accepted value (levels above 50µg/L being considered normal). Iodine content of alimentary salt found at the market of the three villages was in some cases under the prescribed level of 34±8mg/kg. The usage of iodized alimentary salt in households reached 96% in 2004 compared to 53% in the previous years (Goldner, 2005; Stănescu, 2005), but the alimentary salt was insufficient iodized (in 63% of cases, Goldner, 2005). A proportion of 74.5% of the sample of salt tested which was used in the market and for the panification had a standard iodine content of 15-25 mg/kg (Goldner, 2005), which was under the prescribed concentration. In spite of existent legislation to mandatory sale of iodized table salt on the market, about 12% of population consumes not iodized salt (Nanu, 2005), especially in rural environment.

The persistence of moderate iodine deficiency in some zones of Romania was attributed to the insufficient iodization level of the salt and waist during storage, to the uncontrolled selling of industrial salt as alimentary salt, to the lack of control measures in import of salt, to the inadequate monitoring system and the lack of efficient measures to realize entirely the governmental decision, as well as the resistency of alimentary industry (e.g. meat processing industry) to utilize iodized salt (Goldner, 2005).

We must remark the presence of hypothyroidism related to iodine deficiency in 17.7% of the investigated school-children, TPO-Ab being normal in all of them. Although, all cases of hypothyroidism were mildly overt or subclinical forms (15 and 9, respectively), we must take into account that even mild iodine and thyroid hormone deficiencies conduct to psycho-neurological damages, the characteristical complication of latent deficiency being AD-HD syndrome in developed countries. Chronic iodine deficiency leads to suboptimal intellectual development. Recent studies performed in the European countries, known with iodine prevention programs initiated decades ago, and thougth that iodine deficiency was eliminated, sustaine surprisingly the presence of mild iodine deficiency in many countries and implication of this in school performances, psychological and neurological status. These mild deficits probably results from transient hypothyroidism during the first 2-years of life, i.e. during the critical period of brain development (Delange, 2002). Besides iodine deficiency, an increase in iodine intake can also lead to a small but significant increase in the incidence of hypothyroidism, probably attributable to autoregulation of thyroid function.

In conclusion, the rural mountainous zones of Mureş County known before as moderate/ mild iodine-deficient areas, became *mild-deficient*, due to the new measures of iodine prevention. In these areas universal salt iodization is not sufficient, being necessary to apply periodically special prophylactic measures (iodine tablets), too, primarily to prepubertal and pubertal children.

6. Conclusions

This work underlines considerable improvement of iodine nutrition in mountainous rural regions of Mureş County after the implementation in practice of universal salt iodization in Romania since 2003, although these areas remained mildly (some moderately) iodine deficient at about 2.5-3 years after the IDD elimination strategy was intitiated. On one hand the prophylactic measures with higher iodine content of alimentary salt (KIO_3 25.5-42.5mg/kg) might not be sufficient for the full correction of iodine deficiency in these isolated mountainous rural regions, on the other hand special attention is required to monitorize continuously the market and reaching programs, as well as the sustainability of the prophylactic program must be ensured. In these areas special measures, i.e. iodine supplementation to the high-risk populational groups are periodically required in addition to universal salt iodization, especially as iodine deficiency occured with hypothyroidism in 17.7% of school-children. The elimination of mild-moderate iodine deficiency in school-age children living in mountainous rural localities presumes special measures by the daily administration of 0.1-0.2 mg iodine tablets.

Author details

Imre Zoltán Kun[1,2], Zsuzsanna Szántó[1], József Balázs[2], Anisie Năsălean[2] and Camelia Gliga[1,2]

1 University of Medicine and Pharmacy Târgu Mureş, Romania

2 Endocrinology Clinic, Clinical Hospital Mureş County, Romania

References

[1] Andersson M, de Benoist B, Darnton-Hill I, Delange F (2007) WHO, UNICEF: Iodine Deficiency in Europe: A continuing public health problem. World Health Organization, Switzerland, 1-70.

[2] Andersson M (2011) Regional and Global Prevalence of Iodine Deficiency and Burden of Disease Due to Iodine Deficiency. West Central Europe Regional ICCIDD Satellite to 35th Annual ETA Meeting. In: Paschke R & Smyth P (eds.) Thyroid International 5: 14.

[3] Balázs J, Vasilescu Gh, Buksa C, Pintea A, Gliga C, Alexandrescu C, Paşcanu I, Radu C, Balázs A, Puskás A (1998) Guşa endemică, carenţa de iod, condiţia social economică şi indicii de dezvoltare somatometrică şi pubertară la şcolari din localităţi situate în bazinul hidrografic al Mureşului superior şi mijlociu (in Romanian). *Revista de Medicină şi Farmacie* 44(Suppl. 3): 10-11.

[4] Balázs J, Pintea A, Buksa C, Vasilescu G (2000/a) Volumul tiroidian şi aportul de iod la copii de vârstă şcolară din Târgu-Mureş – The thyroid volume and iodine intake in school-children from Târgu-Mureş (in Romanian). *Revista de Medicină şi Farmacie* 46: 60-63.

[5] Balázs J, Kun IZ, Buksa C, Coroş L, Vasilescu G, Năsălean A (2000/b) Studiul privind guşa endemică, tiroidita cronică, funcţia tiroidiană în contextul aportului iodat, la elevi dintr-o localitate de pe cursul superior al Mureşului – Study of endemic goiter, chronic thyroiditis, thyroid function in correlation with iodine intake at school-children living in the superior hydrographic basin of the river Mureş (in Romanian). *Revista de Medicină şi Farmacie* 46: 240-244.

[6] Bernal J (2005) Thyroid hormones and brain development. *Vitamins and Hormones* 71: 95-122.

[7] Bleichrodt N, Born MP (1994) A meta-analysis of research on iodine and its relationship to cognitive development. In: Stanbury JB (ed.) The damaged brain of iodine deficiency. New York, Cognizant Communication: 195-200.

[8] Boyages SC (1994) Primary pediatric hypothyroidism and endemic cretinism. *Current therapy in endocrinology and metabolism* 5: 94-98.

[9] Brook Charles DG, Brown Rosalind S (2008) Handbook of clinical Pediatric Endocrinology. Blackwell Publishing, Oxford.

[10] Cornea GH (1957) Distrofia endemică tireopată pe valea Mureşului, de la izvor până la Târgu-Mureş (in Romanian). In: Milcu SM (ed.) Guşa endemică Editura Academiei, Vol I: 197-201.

[11] de Benoist B, Andersson M, Egli I, Takkouche B, Allen H (2004) Iodine status worldwide. WHO Global Database on Iodine Deficiency. Department of Nutrition for Health and Development World Health Organization Geneva 2004.

[12] Delange F (1994) The disorders induced by iodine deficiency. *Thyroid* 4: 107-128.

[13] Delange F (2000) Endemic cretinism. In: Braverman LE, Utiger RD (eds.) The thyroid. A fundamental and clinical text. 8th Edition. Philadelphia, Lippincott, 743-754.

[14] Delange F (2001) Iodine deficiency as a cause of brain damage. *Postgraduate Medical Journal*: 77:217–220.

[15] Delange F (2002) Iodine deficiency in Europe anno 2002. *Thyroid International* 5: 1-18.

[16] Delange FM, Dunn JT (2005) Iodine deficiency. In: Braverman LE, Utiger RD (eds.): Werner & Ingbar's The Thyroid. A Fundamental and Clinical Text. Ninth Edition. Lippincott Williams & Wilkins, Philadelphia 264-283.

[17] Delange F, Ermans AM (1967) Le métabolisme de l'iode à la pubertè. *Rev Fr Etud Clin Biol* 12: 87-92.

[18] Delange F, Benker G, Caron Ph, Eber O, Ott W, Peter F, Podoba J, Simescu M, Szybinsky Z, Vertongen F, Vitti P, Wiersinga W, Zamrazil V (1997) Thyroid volume and urinary iodine in European school-children: standardization of values for assessment of iodine deficiency. *Eur J Endocrinol* 136: 180-187.

[19] Delange F, Robertson A, McLoughney E, Gerasimov G (1998) Elimination of iodine deficiency disorders (IDD) in central and eastern Europe, the Commonwealth of Independent States, and the Baltic States. World Health Organization. Publication WHO/Eur/NUT/98.1: 1-168.

[20] Delong GR (1989) Observations on the neurology of endemic cretinism. In: Delong GR, Robbins J, Condliffe PG, eds. Iodine and the brain. New York, Plenum Press: 231ff.

[21] Dobbing J & Sands J (1973) Quantitative growth and development of human brain. *Arch Dis Child* 48: 757-767.

[22] Dunn, JT, Crutchfield HE, Gutekunst R, Dunn AD (1993) Methods for measuring iodine in urine. Wageningen: International Council for Control of Iodine Deficiency Disorders (ICCIDD) publ. 1-71.

[23] Fenzi GF, Giusti LF, Aghini-Lombardi F, Bartalena L, Marcocci C, Santini F, Bargagna S, Brizzolara D, Ferretti G, Falciglia G (1990) Neuropsychological assessment in schoolchildren from an area of moderate iodine deficiency. *J Endocrinol Invest* 13(5): 427-431.

[24] Gerasimov G (2002) IDD in eastern Europe and central Asia. IDD Newsletter 18: 33-37.

[25] Glinoer D (2001) Pregnancy and iodine. *Thyroid* 11 471–481.

[26] Goldner T (2005) Tulburările prin deficit de iod - perspectiva naţională - perspectiva regională (in Romanian) Second National Conference for the elimination of Iodine Deficiency Disorders, Bucharest, Bucharest, 14 November 2005.

[27] Gorstein J (2001) Goiter assessment: help or hindrance in tracking progress in iodine deficiency disorders control program *Thyroid* 11: 1201-1202.

[28] Gutekunst R & Teichert HM (1993) Requirements for goiter surveys and the determination of thyroid size. In: Delange F, Dunn JT, Glinoer D (eds.) Iodine deficiency in Europe. A continuing concern. Plenum Press, New York-London 109-115.

[29] Gutekunst R & Scriba PC (1989) Goiter and iodine deficiency in Europe: the European Thyroid Association report as updated in 1988. *J Endocrinol Invest* 12: 209-220.

[30] Hetzel BS (1983) Iodine deficiency disorders (IDD) and their eradication. *Lancet* 2: 1126–1129.

[31] Hetzel BS, Dunn JT, Stanbury JB (1987) The prevention and control of iodine deficiency disorders. Elsevier 257.

[32] Joffe RT & Sokolov ST (1994) Thyroid hormones, the brain, and affective disorders. *Crit Rev Neurobiol* 8: 45-63.

[33] Koibuchi N & Chin WW (2000) Thyroid hormone action and brain development. *Trends Endocrinol Metab* 4: 123-128.

[34] Kun I (2006) Insuficienţa tirodiană în judeţul Mureş (in Romanian) Hypothyroidism in Mureş County Doctoral thesis, University of Medicine and Pharmacy Târgu Mureş, Romania.

[35] Kun I, Szántó Zs, Kun IZ, Szabó B, Coroş L (2007) The evolution of hypothyroidism in pregnant women in County Mureş between 2001-2006. 9th European Congress of Endocrinology, 28 aprilie–2 mai 2007, Budapest, *Endocrine Abstracts* 14: P351.

[36] Kun IZ, Szántó Zs (2003) A pajzsmirigyelégtelenség és szövődményeinek gyakorisága Maros megye területén (in Hungarian) The frequency and complications of hypothyroidism in Mureş County. In: Brassai A (ed.) Orvostudományi Tanulmányok – Sapientia Könyvek. Scientia Cluj-Napoca, pp. 131-206.

[37] Laurberg P, Nohr SB, Pedersen KM, Hreidarsson AB, Andersen S, Bülow Pedersen I, Knudsen N, Perrild H, Jorgensen T, Ovesen L (2000) Thyroid disorders in mild iodine deficiency. *Thyroid* 10: 951-963.

[38] Morreale de Escobar G, Obregon MJ, Escobar del Rey F (2004) Role of thyroid hormone during early brain development. *Eur J Endocrinol* 151 (Suppl. 3): U25-37.

[39] Nanu M (2005) Evaluarea statusului iodului la femeia gravidă. Second National Conference for the elimination of Iodine Deficiency Disorders, Bucharest, 14 November 2005.

[40] Neale DM, Cootauco AC, Burrow G (2007) Thyroid disease in pregnancy. *Clin Perinatol* 34: 543–557.

[41] Pearce EN (2009) What do we know about iodine supplementation in pregnancy? *J Clin Endocrinol Metab* 94: 3188-3190.

[42] Perez C, Scrimshaw S, Munoz A (1960) Technique of endemic goiter surveys. In Endemic Goiter, WHO Geneva, pp. 369-383.

[43] Pop VJ, Brouwers EP, Vader HL, Vulsma T, van Baar AL, de Viljder JJ (2003) Maternal hypothyroxinemia during early pregnancy and subsequent child development: a 3-year follow-up study. *Clin Endocrinol* 59: 282-288.

[44] Simescu M & Ionescu M (1998) Date despre IDD în România în contextul european actual. Consideraţii despre profilaxia iodată şi monitorizarea ei. Hipotiroidismul tranzitoriu neonatal (in Romanian) *Revista de Medicină şi Farmacie* 44(Suppl.3): 8-9.

[45] Simescu M, Zbranca E, Dumitriu L (1999) Monitorizarea profilaxiei guşii endemice în judeţele în care Programul 21 se desfăşoară (in Romanian) The Annual National Congress of Endocrinology, Constanţa, Romania, Book of abstracts: 40.

[46] Stanbury JB (1994) The damaged brain of iodine deficiency. New York, Cognizant Communication.

[47] Stanbury JB, Ermans AE, Bourdoux P, Todd C, Oken E, Tonqlet R, Vidor G, Baverman LE, Medeiros-Neto G (1998) Iodine-induced hyperthyroidism: occurence and epidemiology. *Thyroid* 8(1): 83-100.

[48] Stănescu A (2005) Contextul nutriţional în România. Second National Conference for the elimination of Iodine Deficiency Disorders, Bucharest, 14 November 2005.

[49] Szántó Zs, Kun I, Kun IZ, Coroş L, Cucerea M (2007) The influence of universal salt iodization on the iodine status reflected by TSH serum levels of newborns, in Mureş County, between years 2001-2006. *Acta Endocrinol (Buc)* III(3): 291-301.

[50] Szybinski Z (2011) The WHO Recommendation on Reduction of Daily Salt Intake and its Impact on the USI Program for IDD Prevention. West Central Europe Regional ICCIDD Satellite to 35th Annual ETA Meeting. In: Paschke R & Smyth P (eds.) *Thyroid International* 5: 14.

[51] Vasilescu Gh, Totoianu I, Ismănescu I (1986) Prevalence of endemic goiter in Mureş County. *Rev Roum Med Endocrinol* 24: 27-32.

[52] Vermiglio F, Sidoti M, Finocchiaro MD, Battiato S, Lo Presti VP, Benvenga S, Trimarchi F (1990) Defective neuromotor and cognitive ability in iodine deficient school-children of an endemic goiter region in Sicily. *J Clin Endocrinol Metab* 70: 379-384

[53] Vermiglio F, Lo presti VP, Moleti M, Sidoti M, Tortorella G, Scaffidi G, Castagna MG, Mattina F, Violi MA, Crisa A, Artemisia A, Trimarchi F (2004) Attention deficit and hyperactivity disorders in the offspring of mothers exposed to mild-moderate iodine

deficiency: a possible novel iodine deficiency disorder in developed countries. *J Clin Endocrinol Metab* 89: 6054-6060.

[54] Vulpoi C, Mogoş V, Cojocaru M, Preda C, Ungureanu MC, Brănişteanu DD, Cristea C, Zbranca E (2002) Thyroid volume in a former iodine deficient area. *Revista Română de Endocrinologie şi Metabolism* 1(3): 17-22.

[55] Vitti P, Martino E, Anghini-Lombardi F, Rago T, Antonangeli L, Maccherini D, Nanni P, Loviselli A, Balestrieri A, Araneo G et al (1994) Thyroid volume measurement by ultrasound in children as a tool for the assessment of mild iodine deficiency. J Clin Endocrinol Metab 79(2): 600-603.

[56] Witti P, Delange F, Pinchera A, Zimmermann M, Dunn JT (2003) Europe is iodine deficient. *Lancet* 5: 361.

[57] Zbranca E, Găluscă B, Mogoş V (2008) Tiroida (in Romanian) In: Zbranca E (ed.): Endocrinologie. Ghid de diagnostic şi tratament în bolile endocrine. Third edition. Polirom Iaşi 105-175.

[58] Zimmermann MB, Molinari L, Spehl M, Weidinger-Toth J, Podoba J, Hess S, Delange F (2001) Toward a consensus on reference values for thyroid volume in iodine-replete school-children: results of a workshop on interobserver and inter-equipment variation in sonographic measurement of thyroid volume. *Eur J Endocrinol* 144: 213-220.

[59] Zimmermann MB, Hess SY, Molinari L, de Benoist B, Delange F, Braverman LE, Fujieda K, Ito Y, Jooste PL, Moosa K, Pearce EN, Pretell EA, Shishiba Y (2004) New reference values for thyroid by ultrasound in iodine-sufficient school-children: a World Health Organization/Nutrition for Health and Development Iodine Deficiency Study Group Report. *Am J Clinical Nutrition* 79: 231-237.

[60] Zimmermann MB (2009) Iodine deficiency. *Endocr Rev* 30: 376.

[61] ***Government of Romania (2005) National Strategy on the elimination of iodine deficiency disorders by universal iodization of salt intended for direct human use and for bread baking 2004-2012. UNICEF Romania Bucharest, 1-12.

[62] ***WHO, UNICEF, ICCIDD (1994) Indicators for assessing iodine deficiency disorders and their control through salt iodization. WHO Geneva: WHO/NUT/94.6.

[63] ***WHO, UNICEF, ICCIDD (1999) Progress to wards the elimination of iodine deficiency disorders (IDD). WHO Geneva: WHO/NHD/99.4:1-33.

[64] ***WHO, UNICEF, ICCIDD (2001) Assessment of iodine deficiency disorders and monitoring their elimination. WHO Geneva: WHO/NHD/01.1.

Chapter 5

Diabetes and Its Hepatic Complication

Paola I. Ingaramo, Daniel E. Francés,
María T. Ronco and Cristina E. Carnovale

Additional information is available at the end of the chapter

http://dx.doi.org/10.5772/53684

1. Introduction

After food intake, blood glucose levels rise and insulin is released by the pancreas to maintain homeostasis. In the diabetic state, the absence or deficient action of insulin in target tissues is the cause of hyperglycemia and abnormalities in the metabolism of proteins, fats and carbohydrates. In addition, chronic hyperglycemia, characteristic of diabetes, is responsible for organic dysfunction, being eyes, kidneys, nervous system, heart and blood vessels the most important affected organs. Diabetes mellitus (DM) is a heterogeneous dysregulation of carbohydrate metabolism, characterized by chronic hyperglycemia resulting from impaired glucose metabolism and the subsequent increase in blood serum glucose concentration. The pathogenic equation for DM presents a complex interrelation of metabolic, genetic and environmental factors, as well as inflammatory mediators. Among the latter, it is mostly unclear whether they reflect the disease process or are simply signs of systemic or local responses to the disease [1].

DM affects about 26 million individuals in America and at least 250 million people worldwide (World Health Organization), causing about 5% of all deaths. Besides, the number of affected people is expected to duplicate by 2030 unless urgent measures are taken [2, 3]. Every day, 200 children under 14 years are affected by type 1 diabetes, and this number increases by 3 per cent each year, whereas the analogous increment for preschool children reaches 6 per cent [4]. All these data point out the epidemic character of DM.

2. Animal models for the study of diabetes

Rats and mice are animals commonly used for studying the effects of diabetes. Type 2 DM can be induced in animal models through dietary modification such as the administration of sucrose, fructose, high fat diet and glucose infusion or through genetic manipulation such as db/db mice, ob/ob mice, Goto-Kakizaki rats, Zucker diabetic rats and BHE rats [5].

On the other hand, type 1 diabetes can be replicated in animal models through genetic modifications, i.e. non obese diabetic mice (NOD), which spontaneously develop type 1 diabetes in a manner similar to humans [6]. Other animal models genetically selected are the Bio Breeding rats (BB), in which the pancreatic islets are under the attack of immune T cells, B cells, macrophages and natural killer cells. At approximately 12 weeks of age, these diabetic rats present weight loss, polyuria, polyphagia, hyperglycemia and insulinopenia. As in humans, if these rats are not treated with exogenous insulin, ketoacidosis becomes severe and fatal [7]. Another way to obtain experimental animals with type 1 diabetes is through the administration of chemicals such as alloxan or streptozotocin [8-10]. In our laboratory, we have shown that treatment with streptozotocin causes alterations in biliary excretion during the first seven days post-injection of the drug, becoming normalized 10 days after injection [10, 11]. This is the reason why studies of liver function during streptozotocin-induced diabetic state should be performed fifteen day after injection of the drug. In our work, streptozotocin-induced diabetes (SID) was induced by a single dose of streptozotocin (STZ) (60mg/kg body weight, i.p., in 50 mM citrate buffer, pH 4.5). Control rats were injected with vehicle alone. Fifteen days after STZ injection, a time when the toxic effect of the drug on the liver has disappeared [9, 10], serum glucose levels were tested by means of the glucose oxidase method (Wiener Lab., Rosario, Argentina) in samples obtained from diabetic and control animals. Successful induction of diabetes was defined as a blood glucose level of > 13.2 mmol/l. Between 10 and 12 A.M. the rats were weighed, anesthetized with sodium pentobarbital solution (50 mg/kg body weight, i.p.) and euthanatized. Blood was obtained by cardiac puncture and plasma was separated by centrifugation. Livers were promptly removed and hepatic tissue was either processed for immunohistochemical studies or frozen in liquid nitrogen and stored at −70 °C until analytical assays were performed.

3. Diabetes and inflammation

Inflammation represents a protective response to the control of infections and promotes tissues repair, but it can also contribute to local tissue damage in a broad spectrum of inflammatory disorders. The inflammatory responses are associated with variations of a wide array of plasma proteins and pro-inflammatory cytokines. The acute-phase response is a systemic reaction in which a number of changes in plasma protein concentrations, termed acute-phase proteins, may increase or decrease in response to inflammation [12]. Modifications in the plasma concentration of acute-phase proteins are largely dependent on their biosynthesis in the liver and changes in their production are influenced by the effect of pro-inflammatory cytokines such as IL-1, IL-6 and tumor necrosis factor alpha (TNF-α) on the hepatocytes. These cytokines are produced during the inflammatory process and they are the main stimulators of acute-phase proteins and other markers of chronic inflammation commonly detected in cardiovascular diseases, diabetes mellitus, osteoarthritis, and rheumatoid arthritis [13, 14].

Chronic hyperglycemia can directly promote an inflammatory state where the increase in cytokines can lead to destruction of the pancreatic beta cells and dysfunction of the endocrine pancreas in diabetes type 1 and 2. [15]. There is evidence that autocrine insulin exerts protective anti-apoptotic effects on beta cells and that it inhibits the suppressor of cytokine signaling (SOCS), which is induced by various cytokines and lead to apoptosis of the beta cell [16]. Commonly, DM type 1 and type 2 are considered inflammatory processes [17, 18] as there is a significant increase in interleukin (IL) IL-6, IL-18, IL-1 and TNF-α in blood of patients with this disease [19, 20].

Futhermore, chemokines (ligands 2 and 5 chemokines CCL2, CCL5 and CX3CL1), intercellular adhesion molecule-1 (ICAM-1), vascular cell adhesion molecule -1 (VCAM-1) and nuclear transcription factor κB (NFκB) are involved in the development and progression of the disease [21, 22]. In this connection, we have demonstrated that hyperglycemia increases the production of hydroxyl radical in the liver of streptozotocin-induced diabetic rats [23]. In addition, the increase in oxidative stress induced by hyperglycemia and inflammation conduces to development of associated diseases such as diabetic nephropathy [17, 21].

The role for pro-inflammatory cytokines in regulating insulin action and glucose homeostasis and their function in type 2 diabetes has been suggested by several lines of evidence. High TNF-α levels are related to the pathophysiology of insulin resistance and type 2 diabetes [24]. The mechanisms that govern the association between the increased synthesis of inflammatory factors and type 2 diabetes are still being elucidated. In macrophages, adipocytes, antigen-presenting B-cells, dendritic cells, and Kupffer cells in the liver, a number of germline-encoded pattern recognition receptors (PRRs), such as the toll-like receptors (TLR), are activated upon ligand binding with conserved structural motifs that are either specific patterns of microbial components (eg, bacterial lipopolysaccharide [LPS]) or nutritional factors (eg, free fatty acids [FFAs]) [25]. Binding to PRRs gives rise to inflammatory responses by mediating downstream transcriptional events that activate nuclear factor-κB (NFκB) and activator protein-1 (AP-1) and their pathways [26]. Upon activation, these intracytoplasmic molecular cascades up-regulate the transcription of pro-inflammatory cytokine genes and, consequently, the synthesis of acute-phase inflammatory mediators and activation of c-Jun N-terminal kinase (JNK) and inhibitor of NFκB kinase-β (IKK). In liver and adipose tissue, these two molecules can inactivate the first target of the insulin receptor (INSR), IRS-1, thereby reducing downstream signaling towards metabolic outcomes [27]. Recent data have revealed that the plasma concentration of inflammatory mediators, such as tumor necrosis factor-α (TNF-α) and interleukin-6 (IL-6), is increased in the insulin resistant states of obesity and type 2 diabetes, raising questions about the mechanisms underlying inflammation in these two conditions. Increased concentrations of TNF-α and IL-6, associated with obesity and type 2 diabetes, might interfere with insulin action by suppressing insulin signal transduction. This might interfere with the anti-inflammatory effect of insulin, which in turn might promote inflammation [13].

4. Nitric oxide in TNF-α pathways and apoptosis

As stated above, one of the main cytokines released in these inflammatory processes is TNF-α, which can activate signaling pathways associated with cell survival, apoptosis, inflammatory response and cell differentiation. The induction of the responses mediated by TNF-α occurs through the binding of the cytokine to the receptors TNF-R1 and TNF-R2. Both receptors may mediate cell death, however, TNF-R1 has a death domain while TNF-R2 does not, but it would enhance the cytotoxic effects of TNF-R1. TNF-α is produced primarily by cells of the immune system, such as macrophages and lymphocytes in response to inflammation and infection [28, 29]. The binding of TNF-α to TNF-R1 can promote the activation of NFκB or initiate the activation of caspases, which play a major role in the execution of programmed cell death or apoptosis (Figure 1) [30]. NFκB stimulates the expression of genes encoding cytokines (e.g. TNF-α, IL-1, IL-6, IL-2, IL-12, INF-γ and CM-CSF), cell adhesion molecules (CAMs), chemokine receptors and inducible enzymes (e.g., COX-2, iNOS). It also increases the expression of molecules involved in regulating cell proliferation, apoptosis and cell cycle progression, such as the cellular inhibitor of apoptosis protein 1 and 2 (c-IAP1 and c-IAP2), TNF-receptor-associated factor 1 and 2 (TRAF-1 and TRAF-2), B-cell lymphocyte/leukemia-2 (Bcl-2), Fas, c-myc and cyclin D1 [31, 32]. It was found that high levels of glucose can cause apoptosis, in part, through activation of NFκB [33]. Other authors have shown that high glucose levels activate protein kinase C (PKC) pathway and reactive oxygen species (ROS) [34-36]. Furthermore, cytokines and bacterial pathogens can activate iNOS and generate large concentrations of NO, through activation of nuclear transcription factors [37].

4.1. Hepatic expression of TNF-α and TNF-R1, NFκB activity and iNOS expression

We analyzed the hepatic levels of TNF-α and its receptor TNF-R1 by western blot. As shown in Figure 2 (A and B), hepatic levels of TNF-α and TNF-R1 of the diabetic group were higher than those of the control animals (120 % and 300 %, respectively).

We performed inhibition studies of NO production using a preferential inhibitor of iNOS enzyme, aminoguanidine (AG). Fifteen days after the onset of diabetes, a group of rats was separated into different groups and received injections of AG. The groups were as follows: Control group, injected with the vehicle citrate buffer only, and receiving AG in isotonic saline i.p. (100 mg/kg body weight) once a day, beginning 3 days before euthanized (Control +AG) [38], Diabetic group receiving AG i.p. (100 mg/kg body weight) once a day, beginning 3 days before euthanized (SID+AG). The whole study lasted one month. Six animals from each group (Control+AG and SID+AG) were euthanatized and the samples were promptly processed. We examined the expression of iNOS in liver cytosolic fraction by western blot in all experimental groups. Immunoblot analysis followed by quantitative densitometry from six separate animal sets revealed that iNOS increased by 500% ($p<0.05$) in SID rats compared to the control group (Figure 2 D). Treatment of SID rats with AG markedly decreased the cytosolic protein levels of iNOS, thus reaching the control value.

We also determined the role of TNF-α using ENBREL® (etanercept), a dimeric fusion protein that binds to TNF-α and decreases its role in disorders mediated by excess of TNF-α.

Etanercept mimics the inhibitory effects of naturally occurring soluble TNF-α receptors but has a greatly extended half-life in the bloodstream, and therefore a more profound and long-lasting biologic effect than a naturally occurring soluble TNF-R1 [39]. Etanercept was administered to 6 rats from each group (Control-a-TNF-α and SID-a-TNF-α) in a dose of 8 mg/Kg bw/day twice a week for 15 days.

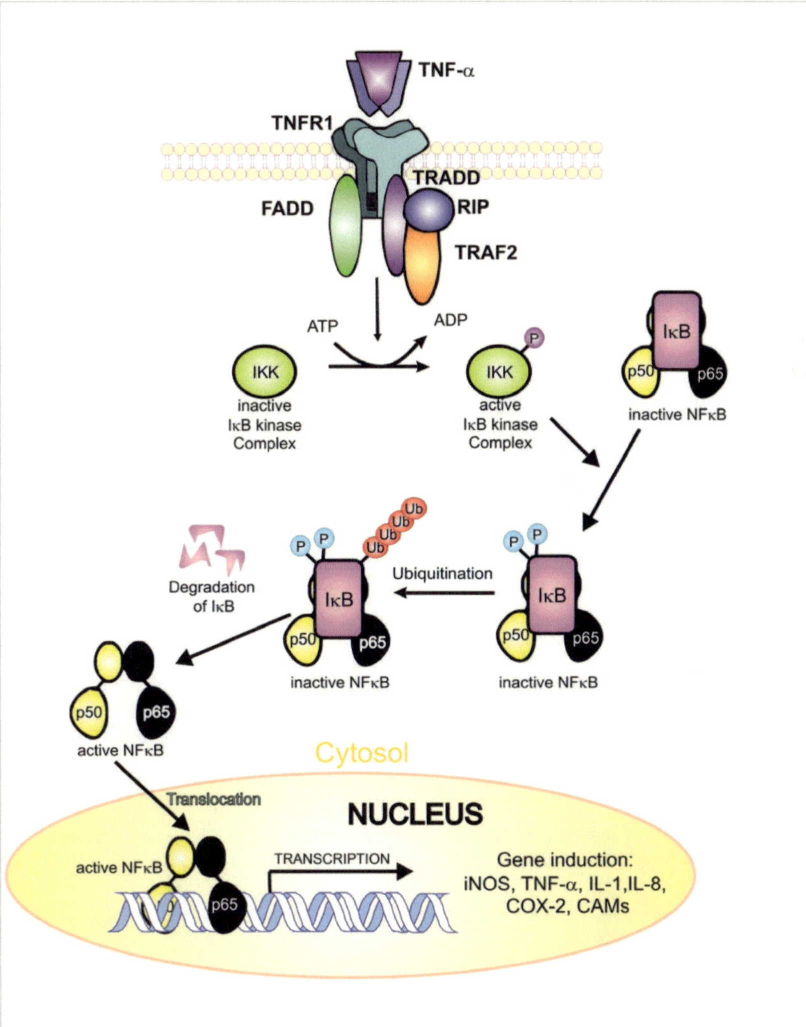

Figure 1. Schematic mechanisms of NFκB activation induced by TNF-α signaling pathways.

Administration of etanercept or AG also produced a significant attenuation of both TNF-α and TNF-R1 when compared to SID, reaching the control values (Figures 2A and 2B). Also, in Figure 2 C we show that the increase of TNF-α levels in the liver of streptozotocin-induced diabetic rats leads to a marked up-regulation of the NFκB pathway. The high levels of

TNF-α due to blood glucose levels increased iNOS expression leading to a high production of NO (see Figure 2 D). Similar findings have been reported in different tissues by other authors [40, 41]. Moreover, we observed that the treatment with etanercept, which blocks TNF-α, leads to a decrease in the expression of iNOS which is increased in the diabetic state. It has been shown that high concentrations of glucose cause an increase in the expression of iNOS induced by cytokines [42] in rat tissues. Consistently, high glucose concentrations do not increase iNOS in the absence of TNF-α [43]. The inhibition of iNOS with a selective inhibitor such as aminoguanidine, also reduced the production of TNF-α, thus evidencing an interaction between TNF-α pathway and the activity of iNOS.

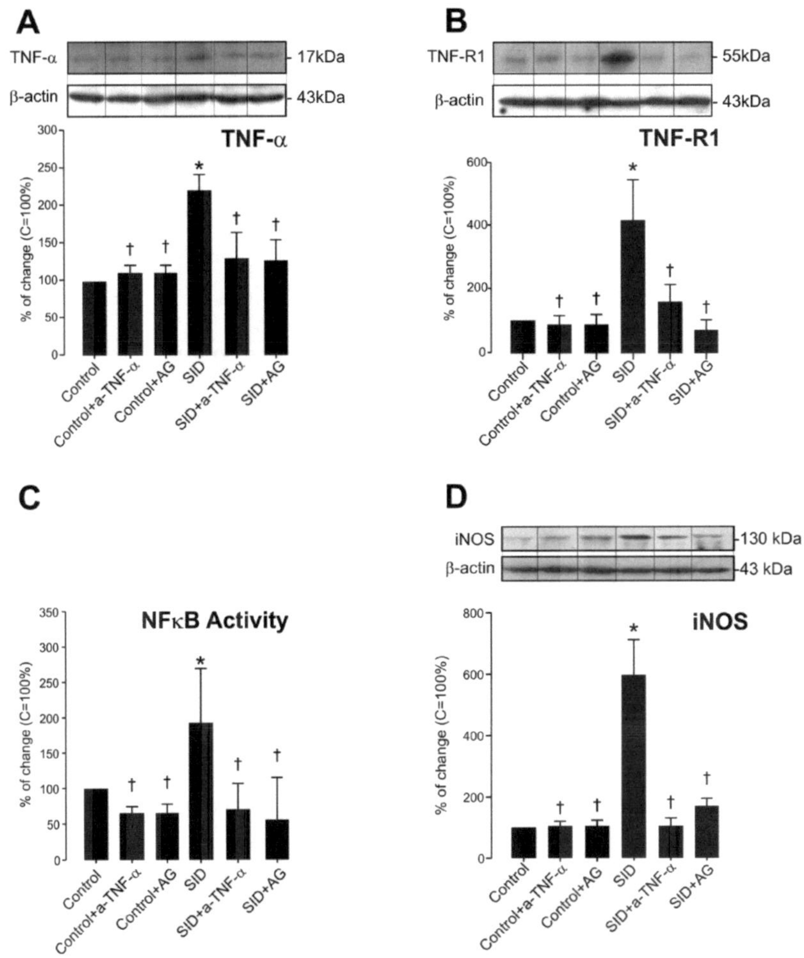

Figure 2. Hepatic TNF-α (Panel A) and TNF-R1 expression (Panel B), NFκB activity (Panel C) and iNOS expression (Panel D). The results obtained for all experimental groups are shown as follows: Lane 1: Control Control group of animals injected with sodium citrate vehicle; Lane 2: Control+a-TNF-α: Etanercept (8 mg/ kg body weight, i.p.) was administered once a day, twice a week, in saline solution starting 15 days after injection of sodium citrate vehicle and for 15 days; Lane 3: Control+AG: Aminoguanidine (100 mg/ kg body weight, i.p.), was administered once a day, in saline sol-

ution starting 15 days after injection of sodium citrate vehicle and for 3 days before euthanasia; Lane 4: SID: Streptozotocin (STZ)-Induced Diabetic rats received an i.p. injection of STZ 60 mg/kg body weight; Lane 5: SID+a-TNF-α: Etanercept (8 mg/ kg body weight, i.p.) was administered once a day, twice a week, in saline solution starting 15 days after injection of STZ and for 15 days Lane 6: SID+AG: Aminoguanidine (100 mg/ kg body weight, i.p.) was administered, once a day, in saline solution starting 15 days after injection of STZ and for 3 days before euthanasia. Immunoblot analysis of TNF-α (Panel A) and TNF-R1 (Panel B) in total liver lysate. Typical examples of Western blots are shown in top panel for each experimental group. The accompanying bars represent the densitometric analysis of the blots as percentage change from six separate animal sets, expressed as arbitrary units considering control as 100%. Data are expressed as means ± SE. Panel C: NFκB activity is showed as follow: Lane 1: Control; Lane 2: Control+a-TNF-α; Lane 3: Control+AG; Lane 4: SID; Lane 5: SID+a-TNF-α; Lane 6: SID+AG.*$p<0.05$ vs Control; †$p<0.05$ vs SID. Panel D: Immunoblot analysis of iNOS expression in total liver lysate. Effect of the treatments on each experimental group described above. Typical examples of Western blots are shown in top panel for each experimental group. The accompanying bars represent the densitometric analysis of the blots expressed as percentage change from six separate animal sets. Data are expressed as means ± SE. *$p<0.05$ vs Control; †$p<0.05$ vs SID.

4.2. Apoptosis induced by TNF-α

Binding of death receptors to their ligands results in the formation of an intracellular death domain (DISC: death-inducing signal complex) generated by the recruitment of two molecules: the death domain-associated TNF-R1 (TRADD: Tumor necrosis factor receptor type 1-associated death domain protein) and protein-associated death domain Fas (FADD: Fas-Associated protein with Death Domain). This complex also recruits procaspase-8 protein, which is activated by proteolysis. Releasing of the active fragment caspase-8 induces the activation of other caspases in the cytosol [44]. Thus, the DISC complex is responsible for the activation of the caspase cascade leading to apoptosis and/or activation of the kinase signaling pathway involved in apoptosis and JNK (c-Jun N- terminal kinase), resulting in the expression of genes through NFκB or AP-1 (activator protein-1) [45, 46]. The activation of caspase-8 that was induced by activation of the death receptor is followed by excision of Bid protein generating an active fragment of 15 kDa, truncated Bid (Bid-t). Bid-t protein is translocated into the mitochondria and interacts with other proteins of the Bcl2 family (Bax and Bak) and induces the release of apoptogenic factors such as SMAC (second mitochondria-derived activator of caspases) / DIABLO (direct IAP protein with low pI), AIF (apoptosis inducing factor) and the release of cytochrome c into the cytosol forming the apoptosome complex with APAF-1 and procaspase-9. In the apoptosome, procaspase-9 is proteolysed to its mature form, which then activates effector caspase-3, ultimately leading to apoptosis [47, 48].

We performed studies in STZ-induced diabetic rats of both, expression of activated caspase-8 and its activity in liver cytosolic fraction. We observed a substantial increase in activated caspase-8 in the diabetic state (Figure 3 A). Administration of etanercept or AG showed a reduction of both activated caspase-8 expression and its activity as compared to STZ-diabetic rats. We also examined the expression of t-Bid in cytosolic fraction and in liver mitochondrial fraction by western blot in all experimental groups. Immunoblot analysis followed by quantitative densitometry revealed that mitochondrial t-Bid protein levels increased by approximately 50% ($p<0.05$) in STZ-diabetic rats when compared to the control group (Figure 3 B). Administration of etanercept or AG produced a significant attenuation of Bid-t in the mitochondrial fraction when compared to SID. According to that described by other authors in different tissues [49, 50] the anti–TNF-α (etanercept) treatment was demonstrated to produce a declination in the response of receptor TNF-R1 to TNF-α (diminished activated caspase-8 expression and activity and mitochondrial protein t-Bid, as compared to SID group). Treatment with the iNOS-inhibitor showed a significant decrease of activated caspase-8 expression and activity when compared to STZ-induced diabetic rats (Figure 3 A). Also, we evaluated the activation of c-Jun N-terminal kinase (JNK), a member of the family of the mitogen-activated protein kinases (MAPK). The administration of both etanercept and AG prevents the hyperglycemia-induced phosphorylation of JNK (Figure 3 C).

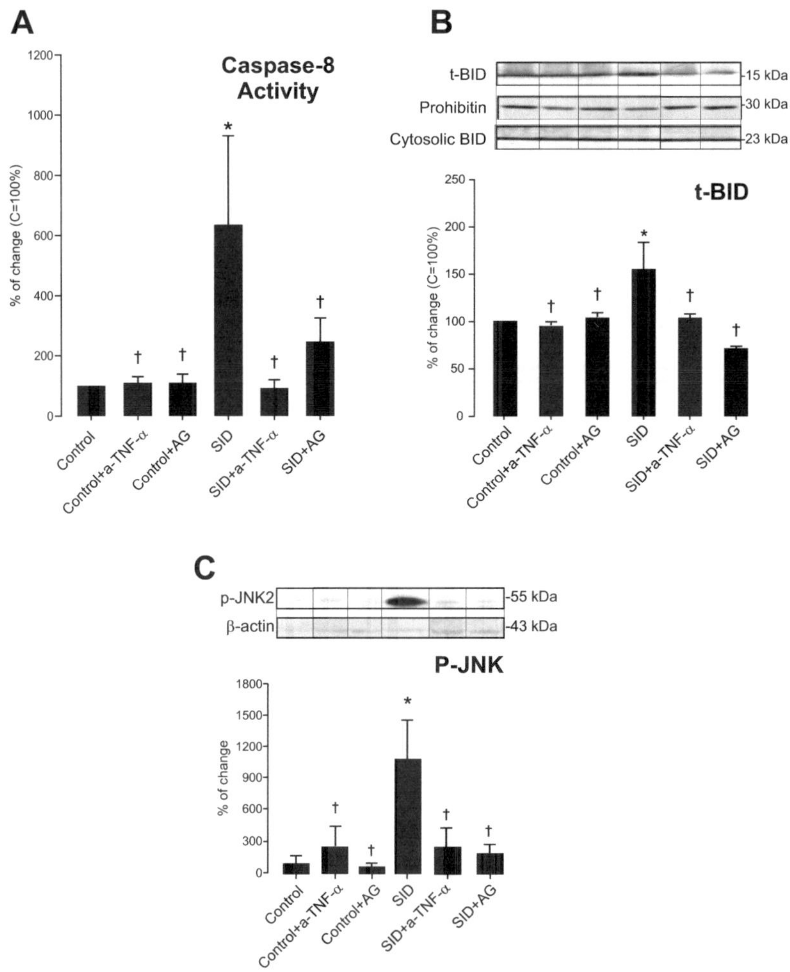

Figure 3. Panel A: Activated Caspase-8 expression and activity in diabetic liver: Protein immunoblot analysis and fluorometric assessment of activity of casapase-8 were performed in cytosolic fraction. Activities represented as bars are shown in arbitrary units. Data are expressed as means ± SE for at least six rats per experimental group. **Panel B:** Immunoblotting of cytosolic BID and t-BID expression in mitochondria-enriched fractions of diabetic liver and effect of different treatments in experimental groups as was described in Figure 2. Typical examples of Western blots are shown

http://dx.doi.org/10.5772/53684

for cytosolic BID and mitochondrial t-BID in top panel for each experimental group. The accompanying bars represent the densitometric analysis of the blots for t-BID expressed as percentage change from six separate animal sets. Data are expressed as mean ± S.E. *p<0.05 vs Control; †p<0.05 vs SID. **Panel C:** Western blot analysis of p-JNK in the liver tissue of diabetic animals and effect of different treatments. Typical examples of Western blots are shown in: Lane 1: Control; Lane 2: Control+a-TNF-α, Lane 3: Control+AG, Lane 4: SID, Lane 5: SID+a-TNF-α, Lane 6: SID+AG. The accompanying bars represent the densitometric analysis of the blots expressed as percentage from six separate animal sets. Data are expressed as means ± SE. *p<0.05 vs Control; †p<0.05 vs SID.

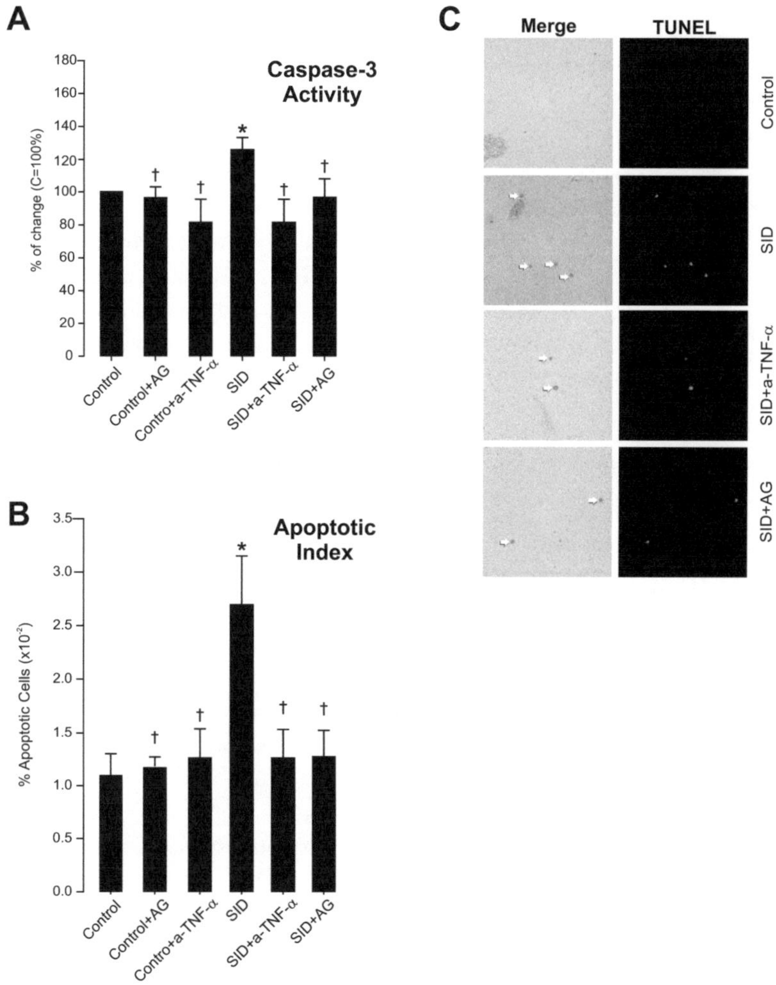

Figure 4. Panel A: Caspase-3 activity in diabetic rats and effect of the different treatments: Caspase-3 activity was fluorometrically determined. The bars represent activity expressed as arbitrary units. Data are expressed as means ± SE for at least six rats per experimental group. *p<0.05 vs Control; †p<0.05 vs SID. **Panel B:** Effect of NO and TNF-α on liver apoptosis of diabetics rats: Bars of apoptotic index (AI) represent the percentage of apoptotic cells scored at least 1000 hepatocytes per field in 10 fields of tissue sections at a magnification of 400X. Data are expressed as means ± SE for at least six rats per experimental group. *p<0.05 vs Control; †p<0.05 vs SID. **Panel C:** TUNEL assay: A representative TUNEL assay was performed on liver slides from the Control group, Control+a-TNF- α, Control+AG, SID, SID+a-TNF-α and SID+AG groups.

An early study had demonstrated that the activation of JNK is associated with increased TNF-induced apoptosis in hepatocytes [51]. In this connection, our results demonstrate that diabetes leads to the activation of JNK, inducing an increase of the apoptotic index. Moreover, we demonstrated that the decrease of TNF-α levels by etanercept treatment seems to completely abolish the observed activation of JNK induced by the diabetic state, thus leading to a decrease of apoptosis (Figures 3 and 4). We assessed apoptotic cell death by determining caspase-3 activity and performing TUNEL assays. There was a significant increase in caspase-3 activity in SID rats when compared to the control group ($p<0.05$). The administration of etanercept or AG to SID rats significantly decreases caspase-3 activity as compared to SID rats ($p<0.05$) (Figure 4 A). Figure 4 B shows Apoptotic Index (AI) expressed as a percentage. Apoptotic cells were identified in all experimental groups. Typical features of apoptosis, such as cellular shrinking with cytoplasmatic acidophilia, condensation and margination of chromatin were corroborated by hematoxylin-eosin staining. The diabetic state significantly increased the AI when compared to the control group ($p<0.05$), while treatments with etanercept or AG significantly attenuated this increment when compared to SID group ($p<0.05$), even reaching the control values (Figure 4 B). In Figure 4 C a representative TUNEL assay for Control, SID, SID+etanercept and SID+AG is showed. TUNEL–positive signal is maximal in the SID group and it is clear that after the different treatments there is a significant reduction of TUNEL-positive cells.

Our results clearly show that in the liver of STZ-induced diabetic rats there is an enlargement of caspase-3 activity with the consequent increase in the AI.

5. Diabetes, inflammation and liver apoptosis

Several studies have shown that TNF-α may be involved in viral hepatitis, alcoholic hepatitis, ischemia/reperfusion liver injury, and fulminant hepatic failure. In human disease, serum levels of TNF-α and hepatic TNF-receptors are frequently increased [52]. A research paper recently published by our group demonstrates that the diabetic state induces an increase of TNF-α and its receptor TNF-R1 in the liver [43]. Data presented in this work show that the increase of TNF-α levels in the liver of streptozotocin-induced diabetic rats leads to a marked up-regulation of the NFκB pathway. NFκB is one of the key transcription factors involved in triggering the cascade of events that allow inflammation and different research groups have demonstrated its activation in the diabetic liver [53, 54]. The expression of iNOS is closely related to stimulation of NFκB, whose recognition sites have been identified in the promoter region of the gene encoding for iNOS.

In the liver of diabetic rats we found an increase of TNF-α due to increased expression of iNOS which led to a high production of NO [43]. Similar results have been reported in different tissues by other authors [40, 41]. In our work, we observed that the treatment with etanercept, which blocks TNF-α, leads to a decrease in the expression of iNOS which is increased in the diabetic state. Furthermore, etanercept treatment reduces the production of NO in the liver of streptozotocin-induced diabetic rats. It has been shown that high concentrations of glucose cause an increase in the expression of iNOS induced by cytokines [42] in rat tissues. Consistent with this, high glucose concentrations do not increase iNOS in the absence of TNF-α [43]. The inhibition of iNOS with a selective inhibitor such as aminoguanidine also reduced the production of TNF-α, thus demonstrating an interaction between TNF-α pathway and the activity of iNOS.

Figure 5 depicts a summary of the apoptotic mechanisms occurring through TNF-α pathway in the liver in the diabetic state.

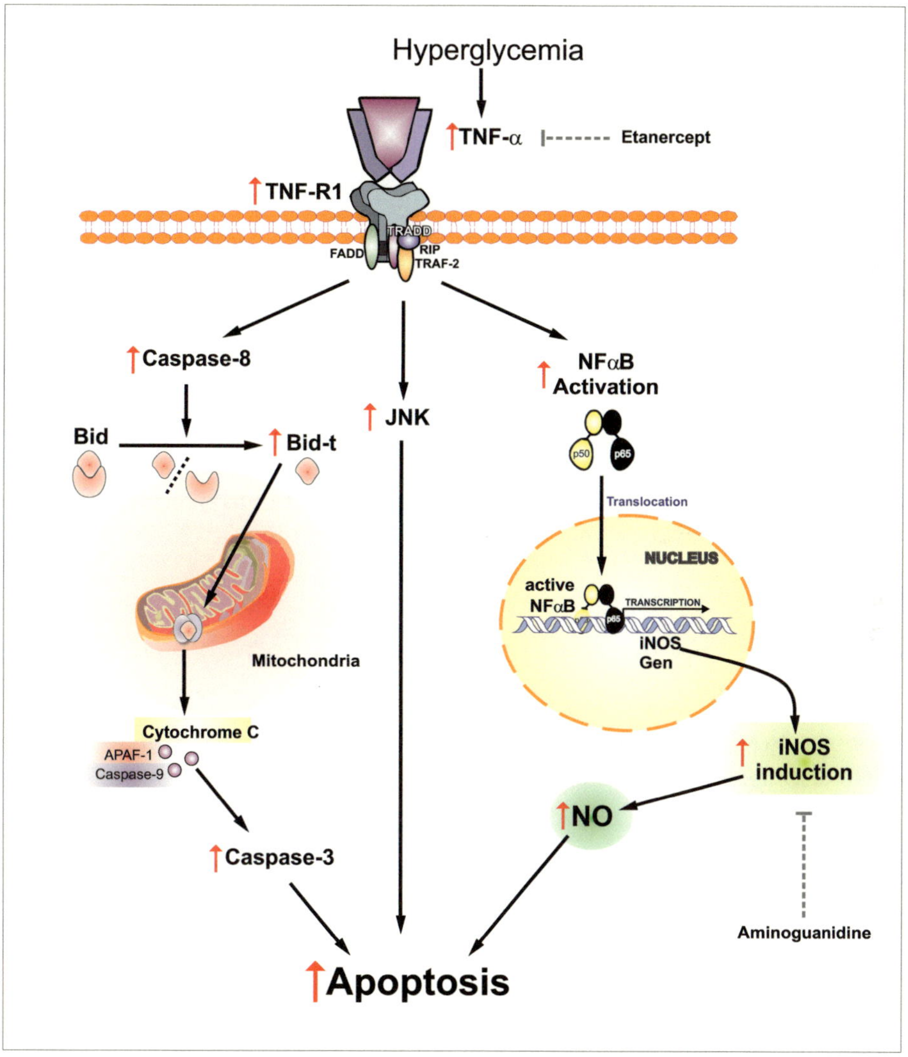

Figure 5. Proposed scheme for the mechanism involved in TNF-α- induced apoptosis in liver disease induced by diabetes type 1. In the diabetic state, hepatic TNF-α elevation induces activation of NFκB, caspase-8 and JNK, thus leading to an increased apoptotic rate.

6. Conclusion

The relevance of the present chapter is to provide further knowledge on the mechanisms underlying the disease process in the liver during an inflammatory process such as type 1 diabetes. The regulation of hepatic TNF-α level and iNOS activity in the diabetic state could be therapeutically relevant for the improvement or delay of the hepatic complications of chronic hyperglycemia.

Acknowledgements

This work was supported by research grants from CONICET. We especially wish to thank PhD Cecilia Basiglio for English revision.

Author details

Paola I. Ingaramo, Daniel E. Francés, María T. Ronco and Cristina E. Carnovale*

*Address all correspondence to: ccarnova@fbioyf.unr.edu.ar

Institute of Experimental Physiology, (CONICET), Faculty of Biochemical and Pharmaceutical Sciences (National University of Rosario), Rosario, Argentina

References

[1] Pietropaolo M, Barinas-Mitchell E, Kuller LH. The heterogeneity of diabetes: unraveling a dispute: is systemic inflammation related to islet autoimmunity? Diabetes 2007; 56 (5) 1189-1197

[2] Kasuga M. Insulin resistance and pancreatic beta cell failure. J.Clin.Invest 2006; 116 (7) 1756-1760

[3] Wild S, Roglic G, Green A et al. Global prevalence of diabetes: estimates for the year 2000 and projections for 2030. Diabetes Care 2004; 27 (5) 1047-1053

[4] Shaw JE, Sicree RA, Zimmet PZ. Global estimates of the prevalence of diabetes for 2010 and 2030. Diabetes Res.Clin.Pract. 2010; 87 (1) 4-14

[5] Srinivasan K, Ramarao P. Animal models in type 2 diabetes research: an overview. Indian J.Med.Res. 2007; 125 (3) 451-472

[6] Kikutani H, Makino S. The murine autoimmune diabetes model: NOD and related strains. Adv.Immunol. 1992; 51 (285-322

[7] Rees DA, Alcolado JC. Animal models of diabetes mellitus. Diabet.Med. 2005; 22 (4) 359-370

[8] Mordes JP, Bortell R, Blankenhorn EP et al. Rat models of type 1 diabetes: genetics, environment, and autoimmunity. ILAR.J. 2004; 45 (3) 278-291

[9] Carnovale CE, Rodriguez Garay EA. Reversible impairment of hepatobiliary function induced by streptozotocin in the rat. Experientia 1984; 40 (3) 248-250

[10] Carnovale CE, Marinelli RA, Rodriguez Garay EA. Bile flow decrease and altered bile composition in streptozotocin-treated rats. Biochem.Pharmacol. 1986; 35 (15) 2625-2628

[11] Carnovale CE, Marinelli RA, Rodriguez Garay EA. Toxic effect of streptozotocin on the biliary secretion of nicotinamide-treated rats. Toxicol.Lett. 1987; 36 (3) 259-265

[12] Wellen KE, Hotamisligil GS. Inflammation, stress, and diabetes. J.Clin.Invest 2005; 115 (5) 1111-1119

[13] Dandona P, Aljada A, Bandyopadhyay A. Inflammation: the link between insulin resistance, obesity and diabetes. Trends Immunol. 2004; 25 (1) 4-7

[14] Willerson JT, Ridker PM. Inflammation as a cardiovascular risk factor. Circulation 2004; 109 (21 Suppl 1) II2-10

[15] Ahrens B. Antibodies in metabolic diseases. N.Biotechnol. 2011; 28 (5) 530-537

[16] Venieratos PD, Drossopoulou GI, Kapodistria KD et al. High glucose induces suppression of insulin signalling and apoptosis via upregulation of endogenous IL-1beta and suppressor of cytokine signalling-1 in mouse pancreatic beta cells. Cell Signal. 2010; 22 (5) 791-800

[17] Alexandraki KI, Piperi C, Ziakas PD et al. Cytokine secretion in long-standing diabetes mellitus type 1 and 2: associations with low-grade systemic inflammation. J.Clin.Immunol. 2008; 28 (4) 314-321

[18] Erbagci AB, Tarakcioglu M, Coskun Y et al. Mediators of inflammation in children with type I diabetes mellitus: cytokines in type I diabetic children. Clin.Biochem. 2001; 34 (8) 645-650

[19] Esposito K, Nappo F, Marfella R et al. Inflammatory cytokine concentrations are acutely increased by hyperglycemia in humans: role of oxidative stress. Circulation 2002; 106 (16) 2067-2072

[20] Foss NT, Foss-Freitas MC, Ferreira MA et al. Impaired cytokine production by peripheral blood mononuclear cells in type 1 diabetic patients. Diabetes Metab 2007; 33 (6) 439-443

[21] Elmarakby AA, Sullivan JC. Relationship between Oxidative Stress and Inflammatory Cytokines in Diabetic Nephropathy. Cardiovasc.Ther. 2012; 30 (1) 49-59

[22] Navarro-Gonzalez JF, Muros M, Mora-Fernandez C et al. Pentoxifylline for renoprotection in diabetic nephropathy: the PREDIAN study. Rationale and basal results. J.Diabetes Complications 2011; 25 (5) 314-319

[23] Frances DE, Ronco MT, Monti JA et al. Hyperglycemia induces apoptosis in rat liver through the increase of hydroxyl radical: new insights into the insulin effect. J.Endocrinol. 2010; 205 (2) 187-200

[24] Pickup JC. Inflammation and activated innate immunity in the pathogenesis of type 2 diabetes. Diabetes Care 2004; 27 (3) 813-823

[25] Shi H, Kokoeva MV, Inouye K et al. TLR4 links innate immunity and fatty acid-induced insulin resistance. J.Clin.Invest 2006; 116 (11) 3015-3025

[26] Takeda K, Akira S. TLR signaling pathways. Semin.Immunol. 2004; 16 (1) 3-9

[27] Aguirre V, Uchida T, Yenush L et al. The c-Jun NH(2)-terminal kinase promotes insulin resistance during association with insulin receptor substrate-1 and phosphorylation of Ser(307). J.Biol.Chem. 2000; 275 (12) 9047-9054

[28] Littlejohn AF, Tucker SJ, Mohamed AA et al. Modulation by caspases of tumor necrosis factor-stimulated c-Jun N-terminal kinase activation but not nuclear factor-kappaB signaling. Biochem.Pharmacol. 2003; 65 (1) 91-99

[29] McFarlane SM, Pashmi G, Connell MC et al. Differential activation of nuclear factor-kappaB by tumour necrosis factor receptor subtypes. TNFR1 predominates whereas TNFR2 activates transcription poorly. FEBS Lett. 2002; 515 (1-3) 119-126

[30] Budihardjo I, Oliver H, Lutter M et al. Biochemical pathways of caspase activation during apoptosis. Annu.Rev.Cell Dev.Biol. 1999; 15 (269-290

[31] Joyce D, Albanese C, Steer J et al. NF-kappaB and cell-cycle regulation: the cyclin connection. Cytokine Growth Factor Rev. 2001; 12 (1) 73-90

[32] Yamamoto Y, Gaynor RB. IkappaB kinases: key regulators of the NF-kappaB pathway. Trends Biochem.Sci. 2004; 29 (2) 72-79

[33] Lim JW, Kim H, Kim KH. NF-kappaB, inducible nitric oxide synthase and apoptosis by Helicobacter pylori infection. Free Radic.Biol.Med. 2001; 31 (3) 355-366

[34] Chen YW, Chenier I, Chang SY et al. High glucose promotes nascent nephron apoptosis via NF-kappaB and p53 pathways. Am.J.Physiol Renal Physiol 2011; 300 (1) F147-F156

[35] Karin M, Greten FR. NF-kappaB: linking inflammation and immunity to cancer development and progression. Nat.Rev.Immunol. 2005; 5 (10) 749-759

[36] Yang WS, Seo JW, Han NJ et al. High glucose-induced NF-kappaB activation occurs via tyrosine phosphorylation of IkappaBalpha in human glomerular endothelial

cells: involvement of Syk tyrosine kinase. Am.J.Physiol Renal Physiol 2008; 294 (5) F1065-F1075

[37] Aktan F. iNOS-mediated nitric oxide production and its regulation. Life Sci. 2004; 75 (6) 639-653

[38] Carnovale CE, Scapini C, Alvarez ML et al. Nitric oxide release and enhancement of lipid peroxidation in regenerating rat liver. J.Hepatol. 2000; 32 (5) 798-804

[39] Madhusudan S, Muthuramalingam SR, Braybrooke JP et al. Study of etanercept, a tumor necrosis factor-alpha inhibitor, in recurrent ovarian cancer. J.Clin.Oncol. 2005; 23 (25) 5950-5959

[40] Powell LA, Warpeha KM, Xu W et al. High glucose decreases intracellular glutathione concentrations and upregulates inducible nitric oxide synthase gene expression in intestinal epithelial cells. J.Mol.Endocrinol. 2004; 33 (3) 797-803

[41] Stadler K, Bonini MG, Dallas S et al. Involvement of inducible nitric oxide synthase in hydroxyl radical-mediated lipid peroxidation in streptozotocin-induced diabetes. Free Radic.Biol.Med. 2008; 45 (6) 866-874

[42] Noh H, Ha H, Yu MR et al. High glucose increases inducible NO production in cultured rat mesangial cells. Possible role in fibronectin production. Nephron 2002; 90 (1) 78-85

[43] Ingaramo PI, Ronco MT, Frances DE et al. Tumor necrosis factor alpha pathways develops liver apoptosis in type 1 diabetes mellitus. Mol.Immunol. 2011; 48 (12-13) 1397-1407

[44] Kruidering M, Evan GI. Caspase-8 in apoptosis: the beginning of "the end"? IUBMB.Life 2000; 50 (2) 85-90

[45] Kiechle FL, Zhang X. Apoptosis: biochemical aspects and clinical implications. Clin.Chim.Acta 2002; 326 (1-2) 27-45

[46] Schattenberg JM, Schuchmann M. Diabetes and apoptosis: liver. Apoptosis. 2009; 14 (12) 1459-1471

[47] Zimmermann KC, Bonzon C, Green DR. The machinery of programmed cell death. Pharmacol.Ther. 2001; 92 (1) 57-70

[48] Zhao Y, Li S, Childs EE et al. Activation of pro-death Bcl-2 family proteins and mitochondria apoptosis pathway in tumor necrosis factor-alpha-induced liver injury. J.Biol.Chem. 2001; 276 (29) 27432-27440

[49] Crisafulli C, Galuppo M, Cuzzocrea S. Effects of genetic and pharmacological inhibition of TNF-alpha in the regulation of inflammation in macrophages. Pharmacol.Res. 2009; 60 (4) 332-340

[50] Fries W, Muja C, Crisafulli C et al. Infliximab and etanercept are equally effective in reducing enterocyte APOPTOSIS in experimental colitis. Int.J.Med.Sci. 2008; 5 (4) 169-180

[51] Wullaert A, Heyninck K, Beyaert R. Mechanisms of crosstalk between TNF-induced NF-kappaB and JNK activation in hepatocytes. Biochem.Pharmacol. 2006; 72 (9) 1090-1101

[52] Ding WX, Yin XM. Dissection of the multiple mechanisms of TNF-alpha-induced apoptosis in liver injury. J.Cell Mol.Med. 2004; 8 (4) 445-454

[53] Boden G, She P, Mozzoli M et al. Free fatty acids produce insulin resistance and activate the proinflammatory nuclear factor-kappaB pathway in rat liver. Diabetes 2005; 54 (12) 3458-3465

[54] Romagnoli M, Gomez-Cabrera MC, Perrelli MG et al. Xanthine oxidase-induced oxidative stress causes activation of NF-kappaB and inflammation in the liver of type I diabetic rats. Free Radic.Biol.Med. 2010; 49 (2) 171-177

Chapter 6

Double Diabetes: The Search for a Treatment Paradigm in Children and Adolescents

Benjamin U. Nwosu

Additional information is available at the end of the chapter

http://dx.doi.org/10.5772/53314

1. Introduction

Diabetes mellitus is one of the most prevalent chronic diseases in children. Diabetes mellitus is classified into four major types. Type 1, type 2, gestational, and other specific types. Type 1 diabetes (T1D) is caused by autoimmune destruction of the insulin-producing beta cells of the pancreas. Type 2 diabetes (T2D) results from a combination of insulin resistance and beta cell insulin secretory defect. The rising prevalence of childhood obesity has made it more difficult to differentiate between these types of diabetes in children. There is a new expression of diabetes in children known as double diabetes, or hybrid diabetes. This is a clinical state where both T1D and T2D co-exist in the same individual as shown in Figure 1 below.

Childhood obesity is one of the most serious public health challenges of the 21st century [1]. According to the National Health and Nutrition Examination Survey data, about 16% of children and adolescents in the United States have a body mass index (BMI) (kg/m^2) ≥95th percentile for age and gender [2]. Body mass index of >95th percentile is classified as overweight by the Center for Disease Control and Prevention [3,4], and as obesity by European criteria [5].

The prevalence of obesity has tripled in the past three decades [6] among male and female adolescents, and across different racial and ethnic groups [6-8]. There has also been a parallel increase in the prevalence of many obesity-related co-morbid conditions [9] such as T2D, dyslipidemia, hypertension, obstructive sleep apnea, poor quality of life and mortality in adulthood [10-13]. Although obesity is associated primarily with T2D due to insulin resistance, [14], it may also impact T1D morbidity.

T1D is caused by autoimmune destruction of the beta cells of the pancreas leading to insulinopenia. It is sub-classified into 2 main categories- type 1A and 1B [15]. In type 1A, individuals have one or more of the anti-islet cell (including glutamic acid decarboxylase, and insulinoma antigen-2) or anti-insulin antibodies. In type 1B these antibodies are absent, but the clinical and biochemical features are similar to 1A. T2D is characterized by insulin resistance and absence of diabetes-associated antibodies in serum.

A new subset of diabetes, called double diabetes is becoming increasingly prevalent as a result of the epidemic of childhood obesity [16-18]. In double diabetes, elements of both T1D and T2D co-exist. In this condition, individuals with T1D have insensitivity to insulin that is most often associated with obesity; and individuals with T2D have antibodies against the pancreatic beta cells [14] (Figure 1). Unlike T1D and T2D, there is no consensus on the therapeutic modalities for double diabetes.

The incidence of both T1D and T2D is rising in children and adolescents [14]. Data from the EURODIAB study indicate that the overall prevalence of T1D among young people under 15 years is increasing by greater than 3% each year, and by more than 6% a year in children aged up to four years [19].Analysis of the 2002 to 2003 data from SEARCH for Diabetes in Youth, a multicenter study funded by the Centers for Disease Control and Prevention and the National Institutes of Health to examine T1D and T2D among children and adolescents in the United States, showed that annually, about 15,000 youth in the United States are newly diagnosed with T1D, and about 3,700 youth with T2D. The reported rate of new cases among youth was 19 per 100,000 each year for T1D, and 5.3 per 100,000 for T2D [20].

2. Prevalence

The prevalence of double diabetes is unknown [16]. However, reports show that about 25% of children with T1D are either overweight or obese [21]. Other reports show that about 35% of children and adolescents with T2D have at least one diabetes-associated antibody [22]. Some authors estimate that about one in three children and adolescents with newly diagnosed diabetes has double diabetes. Pozzilli et al reported a prevalence of 4.96% in their unpublished Italian cohort [1]. The major difficulty with establishing a prevalence rate for double diabetes is that there are no precise definitions for the different types of diabetes presenting in youth [1]. This is because clinical phenotypes frequently overlap at onset of the disease [1]. For example, obesity and ketoacidosis can be found in both T1D and T2D [23], and the age of diagnosis is now a poorly differentiating factor [24]. In other cases, the clinical features of double diabetes are not apparent at diagnosis but evolve over time [18].

3. Etiology and pathophysiology

There are genetic, environmental and behavioral factors that affect the pathophysiological processes of T1D and T2D in such as way to result in double diabetes. Obesity is the central pathophysiological mechanism for double diabetes. Obesity may arise from genetic predisposition or from environmental factors such as the anabolic role of insulin injection in patients with T1D who fail to make the necessary healthy lifestyle changes that are recommended for maintenance of normal weight.

3.1. Genetic factors

Unlike T1D where the *MHC* region of chromosome 6 accounts for approximately 40% of the genetic risk of the disease in concert with other genes [25], and in T2D where genome-wide association studies have identified approximately 50 genetic loci associated with T2D in lean and obese individuals [26-28], there are no distinct genes that are unique to double diabetes. However, it is believed that the major genes that are independently associated with susceptibility to either T1D (e.g., the MHC and cytotoxic T lymphocyte-associated antigen-4 (*CTLA-4*) [29] or T2D (e.g., the genes encoding adiponectin (*APM1*) and transcription factor 7-like 2 (*TCF7L2*) [30] can serve as genetic determinants for double diabetes, such that the frequency of the major T1D genetic susceptibility gene (*MHC*) is reduced, whereas the expression of the genes associated with T2D is enhanced [31].

Apart from the principal genetic determinants of T1D and T2D, there are a number of genes that could potentially lead to an outcome of double diabetes by influencing the pathogenetic processes operating in both T1D and T2D [32]. One of such genes resulting from a genetic variance in insulin receptor substrate 1 (*IRS-1*) plays an important role in insulin resistance, a key component of T2D, and also in β cell apoptosis which is associated with T1D [33]. High mobility group A1 (HMGA1) protein, a product of the Hmga1 gene has been identified as a crucial effector in the control of glucose homeostasis, such that impaired HMGA1 function may contribute to the development of specific forms of diabetes [34]. HMGA1-deficient indiviuduals have reduced insulin receptor expression, reduced insulin signaling and decreased insulin secretion similar to the phenotype of T2D [34].

3.2. Environmental and behavioral factors

The epidemic of childhood obesity has led to increased diagnosis of metabolic syndrome and T2D in all children including those with existing T1D [35]. Obese or overweight children have been reported to develop T1D at younger ages than children of normal weight [35]. The SEARCH for Diabetes in Youth Study [36] reported an obesity prevalence rate of 12.6% in US youth with T1D. The study also reported a higher prevalence of overweight status (BMI 85th – 95th percentile) among youth with T1D than in those without diabetes (22.1% vs. 16.1%) ($P<0.05$). Some children with T1D have either a first- or second-degree relative with T2D [1]. Furthermore, weight gain is prevalent in adolescents with T1D after attainment of adult height, which might further impair insulin sensitivity [37].

Therefore, several enviromental factors could lead to the development of double diabetes by their influence on the disease processes of T1D and T2D. Many of the major genetic factors involved in the etiopathogenesis of T2D appear to promote the development of the disease through their influence on obesity and feeding behavior [38]. There is evidence that rapid growth and obesity in early childhood might increase the risk of T1D [35,39]. The strong environmental basis for this obesity pandemic and influence on feeding behavior was recently outlined in a World Health Organization Technical Report [40] which states that 'Changes in the world food economy have contributed to shifting dietary patterns, for example, increased consumption of energy-dense diets high in fat, particularly saturated fat, and low in unrefined carbohydrates. These patterns are combined with a decline in energy expenditure that is associated with sedentary lifestyle, motorized transport, labor-saving devices at home, the phasing out of physically-demanding manual tasks in the workplace, and leisure time that is preponderantly devoted to physically undemanding pastimes'. However, despite the established association between obesity and the increasing prevalence of T1D, it is unclear how these environmental processes lead to β cell destruction.

Several mechanistic models have been proposed to explain this phenomenon. Some reports have linked high titers of glutamic acid decarboxylase autoantibody to an increase in body mass index (BMI) [41] which suggests that increased BMI might favor the development of an autoimmune response towards β cells. This is in line with other reports indicating that a combination of obesity and insulin resistance speeds up the process of beta cell destruction [35,42]. Other proposed mechanisms for beta cell destruction include the the role of upregulation of autoimmune response by obesity-associated inflammatory cytokines, and hyperleptinemia-associated T-cell activation [43,44].

Other researchers have proposed the following mechanism for obesity-induced insulin resistance : (a) the liberation of large amounts of non-esterified fatty acids by visceral fat which stimulate neoglucogenesis in the liver and diminish glucose uptake in the muscles; (b) the association of obesity with increased activity of the sympathetic nervous system, which in combination with direct release of tumor necrosis factor, resistin and other adipocytokines contribute to insulin resistance; (c) the role of the accummulation of local intramyocellular triglycerides on muscle insulin senstivity [45].

In additon to the above mechanistic models, several hypotheses have been advanced to explain the association between obesity and rising prevlaence of T1D. The most prominent of these hypotheses is the accelerator hypothesis which states that T1D and T2D are the same disease state set in different genetic backgrounds [46]. It originally proposed three major factors as the basis for the development of diabetes: genetic predisposition, insulin resistance and intrinsic rate of beta cell loss. The accelerators have now been reduced to two without altering the premise of the hypothesis [46]. The first is insulin resistance which is believed to accelerate β-cell apoptosis while rendering them more immunogenic. It posits that insulin resistance is the primary driver for the development of diabetes in a susceptible individual and argues that insulin resistance increases through weight gain as does the rate of onset of diabetes [47]. The second accelerator is the hierachy of responsive genes whose reactivity modulates the gradient of β-cell declining function [46].

The central premise of the accelerator hypothesis is based on studies reporting rising incidence of obesity [6,48] and T1D in children [49,50]. These findings were strengthened by reports of an association between weight gain and an increased risk to develop diabetes mellitus [51-53], as well as several reports from Europe indicating that an increasing number of children are being diagnosed with T1D at an earlier age [54-58]. This hypothesis proposes a direct cause and effect relationship between obesity and the development of both T1D and

T2D, and states that as the population becomes heavier (fatter), diabetes appears earlier, thus suggestive of a true acceleration rather than an incidental risk association [59].

The accelerator hypothesis is controversial because studies designed to prove its validity have reached various conclusions [35,60-65]. Reports from the United Kingdom indicated a relationship between younger age at diagnosis of T1D and higher body mass index (BMI) in Middlesbrough [35], and Plymouth [64],but not in Birmingham [61]. Other European studies of large cohorts of German and Austrian children with T1D supported the hypothesis [62,63], although studies from Spain and Australia [66,67] did not. Two studies have been conducted in the United States to examine this hypothesis. Dabelea et al [65] tested the hypothesis in six centers in the US (Cincinnati, Colorado, Hawaii, Seattle, South Carolina, Southern California) and found a significant relationship between BMI standard deviation score (SDS) and age at diagnosis only among patients with low C-peptide values at diagnosis. Evertsen et al [50] reported a significant inverse relationship between age at diagnosis and BMI SDS in their Wisconsin cohort. Thus, there is no consensus on the validity of the hypothesis among children and adolescents with T1D in the United States.

4. Clinical features

Traditionally, a patient with the classic symptoms of diabetes which include polyuria, polydipsia, and polyphagia who also has a family history of T2D, obesity, acanthosis nigricans and lack of both ketosis and diabetes-associated autoantibodies is considered to have T2D [68]. On the other hand, patients with T1D are usually thought to be thin, may present with ketosis, and have diabetes associated autoantibodies. [18] Patients with double diabetes possess the features of both T1D and T2D which could present siimultaneously at the time of diagnosis, or develop sequentially over time [18].

Features of Double Diabetes in Child or Adolescent with Pre-existingType 1 diabetes: The signs and symptoms typical of T2D can develop gradually in a child or adolescent with pre-existing T1D. The rate of the development of these features of increased metabolic load depends on the individual's genetic makeup and his or her degree of weight gain. These patients are usually overweight or obese and require a high dose of insulin to maintain euglycemia because of obesity-related insulin resistance [31,69]. Some of these patients may have hypertension, dyslipidemia, and poor diabetes control. Female adolescent patients may have polycystic ovarian syndrome.

Features of Double Diabetes in Child or Adolescent with Pre-existing Type 2 diabetes: The presence of increased 'autoimmune load' as marked by the presence of diabetes-associated autoantibodies in a child or adolescent with all of the typical clinical features of T2D - excess body weight, acanthosis nigricans, high blood pressure, dyslipidemia, polycystic ovary syndrome, positive family history of T2D, belonging to ethnic/racial minority group – is consistent with a diagnosis of double diabetes [31,69].

5. Diagnosis

There is the need to formulate universal diagnostic criteria to facilitate the recognition of double diabetes either at the time of onset of hyperglycemia or in the course of the disease process. Pozzilli et al [16,31] recently introduced the concept of 'metabolic load' to describe the features of T2D and 'autoimmune load' to describe the features of T1D. They stated that in an obese child or adolescent with hyperglycemia, an increased 'metabolic load' and a reduced 'autoimmune load' are features of double diabetes (Figure 1). Based on this principle, they advanced the following clinical and biochemical guidelines to facilitate the diagnosis of double diabetes:

i. The presence of clinical features of T2D, hypertension, dyslipidemia, increased body mass index with increased cardiovascular risk, compared with children with classical T1D. Family history for T2D and T1D might be present.

ii. The presence of a reduced number of clinical features typical of T1D, such as weight loss, polyuria and polydipsia, development of ketoacidosis; insulin therapy is not the first line of therapy, by contrast to the situation in subjects with classical T1D.

iii. The presence of autoantibodies to islet cells, although with a reduced number and titer compared with T1D, and probably a reduced risk associated with the *MHC* locus compared with subjects with T1D. As compared with T1D, where insulin resistance and obesity are not common features, double diabetes is always characterized by an obese phenotype, with the additional coexistence of β cell autoimmunity.

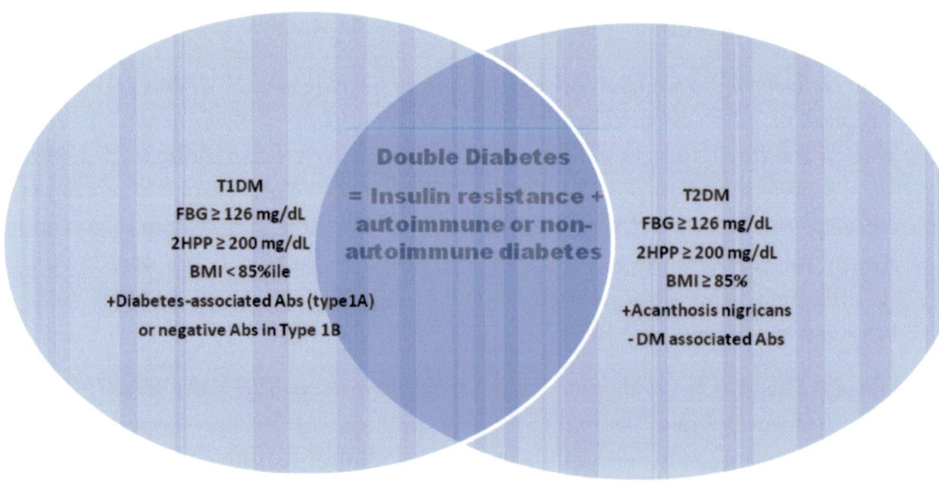

Figure 1. The relationship between T1D, T2D and Double Diabetes, TID = type 1 diabetes, T2D = type 2 diabetes, FBG = fasting blood glucose, 2HPP = 2 hour post prandial glucose level; BMI = body mass index; Abs = antibodies

6. Treatment

There is no consensus on the best therapeutic regimen for double diabetes. However, because insulin resistance is central to the pathophysiological mechanism of double diabetes, optimal management of this condition necessitates the addition of insulin sensitizers to the patient's therapeutic regimen under appropriate clinical circumstances [18]. Intensification of lifestyle modification strategies should be encouraged to maintain normal weight and attenuate insulin resistance. Finally, because these patients require increased doses of insulin to maintain euglycemia, it is necessary to develop an insulin titration regimen that would ensure adequate glycemic control.

6.1. The burden of poor glycemic control in children and adolescents

The availability of insulin analogs and diabetes monitoring devices has improved diabetes care around the world. However, according to recent studies, the prevalence of poorly-controlled diabetes in youth is still high [70]. This poor glycemic control predisposes the youth to acute and chronic complications of diabetes.

A report by the SEARCH for Diabetes in Youth Study group showed that a high proportion of youth with diabetes had high HbA1c values, with 17% of the youth with TIDM, and 27% of those with T2D showing poor control, defined as HbA1c ≥ 9.5% [70]. The American Diabetes Association target values for HbA1c in relation to age are as follows: 7.5-8.5% at age < 6 years, <8% at age 6-12 years, <7.5% at age 13-18 years, and <7.0% at age 19+ years [68]. Thus only a minority of children and adolescents meet the recommended glycemic targets.

The physiological factors that contribute to poor glycemic control in youth are in part related to the hormonal changes in puberty. Puberty is associated with relative insulin resistance, reflected in a two- to threefold increase in the peak insulin response to oral or intravenous glucose [71]; insulin-mediated glucose disposal is approximately 30% lower in adolescents than in prepubertal children or young adults [72]. This physiologic insulin resistance of puberty is of minimal consequence in the presence of adequate beta-cell function [73]. The cause of this physiologic resistance is likely the transitory increased activity of the growth hormone-insulin growth factor axis, as well as sex steroids, which coincides with the physiologic insulin resistance of adolescence [74] and act as counter-regulatory hormones. As a result of these physiological changes, insulin dosages are often increased to overcome the resistance to insulin, but metabolic control still frequently worsens during the later stages of pubertal development [37].

6.2. Alternative therapeutic strategies

The increasing insulin resistance and deterioration of glycemic control in adolescents create a great need for alternative therapeutic strategies in adolescents with T1D. One such strategy is the addition of a drug that improves insulin sensitivity such as metformin, a biguanide that acts principally by increasing insulin sensitivity in the liver by inhibiting hepatic gluconeogenesis and thereby reducing hepatic glucose production [75]. Other minor mechanisms include decreasing fatty acid oxidation and intestinal glucose absorption [76], and increasing peripheral insulin sensitivity by enhancing glucose uptake in the muscles [77]. Metformin has mainly been used in adult patients with T2D and several studies have shown beneficial effects on body weight, blood lipid levels and metabolic control [78-80]. Randomized controlled trials with metformin in adolescents with T2D reported an improvement in fasting plasma glucose level [81]. However, there have been conflicting reports from studies in adolescents with T1D [75-77,82,83]. The benefit was transient in one study [83] and negative in another [82]. The main drawback of these studies was the small sample size and lack of reporting on long term benefit and safety of adjunctive therapy in many of them [84].

Evidence for the coexistence of insulin resistance and insulin deficiency in childhood-onset T1D adults has been demonstrated by the insulin-glucose clamp technique [85,86]. Furthermore, two randomized, placebo-controlled trials have investigated the role of adjunctive metformin therapy in adolescents with T1D. In a randomized placebo controlled trial in children with T1D who were treated for 3 months with adjunctive metformin, Sarnblad et al [77] reported a significant decrease in A1c from 9.6% to 8.7%($p<0.05$) in the metformin group, compared to 9.5 to 9.2% (p=NS) in the placebo group. In another study, Hamilton et al [75] reported an HbA1c 0.6% lower in the metformin group than in the placebo group ($P<0.035$), after 3 months of therapy. Mean HbA1c at the end of the study was decreased by 0.3% in the metformin group, while it increased by 0.3% in the placebo group ($p=0.03$). Both studies reported no difference in mean body mass index and serum lipids in the metformin versus placebo group after 3 months of therapy. Hamilton et al [75] reported no significant changes in mean insulin sensitivity, measured by frequently sampled glucose after intravenous glucose tolerance test, after 3 months of metformin therapy in the metformin versus placebo group. Sarnblad et al [77], using hyperinsulinemic euglycemic clamp study, demonstrated no significant change in insulin sensitivity after 3 months between the groups, but they did report an increase in insulin sensitivity in the metformin group during the study ($P<0.05$). Hamilton et al [75] reported a significant change in the mean daily insulin dose in the metformin group in comparison to the placebo group after 3 months of metformin therapy of -0.14 vs. 0.02, $P=0.01$. However, Sarnblad [77] did not find a significant difference in the daily insulin dosage between the metformin and placebo groups after 3 months of therapy (1.1 vs. 1.3).

The two randomized, controlled studies by Hamilton and Sarnblad did not categorically recruit children and adolescents with double diabetes. This is important because this sub-set of diabetic youth is known to be insulin resistant and may require a careful titration of insulin doses. Adjunctive metformin therapy to achieve glycemic control may also be more effective in this subset of diabetes patients.

Furthermore, even though these randomized controlled trials were designed to investigate the effectiveness of adjunctive metformin therapy compared to insulin therapy alone, they were not designed to compare metformin adjunctive therapy to protocol-driven, optimized insulin therapy. Neither study demonstrated a strong head-to-head comparison of adjunctive metformin to patient-directed, treat to target insulin regimen to ensure optimal insulin delivery during the study. Such a comparison is critical because poor glycemic control contributes to insulin resistance [87] as there is an inverse relationship between glycemic control (as determined by HbA1c) and insulin sensitivity (estimated by glucose infusion rate during euglycemic-hyperinsulinemic clamp) [88].

6.3. The need for an insulin titration regimen for double diabetes

In general, patients with double diabetes are overweight or obese and the resultant insulin resistance increases their insulin requirement [1]. However, in addition to requiring a high insulin dose, evidence suggests that many patients often do not have insulin doses titrated sufficiently to achieve target levels of glucose control [89,90]. These patients remain on suboptimal doses of insulin and fail to reach treatment targets [91]. In a recent study Blonde et al [91] demonstrated the efficacy of algorithm-guided, patient titration of once daily long acting insulin in normalizing HbA1c in adult patients with T2D. They conducted a 20-week, randomized, controlled, open label, multicenter, parallel-group study comparing the safety and efficacy of insulin detemir administered once daily in combination with oral antidiabetic agents when titrated to two fasting plasma glucose targets (3.0-5.0 mmol/L versus 4.4.-6.1 mmol/L) for the treatment of T2D in adults. In that study, fasting plasma glucose level decreased throughout the first 8 weeks of the study and then generally remained flat for each treatment group. The combined treatment groups achieved a mean HbA1c level of 6.9% at the end of the study. There were significant reductions in HbA1c in both titration groups: in the 3.9-5.0 mmol/L fasting plasma glucose target group, HbA1c values decreased from a baseline mean of 8% to 6.8% at 20 weeks. In the 4.4-6.1 mmol/L fasting plasma glucose target group, HbA1c values decreased from a 7.9% at baseline to 7.0% at 20 weeks. Overall rates of hypoglycemia episodes were low and were comparable between treatment groups: 7.73 and 5.27 events/subject/year for the 3.9-5 mmol/L and 4.4-6.1 mmol/L groups, respectively. Mean weight changes from baseline to the end of the study were small and did not differ significantly between groups.

Our group is conducting a randomized control trial to explore the role of protocol-driven treat-to-target regimen in children and adolescents with double diabetes. Given the rising prevalence of obesity in the general population we speculate that many children with T1D will eventually develop double diabetes. Thus, it is timely to devise an appropriate management protocol to treat this burgeoning sub-population. Our aim is to primarily study this group of patients to determine the role of protocol-driven, treat-to-target regimen alone or in combination with metformin therapy in their care. Metformin is approved by the Food and Drug Administration for use in children with T2D, and recently it has been recommended that metformin added to insulin therapy might be used in clinical practice in adolescents with T1D who are poorly controlled and show evidence of insulin resistance (double diabetes) as noted in T2D [84]. Given the conflicting reports on the efficacy of adjunctive metformin therapy in adolescents with T1D, this double blind, randomized, placebo controlled trial will demonstrate the effect of meformin on HbA1c reduction under optimized insulin titration regimen. Secondly, we will investigate whether a titrated insulin regimen alone would have a superior-, or similar effect to combined metformin and titrated insulin regimen in children and adolescents with double diabetes and how this modality of treatment compares to standard insulin therapy.

Blonde et al [91] demonstrated that self-titration regimens facilitate empowerment of patients, allowing them to become more involved in their treatment, which can result in improved glycemic control. Patient-directed insulin titration is increasingly important as health care practitioners often do not have the resources to advise patients with the frequency needed to effectively titrate their insulin doses to maintain euglycemia. Optimal patient empowerment through self-titration regimens is critical for the motivation to reach treatment targets.

7. Prognosis

The coexistence of both T1D and T2D in an individual should in principle denote an increased risk for the complications of both diseases [32]. Therefore, it is possible that these individuals are at higher risk for the microvascular and metabolic complications of T1D and the macrovascular complications of T2D [18]. This is supported by investigations by Orchard et al [85,92], in the Epidemiology of Diabetes Complications Study, who reported that patients with T1D who have a positive family history of T2D were at greater risk for cardiovascular disease than those who did not. Furthermore, data from the Diabetes Control and Complications Trial (DCCT) show that weight gain and central obesity are associated with insulin resistance, hypertension, and dyslipidemia in T1D [93], and data from Epidemiology of Diabetes Interventions and Complications (EDIC) Study show that central obesity is an independent risk factor for incident microalbuminuria in individuals with T1D [94]. However, both DCCT and EDIC follow up studies show that intensive diabetes therapy results in a uniform, major reduction in (and significant protection from) microvascular disease [95], even in overweight or obese T1D patients [92]. Thus, there is the need to devise a consensus treatment regimen that would ensure the best glycemic and metabolic outcome for patients with double diabetes.

8. Conclusions

The global pandemic of obesity in children and adolescents has resulted in a new expression of diabetes mellitus known as double diabetes. The entity encompasses the autoimmune load of T1D and the metabolic load of T2D. There is no consensus on the best therapeutic modality for this new expression of diabetes mellitus. However, optimal therapeutic options must address the coexistence of both metabolic and autoimmune components of diabetes mellitus in the patient. There have also been calls to revise the current classification of diabetes mellitus to take into account the surging prevalence of double diabetes in children and adolescents.

Author details

Benjamin U. Nwosu

University of Massachusetts Medical School, Worcester, Massachusetts, USA

References

[1] Pozzilli P, Guglielmi C, Caprio S, Buzzetti R: Obesity, autoimmunity, and double diabetes in youth. Diabetes Care;34 Suppl 2:S166-170.

[2] Hedley AA, Ogden CL, Johnson CL, Carroll MD, Curtin LR, Flegal KM: Prevalence of overweight and obesity among US children, adolescents, and adults, 1999-2002. Jama 2004;291:2847-2850.

[3] Flegal KM, Wei R, Ogden C: Weight-for-stature compared with body mass index-for-age growth charts for the United States from the Centers for Disease Control and Prevention. Am J Clin Nutr 2002;75:761-766.

[4] Himes JH, Dietz WH: Guidelines for overweight in adolescent preventive services: recommendations from an expert committee. The Expert Committee on Clinical Guidelines for Overweight in Adolescent Preventive Services. Am J Clin Nutr 1994;59:307-316.

[5] Flodmark CE, Lissau I, Moreno LA, Pietrobelli A, Widhalm K: New insights into the field of children and adolescents' obesity: the European perspective. Int J Obes Relat Metab Disord 2004;28:1189-1196.

[6] Ogden CL, Flegal KM, Carroll MD, Johnson CL: Prevalence and trends in overweight among US children and adolescents, 1999-2000. Jama 2002;288:1728-1732.

[7] Ogden CL, Carroll MD, Curtin LR, McDowell MA, Tabak CJ, Flegal KM: Prevalence of overweight and obesity in the United States, 1999-2004. Jama 2006;295:1549-1555.

[8] Troiano RP, Flegal KM, Kuczmarski RJ, Campbell SM, Johnson CL: Overweight prevalence and trends for children and adolescents. The National Health and Nutrition Examination Surveys, 1963 to 1991. Arch Pediatr Adolesc Med 1995;149:1085-1091.

[9] Must A, Strauss RS: Risks and consequences of childhood and adolescent obesity. Int J Obes Relat Metab Disord 1999;23 Suppl 2:S2-11.

[10] Daniels SR, Arnett DK, Eckel RH, Gidding SS, Hayman LL, Kumanyika S, Robinson TN, Scott BJ, St Jeor S, Williams CL: Overweight in children and adolescents: pathophysiology, consequences, prevention, and treatment. Circulation 2005;111:1999-2012.

[11] Ebbeling CB, Pawlak DB, Ludwig DS: Childhood obesity: public-health crisis, common sense cure. Lancet 2002;360:473-482.

[12] Williams J, Wake M, Hesketh K, Maher E, Waters E: Health-related quality of life of overweight and obese children. Jama 2005;293:70-76.

[13] Schwimmer JB, Burwinkle TM, Varni JW: Health-related quality of life of severely obese children and adolescents. Jama 2003;289:1813-1819.

[14] Kaufman F: 'Double diabetes' in young people and how to treat it. Diabetes Voice 2006;51:19-22.

[15] Pickup JC, Williams, G.: Textbook of Diabetes. ed 3rd, Blackwell Publishing, 2002.

[16] Pozzilli P, Guglielmi C: Double diabetes: a mixture of type 1 and type 2 diabetes in youth. Endocr Dev 2009;14:151-166.

[17] Reinehr T, Schober E, Wiegand S, Thon A, Holl R: Beta-cell autoantibodies in children with type 2 diabetes mellitus: subgroup or misclassification? Arch Dis Child 2006;91:473-477.

[18] Libman IM, Becker DJ: Coexistence of type 1 and type 2 diabetes mellitus: "double" diabetes? Pediatr Diabetes 2003;4:110-113.

[19] Variation and trends in incidence of childhood diabetes in Europe. EURODIAB ACE Study Group. Lancet 2000;355:873-876.

[20] CDC: Epidemiology of Type 1 and Type 2 Diabetes Mellitus Among North American Children and Adolescents. In, Center For Disease Control and Prevention, 2008.

[21] Yki-Jarvinen H: Acute and chronic effects of hyperglycaemia on glucose metabolism: implications for the development of new therapies. Diabet Med 1997;14 Suppl 3:S32-37.

[22] Hathout EH, Thomas W, El-Shahawy M, Nahab F, Mace JW: Diabetic autoimmune markers in children and adolescents with type 2 diabetes. Pediatrics 2001;107:E102.

[23] Rosenbloom AL, Joe JR, Young RS, Winter WE: Emerging epidemic of type 2 diabetes in youth. Diabetes Care 1999;22:345-354.

[24] Dabelea D, Pettitt DJ, Jones KL, Arslanian SA: Type 2 diabetes mellitus in minority children and adolescents. An emerging problem. Endocrinol Metab Clin North Am 1999;28:709-729, viii.

[25] Laine AP, Nejentsev S, Veijola R, Korpinen E, Sjoroos M, Simell O, Knip M, Akerblom HK, Ilonen J: A linkage study of 12 IDDM susceptibility loci in the Finnish population. Diabetes Metab Res Rev 2004;20:144-149.

[26] Voight BF, Scott LJ, Steinthorsdottir V, Morris AP, Dina C, Welch RP, Zeggini E, Huth C, Aulchenko YS, Thorleifsson G, McCulloch LJ, Ferreira T, Grallert H, Amin N, Wu G, Willer CJ, Raychaudhuri S, McCarroll SA, Langenberg C, Hofmann OM,

Dupuis J, Qi L, Segre AV, van Hoek M, Navarro P, Ardlie K, Balkau B, Benediktsson R, Bennett AJ, Blagieva R, Boerwinkle E, Bonnycastle LL, Bengtsson Bostrom K, Bravenboer B, Bumpstead S, Burtt NP, Charpentier G, Chines PS, Cornelis M, Couper DJ, Crawford G, Doney AS, Elliott KS, Elliott AL, Erdos MR, Fox CS, Franklin CS, Ganser M, Gieger C, Grarup N, Green T, Griffin S, Groves CJ, Guiducci C, Hadjadj S, Hassanali N, Herder C, Isomaa B, Jackson AU, Johnson PR, Jorgensen T, Kao WH, Klopp N, Kong A, Kraft P, Kuusisto J, Lauritzen T, Li M, Lieverse A, Lindgren CM, Lyssenko V, Marre M, Meitinger T, Midthjell K, Morken MA, Narisu N, Nilsson P, Owen KR, Payne F, Perry JR, Petersen AK, Platou C, Proenca C, Prokopenko I, Rathmann W, Rayner NW, Robertson NR, Rocheleau G, Roden M, Sampson MJ, Saxena R, Shields BM, Shrader P, Sigurdsson G, Sparso T, Strassburger K, Stringham HM, Sun Q, Swift AJ, Thorand B, Tichet J, Tuomi T, van Dam RM, van Haeften TW, van Herpt T, van Vliet-Ostaptchouk JV, Walters GB, Weedon MN, Wijmenga C, Witteman J, Bergman RN, Cauchi S, Collins FS, Gloyn AL, Gyllensten U, Hansen T, Hide WA, Hitman GA, Hofman A, Hunter DJ, Hveem K, Laakso M, Mohlke KL, Morris AD, Palmer CN, Pramstaller PP, Rudan I, Sijbrands E, Stein LD, Tuomilehto J, Uitterlinden A, Walker M, Wareham NJ, Watanabe RM, Abecasis GR, Boehm BO, Campbell H, Daly MJ, Hattersley AT, Hu FB, Meigs JB, Pankow JS, Pedersen O, Wichmann HE, Barroso I, Florez JC, Frayling TM, Groop L, Sladek R, Thorsteinsdottir U, Wilson JF, Illig T, Froguel P, van Duijn CM, Stefansson K, Altshuler D, Boehnke M, McCarthy MI: Twelve type 2 diabetes susceptibility loci identified through large-scale association analysis. Nat Genet;42:579-589.

[27] Cho YS, Chen CH, Hu C, Long J, Ong RT, Sim X, Takeuchi F, Wu Y, Go MJ, Yamauchi T, Chang YC, Kwak SH, Ma RC, Yamamoto K, Adair LS, Aung T, Cai Q, Chang LC, Chen YT, Gao Y, Hu FB, Kim HL, Kim S, Kim YJ, Lee JJ, Lee NR, Li Y, Liu JJ, Lu W, Nakamura J, Nakashima E, Ng DP, Tay WT, Tsai FJ, Wong TY, Yokota M, Zheng W, Zhang R, Wang C, So WY, Ohnaka K, Ikegami H, Hara K, Cho YM, Cho NH, Chang TJ, Bao Y, Hedman AK, Morris AP, McCarthy MI, Takayanagi R, Park KS, Jia W, Chuang LM, Chan JC, Maeda S, Kadowaki T, Lee JY, Wu JY, Teo YY, Tai ES, Shu XO, Mohlke KL, Kato N, Han BG, Seielstad M: Meta-analysis of genome-wide association studies identifies eight new loci for type 2 diabetes in east Asians. Nat Genet; 44:67-72.

[28] Dupuis J, Langenberg C, Prokopenko I, Saxena R, Soranzo N, Jackson AU, Wheeler E, Glazer NL, Bouatia-Naji N, Gloyn AL, Lindgren CM, Magi R, Morris AP, Randall J, Johnson T, Elliott P, Rybin D, Thorleifsson G, Steinthorsdottir V, Henneman P, Grallert H, Dehghan A, Hottenga JJ, Franklin CS, Navarro P, Song K, Goel A, Perry JR, Egan JM, Lajunen T, Grarup N, Sparso T, Doney A, Voight BF, Stringham HM, Li M, Kanoni S, Shrader P, Cavalcanti-Proenca C, Kumari M, Qi L, Timpson NJ, Gieger C, Zabena C, Rocheleau G, Ingelsson E, An P, O'Connell J, Luan J, Elliott A, McCarroll SA, Payne F, Roccasecca RM, Pattou F, Sethupathy P, Ardlie K, Ariyurek Y, Balkau B, Barter P, Beilby JP, Ben-Shlomo Y, Benediktsson R, Bennett AJ, Bergmann S, Bochud M, Boerwinkle E, Bonnefond A, Bonnycastle LL, Borch-Johnsen K, Bottcher

Y, Brunner E, Bumpstead SJ, Charpentier G, Chen YD, Chines P, Clarke R, Coin LJ, Cooper MN, Cornelis M, Crawford G, Crisponi L, Day IN, de Geus EJ, Delplanque J, Dina C, Erdos MR, Fedson AC, Fischer-Rosinsky A, Forouhi NG, Fox CS, Frants R, Franzosi MG, Galan P, Goodarzi MO, Graessler J, Groves CJ, Grundy S, Gwilliam R, Gyllensten U, Hadjadj S, Hallmans G, Hammond N, Han X, Hartikainen AL, Hassanali N, Hayward C, Heath SC, Hercberg S, Herder C, Hicks AA, Hillman DR, Hingorani AD, Hofman A, Hui J, Hung J, Isomaa B, Johnson PR, Jorgensen T, Jula A, Kaakinen M, Kaprio J, Kesaniemi YA, Kivimaki M, Knight B, Koskinen S, Kovacs P, Kyvik KO, Lathrop GM, Lawlor DA, Le Bacquer O, Lecoeur C, Li Y, Lyssenko V, Mahley R, Mangino M, Manning AK, Martinez-Larrad MT, McAteer JB, McCulloch LJ, McPherson R, Meisinger C, Melzer D, Meyre D, Mitchell BD, Morken MA, Mukherjee S, Naitza S, Narisu N, Neville MJ, Oostra BA, Orru M, Pakyz R, Palmer CN, Paolisso G, Pattaro C, Pearson D, Peden JF, Pedersen NL, Perola M, Pfeiffer AF, Pichler I, Polasek O, Posthuma D, Potter SC, Pouta A, Province MA, Psaty BM, Rathmann W, Rayner NW, Rice K, Ripatti S, Rivadeneira F, Roden M, Rolandsson O, Sandbaek A, Sandhu M, Sanna S, Sayer AA, Scheet P, Scott LJ, Seedorf U, Sharp SJ, Shields B, Sigurethsson G, Sijbrands EJ, Silveira A, Simpson L, Singleton A, Smith NL, Sovio U, Swift A, Syddall H, Syvanen AC, Tanaka T, Thorand B, Tichet J, Tonjes A, Tuomi T, Uitterlinden AG, van Dijk KW, van Hoek M, Varma D, Visvikis-Siest S, Vitart V, Vogelzangs N, Waeber G, Wagner PJ, Walley A, Walters GB, Ward KL, Watkins H, Weedon MN, Wild SH, Willemsen G, Witteman JC, Yarnell JW, Zeggini E, Zelenika D, Zethelius B, Zhai G, Zhao JH, Zillikens MC, Borecki IB, Loos RJ, Meneton P, Magnusson PK, Nathan DM, Williams GH, Hattersley AT, Silander K, Salomaa V, Smith GD, Bornstein SR, Schwarz P, Spranger J, Karpe F, Shuldiner AR, Cooper C, Dedoussis GV, Serrano-Rios M, Morris AD, Lind L, Palmer LJ, Hu FB, Franks PW, Ebrahim S, Marmot M, Kao WH, Pankow JS, Sampson MJ, Kuusisto J, Laakso M, Hansen T, Pedersen O, Pramstaller PP, Wichmann HE, Illig T, Rudan I, Wright AF, Stumvoll M, Campbell H, Wilson JF, Bergman RN, Buchanan TA, Collins FS, Mohlke KL, Tuomilehto J, Valle TT, Altshuler D, Rotter JI, Siscovick DS, Penninx BW, Boomsma DI, Deloukas P, Spector TD, Frayling TM, Ferrucci L, Kong A, Thorsteinsdottir U, Stefansson K, van Duijn CM, Aulchenko YS, Cao A, Scuteri A, Schlessinger D, Uda M, Ruokonen A, Jarvelin MR, Waterworth DM, Vollenweider P, Peltonen L, Mooser V, Abecasis GR, Wareham NJ, Sladek R, Froguel P, Watanabe RM, Meigs JB, Groop L, Boehnke M, McCarthy MI, Florez JC, Barroso I: New genetic loci implicated in fasting glucose homeostasis and their impact on type 2 diabetes risk. Nat Genet; 42:105-116.

[29] Barker JM: Clinical review: Type 1 diabetes-associated autoimmunity: natural history, genetic associations, and screening. J Clin Endocrinol Metab 2006;91:1210-1217.

[30] Freeman H, Cox RD: Type-2 diabetes: a cocktail of genetic discovery. Hum Mol Genet 2006;15 Spec No 2:R202-209.

[31] Pozzilli P, Buzzetti R: A new expression of diabetes: double diabetes. Trends Endocrinol Metab 2007;18:52-57.

[32] Pozzilli P, Guglielmi C, Pronina E, Petraikina E: Double or hybrid diabetes associated with an increase in type 1 and type 2 diabetes in children and youths. Pediatr Diabetes 2007;8 Suppl 9:88-95.

[33] Sesti G, Federici M, Hribal ML, Lauro D, Sbraccia P, Lauro R: Defects of the insulin receptor substrate (IRS) system in human metabolic disorders. Faseb J 2001;15:2099-2111.

[34] Foti D, Chiefari E, Fedele M, Iuliano R, Brunetti L, Paonessa F, Manfioletti G, Barbetti F, Brunetti A, Croce CM, Fusco A, Brunetti A: Lack of the architectural factor HMGA1 causes insulin resistance and diabetes in humans and mice. Nat Med 2005;11:765-773.

[35] Kibirige M, Metcalf B, Renuka R, Wilkin TJ: Testing the accelerator hypothesis: the relationship between body mass and age at diagnosis of type 1 diabetes. Diabetes Care 2003;26:2865-2870.

[36] Liu LL, Lawrence JM, Davis C, Liese AD, Pettitt DJ, Pihoker C, Dabelea D, Hamman R, Waitzfelder B, Kahn HS: Prevalence of overweight and obesity in youth with diabetes in USA: the SEARCH for Diabetes in Youth Study. Pediatr Diabetes 2009.

[37] Mortensen HB, Robertson KJ, Aanstoot HJ, Danne T, Holl RW, Hougaard P, Atchison JA, Chiarelli F, Daneman D, Dinesen B, Dorchy H, Garandeau P, Greene S, Hoey H, Kaprio EA, Kocova M, Martul P, Matsuura N, Schoenle EJ, Sovik O, Swift PG, Tsou RM, Vanelli M, Aman J: Insulin management and metabolic control of type 1 diabetes mellitus in childhood and adolescence in 18 countries. Hvidore Study Group on Childhood Diabetes. Diabet Med 1998;15:752-759.

[38] Frayling TM, Timpson NJ, Weedon MN, Zeggini E, Freathy RM, Lindgren CM, Perry JR, Elliott KS, Lango H, Rayner NW, Shields B, Harries LW, Barrett JC, Ellard S, Groves CJ, Knight B, Patch AM, Ness AR, Ebrahim S, Lawlor DA, Ring SM, Ben-Shlomo Y, Jarvelin MR, Sovio U, Bennett AJ, Melzer D, Ferrucci L, Loos RJ, Barroso I, Wareham NJ, Karpe F, Owen KR, Cardon LR, Walker M, Hitman GA, Palmer CN, Doney AS, Morris AD, Smith GD, Hattersley AT, McCarthy MI: A common variant in the FTO gene is associated with body mass index and predisposes to childhood and adult obesity. Science 2007;316:889-894.

[39] Hypponen E, Virtanen SM, Kenward MG, Knip M, Akerblom HK: Obesity, increased linear growth, and risk of type 1 diabetes in children. Diabetes Care 2000;23:1755-1760.

[40] Diet, nutrition and the prevention of chronic diseases. World Health Organ Tech Rep Ser 2003;916:i-viii, 1-149, backcover.

[41] Rolandsson O, Hagg E, Hampe C, Sullivan EP, Jr., Nilsson M, Jansson G, Hallmans G, Lernmark A: Glutamate decarboxylase (GAD65) and tyrosine phosphatase-like protein (IA-2) autoantibodies index in a regional population is related to glucose intolerance and body mass index. Diabetologia 1999;42:555-559.

[42] Libman IM, Pietropaolo M, Arslanian SA, LaPorte RE, Becker DJ: Changing prevalence of overweight children and adolescents at onset of insulin-treated diabetes. Diabetes Care 2003;26:2871-2875.

[43] Matarese G, Moschos S, Mantzoros CS: Leptin in immunology. J Immunol 2005;174:3137-3142.

[44] Matarese G, Sanna V, Lechler RI, Sarvetnick N, Fontana S, Zappacosta S, La Cava A: Leptin accelerates autoimmune diabetes in female NOD mice. Diabetes 2002;51:1356-1361.

[45] Kahn BB, Flier JS: Obesity and insulin resistance. J Clin Invest 2000;106:473-481.

[46] Wilkin TJ: The accelerator hypothesis: a review of the evidence for insulin resistance as the basis for type I as well as type II diabetes. Int J Obes (Lond) 2009.

[47] Wilkin TJ: The accelerator hypothesis: weight gain as the missing link between Type I and Type II diabetes. Diabetologia 2001;44:914-922.

[48] Strauss RS, Pollack HA: Epidemic increase in childhood overweight, 1986-1998. Jama 2001;286:2845-2848.

[49] Onkamo P, Vaananen S, Karvonen M, Tuomilehto J: Worldwide increase in incidence of Type I diabetes--the analysis of the data on published incidence trends. Diabetologia 1999;42:1395-1403.

[50] Evertsen J, Alemzadeh R, Wang X: Increasing incidence of pediatric type 1 diabetes mellitus in Southeastern Wisconsin: relationship with body weight at diagnosis. PLoS One 2009;4:e6873.

[51] Baum JD, Ounsted M, Smith MA: Letter: Weight gain in infancy and subsequent development of diabetes mellitus in childhood. Lancet 1975;2:866.

[52] Forsen T, Eriksson J, Tuomilehto J, Reunanen A, Osmond C, Barker D: The fetal and childhood growth of persons who develop type 2 diabetes. Ann Intern Med 2000;133:176-182.

[53] Hypponen E, Kenward MG, Virtanen SM, Piitulainen A, Virta-Autio P, Tuomilehto J, Knip M, Akerblom HK: Infant feeding, early weight gain, and risk of type 1 diabetes. Childhood Diabetes in Finland (DiMe) Study Group. Diabetes Care 1999;22:1961-1965.

[54] Pundziute-Lycka A, Dahlquist G, Nystrom L, Arnqvist H, Bjork E, Blohme G, Bolinder J, Eriksson JW, Sundkvist G, Ostman J: The incidence of Type I diabetes has not increased but shifted to a younger age at diagnosis in the 0-34 years group in Sweden 1983-1998. Diabetologia 2002;45:783-791.

[55] Charkaluk ML, Czernichow P, Levy-Marchal C: Incidence data of childhood-onset type I diabetes in France during 1988-1997: the case for a shift toward younger age at onset. Pediatr Res 2002;52:859-862.

[56] Karvonen M, Pitkaniemi J, Tuomilehto J: The onset age of type 1 diabetes in Finnish children has become younger. The Finnish Childhood Diabetes Registry Group. Diabetes Care 1999;22:1066-1070.

[57] Weets I, De Leeuw IH, Du Caju MV, Rooman R, Keymeulen B, Mathieu C, Rottiers R, Daubresse JC, Rocour-Brumioul D, Pipeleers DG, Gorus FK: The incidence of type 1 diabetes in the age group 0-39 years has not increased in Antwerp (Belgium) between 1989 and 2000: evidence for earlier disease manifestation. Diabetes Care 2002;25:840-846.

[58] Weets I, Rooman R, Coeckelberghs M, De Block C, Van Gaal L, Kaufman JM, Keymeulen B, Mathieu C, Weber E, Pipeleers DG, Gorus FK: The age at diagnosis of type 1 diabetes continues to decrease in Belgian boys but not in girls: a 15-year survey. Diabetes Metab Res Rev 2007;23:637-643.

[59] Wilkin TJ: Diabetes: 1 and 2, or one and the same? Progress with the accelerator hypothesis. Pediatr Diabetes 2008;9:23-32.

[60] Feltbower RG, McKinney PA, Parslow RC, Stephenson CR, Bodansky HJ: Type 1 diabetes in Yorkshire, UK: time trends in 0-14 and 15-29-year-olds, age at onset and age-period-cohort modelling. Diabet Med 2003;20:437-441.

[61] Porter JR, Barrett TG: Braking the accelerator hypothesis? Diabetologia 2004;47:352-353.

[62] Kordonouri O, Hartmann R: Higher body weight is associated with earlier onset of Type 1 diabetes in children: confirming the 'Accelerator Hypothesis'. Diabet Med 2005;22:1783-1784.

[63] Knerr I, Wolf J, Reinehr T, Stachow R, Grabert M, Schober E, Rascher W, Holl RW: The 'accelerator hypothesis': relationship between weight, height, body mass index and age at diagnosis in a large cohort of 9,248 German and Austrian children with type 1 diabetes mellitus. Diabetologia 2005;48:2501-2504.

[64] Betts P, Mulligan J, Ward P, Smith B, Wilkin T: Increasing body weight predicts the earlier onset of insulin-dependant diabetes in childhood: testing the 'accelerator hypothesis' (2). Diabet Med 2005;22:144-151.

[65] Dabelea D, D'Agostino RB, Jr., Mayer-Davis EJ, Pettitt DJ, Imperatore G, Dolan LM, Pihoker C, Hillier TA, Marcovina SM, Linder B, Ruggiero AM, Hamman RF: Testing the accelerator hypothesis: body size, beta-cell function, and age at onset of type 1 (autoimmune) diabetes. Diabetes Care 2006;29:290-294.

[66] Gimenez M, Aguilera E, Castell C, de Lara N, Nicolau J, Conget I: Relationship between BMI and age at diagnosis of type 1 diabetes in a Mediterranean area in the period of 1990-2004. Diabetes Care 2007;30:1593-1595.

[67] O'Connell MA, Donath S, Cameron FJ: Major increase in Type 1 diabetes: no support for the Accelerator Hypothesis. Diabet Med 2007;24:920-923.

[68] Type 2 diabetes in children and adolescents. American Diabetes Association. Diabetes Care 2000;23:381-389.

[69] Double Diabetes Summary. In, Children With Diabetes, 2009.

[70] Petitti DB, Klingensmith GJ, Bell RA, Andrews JS, Dabelea D, Imperatore G, Marcovina S, Pihoker C, Standiford D, Waitzfelder B, Mayer-Davis E: Glycemic Control in Youth with Diabetes: The SEARCH for Diabetes in Youth Study. J Pediatr 2009;155:668-672.

[71] Rosenbloom AL, Wheeler L, Bianchi R, Chin FT, Tiwary CM, Grgic A: Age-adjusted analysis of insulin responses during normal and abnormal glucose tolerance tests in children and adolescents. Diabetes 1975;24:820-828.

[72] Caprio S, Tamborlane WV: Metabolic impact of obesity in childhood. Endocrinol Metab Clin North Am 1999;28:731-747.

[73] Miller J SJ, Rosenbloom AL.: Pediatric Endocrinology. ed 5th, New York, Informa Healthcare USA, Inc., 2007.

[74] Miller J, Silverstein, J.H., Rosenbloom, A.L.: Pediatric Endocrinology. ed 5th, New York, Informa Healthcare USA, Inc., 2007.

[75] Hamilton J, Cummings E, Zdravkovic V, Finegood D, Daneman D: Metformin as an adjunct therapy in adolescents with type 1 diabetes and insulin resistance: a randomized controlled trial. Diabetes Care 2003;26:138-143.

[76] Meyer L, Bohme P, Delbachian I, Lehert P, Cugnardey N, Drouin P, Guerci B: The benefits of metformin therapy during continuous subcutaneous insulin infusion treatment of type 1 diabetic patients. Diabetes Care 2002;25:2153-2158.

[77] Sarnblad S, Kroon M, Aman J: Metformin as additional therapy in adolescents with poorly controlled type 1 diabetes: randomised placebo-controlled trial with aspects on insulin sensitivity. Eur J Endocrinol 2003;149:323-329.

[78] Howlett HC, Bailey CJ: A risk-benefit assessment of metformin in type 2 diabetes mellitus. Drug Saf 1999;20:489-503.

[79] Mehnert H: Metformin, the rebirth of a biguanide: mechanism of action and place in the prevention and treatment of insulin resistance. Exp Clin Endocrinol Diabetes 2001;109 Suppl 2:S259-264.

[80] Effect of intensive blood-glucose control with metformin on complications in overweight patients with type 2 diabetes (UKPDS 34). UK Prospective Diabetes Study (UKPDS) Group. Lancet 1998;352:854-865.

[81] Jones KL, Arslanian S, Peterokova VA, Park JS, Tomlinson MJ: Effect of metformin in pediatric patients with type 2 diabetes: a randomized controlled trial. Diabetes Care 2002;25:89-94.

[82] Desmangles J BJ, Shine B, Quattrin T.: Is Metformin a useful adjunct to insulin therapy in adolescents with type 1 diabetes in poor control? In Endocrine Society Meeting. 2000.

[83] Walravens PA CP, Klingensmith GJ, Essison M, Cornell C, Monahan K.: Low Dose Metformin in adolescents type 1 diabetes mellitus: a double blind, controlled study. In American Diabetes Association 60th Scientific Sessions. 2000.

[84] Abdelghaffar S, Attia AM: Metformin added to insulin therapy for type 1 diabetes mellitus in adolescents. Cochrane Database Syst Rev 2009:CD006691.

[85] Erbey JR, Kuller LH, Becker DJ, Orchard TJ: The association between a family history of type 2 diabetes and coronary artery disease in a type 1 diabetes population. Diabetes Care 1998;21:610-614.

[86] Williams KV, Erbey JR, Becker D, Arslanian S, Orchard TJ: Can clinical factors estimate insulin resistance in type 1 diabetes? Diabetes 2000;49:626-632.

[87] Scarlett JA, Gray RS, Griffin J, Olefsky JM, Kolterman OG: Insulin treatment reverses the insulin resistance of type II diabetes mellitus. Diabetes Care 1982;5:353-363.

[88] Yki-Jarvinen H, Koivisto VA: Natural course of insulin resistance in type I diabetes. N Engl J Med 1986;315:224-230.

[89] Intensive blood-glucose control with sulphonylureas or insulin compared with conventional treatment and risk of complications in patients with type 2 diabetes (UKPDS 33). UK Prospective Diabetes Study (UKPDS) Group. Lancet 1998;352:837-853.

[90] Davies M, Storms F, Shutler S, Bianchi-Biscay M, Gomis R: Improvement of glycemic control in subjects with poorly controlled type 2 diabetes: comparison of two treatment algorithms using insulin glargine. Diabetes Care 2005;28:1282-1288.

[91] Blonde L, Merilainen M, Karwe V, Raskin P: Patient-directed titration for achieving glycaemic goals using a once-daily basal insulin analogue: an assessment of two different fasting plasma glucose targets - the TITRATE study. Diabetes Obes Metab 2009;11:623-631.

[92] Williams KV, Erbey JR, Becker D, Orchard TJ: Improved glycemic control reduces the impact of weight gain on cardiovascular risk factors in type 1 diabetes. The Epidemiology of Diabetes Complications Study. Diabetes Care 1999;22:1084-1091.

[93] Effect of intensive diabetes treatment on the development and progression of long-term complications in adolescents with insulin-dependent diabetes mellitus: Diabetes Control and Complications Trial. Diabetes Control and Complications Trial Research Group. J Pediatr 1994;125:177-188.

[94] de Boer IH, Sibley SD, Kestenbaum B, Sampson JN, Young B, Cleary PA, Steffes MW, Weiss NS, Brunzell JD: Central obesity, incident microalbuminuria, and change in

creatinine clearance in the epidemiology of diabetes interventions and complications study. J Am Soc Nephrol 2007;18:235-243.

[95] Effect of intensive diabetes management on macrovascular events and risk factors in the Diabetes Control and Complications Trial. Am J Cardiol 1995;75:894-903.

Chapter 7

Glucagon-Like Peptide-1 and Its Implications in Obesity

Veronica Hurtado, Isabel Roncero,
Enrique Blazquez, Elvira Alvarez and Carmen Sanz

Additional information is available at the end of the chapter

http://dx.doi.org/10.5772/54221

1. Introduction

Glucagon-like peptide (GLP-1) is derived from the processing of the proglucagon gene. This peptide has diverse biological activities affecting peripheral tissues and the central nervous system. Thus, for example, GLP-1 stimulates pancreas insulin secretion in a glucose-dependent manner after eating, hence its denomination as an "incretin". GLP-1 has also been considered an anorexigenic peptide, while also reducing cerebral glucose metabolism in the human hypothalamus and brain stem. These GLP-1 actions in the pancreas and central nervous system are achieved through GLP-1 receptors (GLP-1R) that share the same gene sequence in both tissues. In short, GLP-1 is an antidiabetogenic agent due to its action in the pancreas while acting in hypothalamic areas, helping to generate a state of satiety. Interestingly, GLP-1/exendin-4 administration in obese Zucker rats, which also develop insulin resistance, hyperinsulinemia and hyperlipidemia, reduces food intake and induced weight loss, which applies to lean rats, too.

The mid 20th century recorded the first indications that the hypothalamus plays a major role in feeding behaviour and energy homeostasis, whereby the electrical stimulation of the ventromedial hypothalamus (VMH) suppresses food intake, and the bilateral lesions of these structures induce hyperphagia and obesity. The VMH was therefore called the satiety centre. In contrast, alterations in the lateral hypothalamic area (LH) induced the opposite set of responses, and the LH was hence called the hunger centre. At least two kinds of glucose sensor neurons have been described in the brain: glucose-excited neurons are located mainly in the VMH and are excited by increased glucose levels in the extracellular space, while glucose-inhibited neurons (mainly present in the LH) are excited by decreases in glucose concentrations. A direct relationship has also been established between the regulation of food intake and energy homeostasis and hypothalamic metabolic sensor activities.

Both AMP-activated protein kinase (AMPK) and the mammalian target of rapamycin (mTOR) and its downstream target p70 ribosomal protein S6 Kinase 1 (S6K1) contribute to detecting cellular energy and integrate nutrient and hormonal signals in order to maintain energy homeostasis in the organism. Thus, the Ser/Thr kinase AMPK is activated during energy depletion, when the AMP/ATP ratio increases and triggers a large number of downstream effectors by stimulating ATP-generating catabolic pathways and inhibiting anabolic pathways in order to restore the energy balance. Specifically, it has been reported that fasting increases, and re-feeding decreases, AMPK activity in several hypothalamic areas. Likewise, the hypothalamic mTOR/S6K1 pathway has also been involved in the control of feeding and in the regulation of energy balances. Thus, mTOR is activated by glucose and amino acids and, therefore, hypothalamic AMPK and mTOR/S6K1 respond to changes in glucose and other nutrients in the opposite way, and their effects on the regulation of food intake may overlap. Our recent results indicate that AMPK and S6K1 are functionally expressed in the VMH and LH areas, with differential activation in response to glucose fluctuations, in both in vitro models of hypothalamic organotypic slice cultures and animals in response to fasting and re-feeding, as well as in Zucker obese rats with a lower activation degree of hypothalamic AMPK in response to fasting.

In addition, we have reported that GLP-1/exendin-4 treatment inhibits the activities of AMPK and S6K1 when the activation of these protein kinases peak in both the VMH and LH areas. In pathophysiological situations, as occurs in Zucker obese rats, exendin-4 seems to act as a compensator for the variations in AMPK activity produced either by oscillations in glucose levels or by pathologies such as obesity or episodes of hyperinsulinemia.

In conclusion, it seems that GLP-1/exendin-4 acts in the VMH and LH, modulating the activation status of AMPK and S6K1 in response to glucose fluctuations, helping to improve pathophysiological states such as obesity and insulin resistance. The effects of these peptides in the hypothalamus are mediated through the activation of PKA, PKC and PI3K, as well as the phosphatase PP2.

2. Glucagon-like peptide-1: Dual role as an incretin and anorexigenic peptide

Glucagon and related peptides constitute a family derived from the proglucagon molecule, which is identical in sequence in the pancreas, intestine and brain [1], although post-translational processing of the precursor yields different products in these organs [2]. (Figure 1)

In gut L-cells, the C–terminal portion of proglucagon is predominantly processed to glucagon-like peptide-1 (GLP-1) and GLP-2. Further processing of GLP-1 in these cells produces the amidated and truncated forms of the peptide: GLP-1 [7-36] amide, GLP-1 [7-37] and GLP-1 [1-36] amide, with the first two being the biologically active forms, which are cited in the rest of the test as GLP-1. Although the truncated forms of GLP-1 are reported to have strong incretin activity, it is currently known that they are also important in the functioning of other peripheral tissues and the central nervous system. Both forms of the peptide are in-

http://dx.doi.org/10.5772/54221

distinguishable in their ability to produce biological effects through GLP-1 receptors located in pancreatic cells [3], gastric glands [4] and in adipocytes [5], lung [6] and brain [7-10].

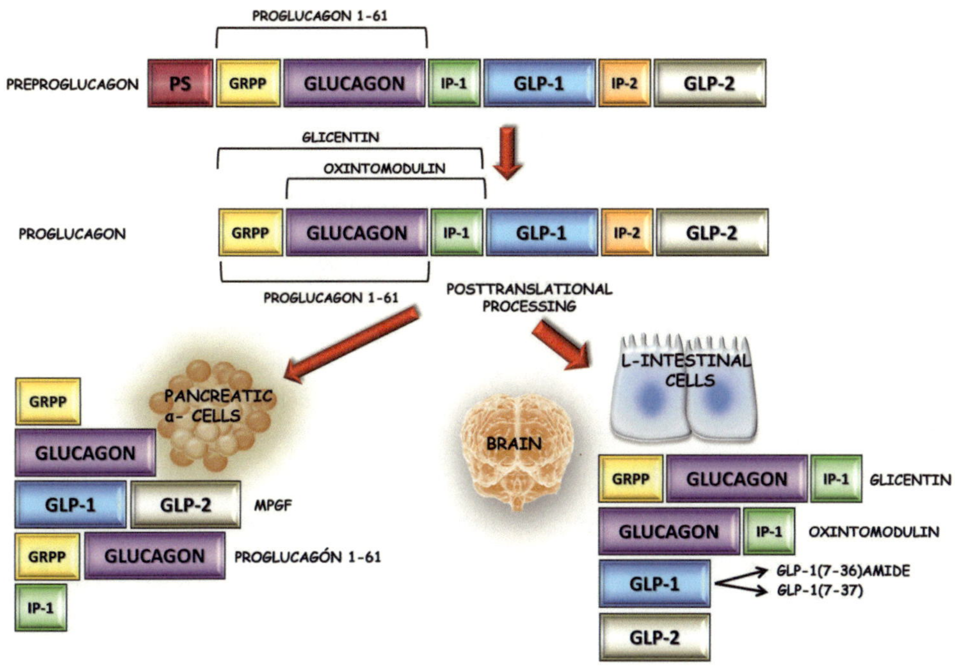

Figure 1. Posttranslational processing of preproglucagon. GLP: Glucagon-like peptide; GRPP: Glicentin-related pancreatic peptide; IP: Intermediate peptide; MPGF: the major proglucagon fragment; PS: Signal peptide.

In addition, GLP-1 and its own receptors are synthesized in the same brain regions, strongly supporting the actions of this peptide on the CNS. Thus, the perfusion of several brain nuclei with GLP-1 produces a selective release of neurotransmitters [11, 12], and the central and peripheral administration of this peptide inhibits food and drink intake [13-15]. The co-expression of GLP-1R, glucokinase, and glucose transporter protein 2 (GLUT-2) in the neurons involved in the control of food intake suggests that these cells may play a role in glucose sensing in the brain [14, 16-19]. Furthermore, GLP-1 has beneficial cardiovascular effects in humans by lowering blood pressure and improving myocardial function [20, 21], although in rats this peptide significantly increases arterial blood pressure and heart rate [22, 23]. Interestingly, GLP-1 has proliferative and antiapoptotic actions on pancreatic β-cells [24, 25], and has neurotrophic and neuroprotective features [21]. Considering the functions of GLP-1, its exendin-4 analogue is used in the treatment of type 2 diabetes [26].

Within the multiple functions of GLP-1, we have selected two important ones, namely, an incretin and an anorexigenic peptide.

2.1. GLP-1 actions as incretin hormone

The proposals made in 1906 by Moore et al. [27] on the antidiabetogenic effect of intestinal factors, and in 1929 by Zung & La Barre [28] on the release of a substance from intestinal mucosa with properties to decrease glycaemia, signalled the start of the development of the incretin concept and the study of the relationships between the gut and the endocrine pancreas. However, for many years these suggestions were ignored, until the development of radioimmunoassays, when Elrich et al. [29] demonstrated that the insulin secretion response to an oral glucose overload was greater to that obtained after intravenous perfusion with the same amount of glucose. This lends support to the belief that substances from the intestine were involved in the postprandial control of insulin secretion, which was referred to accordingly as the incretin effect. It is accepted that 20% to 60% of the increase in postprandial insulin secretion is due to this effect; with the broad oscillation being explained by the amount and composition of food intake.

The functional relationships between the intestine and the pancreatic islet were named by Unger and Eisentraut in 1969 [30] as the enteroinsular axis, while the criteria formulated by Creutzfeldt [31] considered a molecule to be incretin when it is secreted in response to nutrients, and that physiological concentrations increased the secretion of insulin in the presence of high glucose concentrations.

The first peptide described with incretin activity was the gastric inhibitory polypeptide (GIP) that went on to be referred to also as the glucose-dependent insulinotropic polypeptide GIP). Thereafter, the observation of incretin activity after the inactivation of GIP suggested the existence of other molecules with an incretin effect. Thus, in experimental models where GIP was blocked by its own antibodies 50-80% of incretin activity was still observed. We now know that GLP-1 has a greater incretin effect than GIP, being considered the most powerful incretin molecule of all those known. In other words, a molecule with incretin activity may be defined as a hormone of intestinal origin that potentiates the secretion of insulin after the oral ingestion of nutrients. Knowledge of incretins has been very useful for a better understanding of certain pathophysiological entities [32]. In 1986, Nauck et al. [33] first documented a reduced incretin effect in patients, with type 2 diabetes. It is important to note that Nauck et al. described this reduced effect with GIP and not with GLP-1, because at that time GIP was the only incretin known. However, a year later [34], GLP-1 was identified as an incretin hormone and shown to be more effective than GIP to stimulate insulin secretion on a molar basis and at an equivalent level of glucose concentration [35]. Both in non-diabetic and type 2 diabetic subjects, GLP-1 was more effective than GIP at enhancing insulin secretion and lowering glucagon concentrations [36].

The recognition that native GLP-1 is quickly degraded by the protease dipeptidyl peptidase IV (DPP-4) led to the development of GLP-1 agonists that are resistant to this enzyme [37]. The degradation by DPP-4 of exenatide and liraglutide and DPP-4 inhibitors (sitagliptin, saxagliptin, vildagliptin and linagliptin) currently represents an effective therapeutic option for patients with type 2 diabetes. Furthermore, several agents have been developed in recent years, including longer acting DPP-4 resistant GLP-1 agonists.

In addition, many biological effects of GLP-1, other than incretin actions, have been reported in recent decades, representing a good tool for several therapeutic treatments. These GLP-1 effects include properties such as an anorexic peptide, beneficial cardiovascular actions in humans, increased pulmonary surfactant formation in human and experimental animals, pancreatic islet neogenesis and proliferative and antiapoptotic actions. GLP-1 receptors are also widely expressed in the brain [9, 10], where their agonists produce a selective release of neurotransmitters [11, 12] and increase GLP-1 receptor expression in glia after a mechanical lesion of the rat brain has been reported [38]. Accordingly pre-clinical data suggest a neuroprotective/neurotrophic function of GLP-1, and some authors have proposed that this peptide may have a positive potential role for reversing neurodegenerative disorders [21].

2.2. GLP-1 actions in the control of food intake

A number of peptide hormones, previously thought to be specific to the gastroenteropancreatic system and later found also in the mammalian brain, have been shown to modulate appetite, energy homeostasis and body weight. They have these physiological effects together with other neuropeptides, such as neuropeptide Y (NPY), opioid peptides, galanin, vasopressin, and GHRH. Peptide Y (Y_{3-36}) is also released from the gastrointestinal tract postprandially, and acts on the NPY Y_2 receptor in the arcuate nucleus to inhibit feeding, with a long–term effect [39]. Conversely, other satiety signals induced by gut-brain peptides such as GLP-1 [13-15], GLP-2 [40] and cholecystokinin produced a short-term effect, while insulin and leptin [41] inhibit the appetite by increasing the formation of pro-opiomelanocortin (POMC) and reducing NPY action. In addition, ghrelin, a peptide released by the stomach, is stimulated before meals to facilitate NPY action.

GLP-1 and GLP-2 significantly modify feeding behaviour. The intracerebroventricular (icv) or subcutaneous administration (sc) of GLP-1 produced a marked reduction in food intake and water ingestion [13-15]. Exendin-4 proved also to be a potent agonist of GLP-1 by decreasing both food and water intake in a dose-dependent manner. Pre-treatment with exendin [9-39], an inhibitor of the GLP-1 receptor, reversed the inhibitory effects of GLP-1 and exendin-4. These findings suggest that GLP-1 may modulate both food and water intake through either a central or peripheral mechanism. Similar results have been found in humans when the peptide was administered in the periphery [42]. After the subcutaneous administration of GLP-1, it could enter the brain by binding to blood–brain–barrier-free organs such as the subfornical organ and the area postrema [43], or through the choroid plexus, which has a high density of GLP-1 receptors [17].

Several observations suggest a possible action of GLP-1 on thirst-regulatory mechanisms, since GLP-1R mRNA has been located in brain areas related to the control of thirst, such as the preoptic area, glial cells lining the third ventricle and, especially, the neurons of the PVN, which is a key station for water balance regulation through the antidiuretic effects of vasopressin released by its projection to the neurohypophysis [44]. In addition, the icv administration of GLP-1 significantly increases the circulating levels of vasopressin, and the colocalization of the mRNA of the GLP-1 receptor, and vasopressin has been found in the neurons of the PVN [45].

The control of feeding behaviour by GLP-1 and exendin-4 has been explored in Zucker obese rats, resulting in a reduction in food intake, with exendin-4 being much more potent than GLP-1. The long-term sc administration of exendin-4 decreased daily food intake and practically blocked weight gain in obese rats. These observations highlight the potential usefulness of exendin-4 as a tool for treating obesity and/or diabetes. Both GLP-1 and exendin-4 control blood glucose through the stimulation of glucose-dependent insulin secretion, the inhibition of glucagon secretion, and delayed gastric emptying [34, 46, 47], which facilitate the decrease in blood glucose in type 1 and type 2 diabetic patients [48]. In the light of these results, different N-terminal substituted GLP-1 analogues resistant to DPP-IV have recently been developed. These resistant analogues have a prolonged metabolic stability in vivo and improved biological activity, which is of great interest in the treatment of type 2 diabetes and/or obesity.

On the other hand, the icv administration of GLP-2 to mice and rats produced a marked decrease in food intake but not in water ingestion [43]. Surprisingly, this effect was avoided by the administration of exendin [9-39], an antagonist of GLP-1.

3. Importance of the VMH and LH in the control of food intake

In recent years, researchers have been focusing on the relationship between gut hormones and the brain areas controlling appetite, ingestion, food reward and body weight [49, 50].

Both gut and brain are considered the main organs responsible for controlling body weight. The hypothalamus is the focus of many of the peripheral signals and neural pathways that control energy homeostasis and body weight. However, new evidence has been forthcoming in recent years to suggest that human food intake is also controlled by other areas in the central nervous system, such as subcortical and cortical areas.

The hypothalamus regulates body weight by precisely balancing the intake of food, energy expenditure and body fat tissue. The role of the hypothalamus in regulating food intake and body weight was established in 1940 [51] through the classical experiments by Hetherington and Ranson. They placed bilateral electrolytic lesions in a vast region of the hypothalamus, occupied by the dorsomedial and ventromedial areas, the arcuate nucleus, the fornix and a portion of the lateral hypothalamic area (without disturbing the pituitary gland). The results were a marked adiposity characterized by a doubling of body weight and a huge increase in body lipids. A few years later, Anand and Brobeck [52] continued these experiments in greater detail, demonstrating that lesions of the lateral hypothalamus at the level adjacent to the ventromedial nucleus caused loss of appetite, inanition, and even death by starvation. Thus, the lateral hypothalamic area acted as a "feeding centre" and the ventromedial nucleus as a "satiety centre". Since then, it has been established that the "dual centre model" regulates feeding [53], that the proposed lesioning of the VMH increases appetite, while stimulating the VMH decreases it. By contrast, lesioning or stimulating the LH decreases or induces appetite, respectively.

http://dx.doi.org/10.5772/54221

The dual control theory of feeding is based on the homeostatic view of hunger and satiety, together with the consideration of glucose not only as a metabolic fuel, but also as a signalling molecule, and the existence of specialized neurons containing glucose sensors that activate or inhibit feeding when blood glucose levels change. A fall in glucose would activate the LH and, consequently, give rise to hunger. Hunger leads to the consumption of food and thus to an elevation of glucose levels that would activate the VMH, leading to a feeling of satiety that will stop the feeding, and eventually glucose levels would fall again.

Over the last 25 years, there has been a dramatic increase in studies on the hypothalamus. Knowledge of the hypothalamus has only recently evolved from anatomical concepts (nuclei, 'areas' and fibre tracts) to neurochemicals (characterizing the distributions of neuropeptides and transmitters and their receptors), focusing on the modulation of feeding behaviour and energy expenditure. We are now beginning to reach the stage of functionally understanding the molecular mechanisms, defining exactly which neuronal populations respond to specific nutritional and related signals, and how they pass on that information. At least 25 transmitters have been suggested to play key roles in feeding behaviour [54]. Accordingly, the dorsomedial and paraventricular regions are important within the hypothalamus, along with the well-established VMH and LH [55]. The VMH, which consists of the ventromedial and arcuate nuclei, respectively, is a key region for integrating the peripheral signals of nutrient status and adiposity. The arcuate nucleus contains neurons with NPY/AgRP and POMC, which have opposing effects on energy homeostasis. Thus, NPY increases food intake and activates energy sparing mechanisms, while melanocortins decrease food intake and increase energy expenditure [56]. On the other hand, the LH, the classical "feeding centre", is a heterogeneous area that receives a multitude of neuronal inputs from many areas known to be important in the regulation of energy homeostasis: LH encompassing neurons and terminals containing orexigenic peptides. Basically, the LH contains two distinct neuronal cell populations that regulate feeding behaviour: containing hypocretin/orexin [57, 58] and a melanin-concentrating hormone (MCH) [59] (Figure 2).

In addition to its response to circulating peptides and hormones that reflect energy status, the brain, and specifically the hypothalamus, also senses and responds to changes in blood glucose levels [14, 16, 18, 19, 60]. There are several areas in the brain acting as a glucose sensor. Examples of these are the hypothalamus [60, 61], nucleus solitarius [62] and amygdala [63]. The glucose sensing neurons located in these areas monitor energy status and initiate the responses to maintain glucose and energy homeostasis. Besides the brain glucose sensors, there are also glucose sensors located in peripheral tissues including the intestine [64], the carotid body [65] and mesenteric veins [66]. In fact, glucose sensors in the hypothalamus were first discovered in the VMH and LH [57, 58]. Moreover, interstitial glucose levels in the VMH and LH vary with blood glucose concentration [67], and these changes in glucose have been postulated to trigger meal initiation. Since glucose is the brain's primary fuel, it should respond to a severe glucose deficiency. In this way, VMH glucose sensors may play a role in detecting and countering severe glucose deficiency [68]. However, Levin et al. recently showed there was no correlation between VMH glucose levels and spontaneous feeding

[69]. It is therefore unlikely that VMH glucose sensors regulate meal-to-meal food intake, although it does not rule out a role for glucose sensors in the LH or other brain regions.

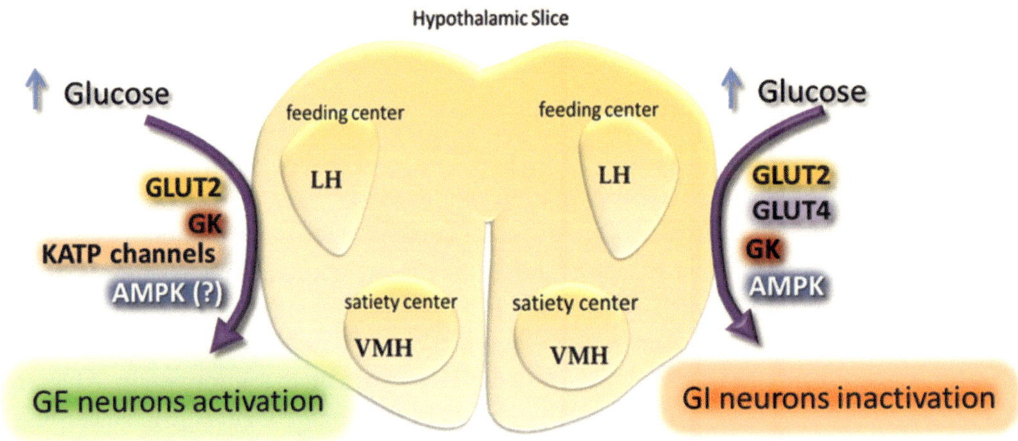

Figure 2. Schematic representation of a hypothalamic slice. Localization of the VMH and LH are indicated. GE and GI neurons are activated or inactivated by a rise in glucose, respectively. The putative components responsible for glucose sensing in GE and GI are shown.

Glucose sensing neurons are those that alter their frequency of potential actions in response to changes in interstitial glucose levels [60, 70]. There are mainly two neurons whose activity is regulated by alterations in glucose levels [60]: Glucose-excited (GE) neurons that increase their potential frequency in response to increases in interstitial glucose from 0.1 to 2.5 mM glucose. The other kind of neurons (GI) are those that decrease their frequency of potential actions when glucose rises. More recently [71], other neurons have been described that respond to an increase of more than 5 mM glucose. Thus, high GE (HGE) and high GI (HGI) neurons increase or decrease their frequency of potential actions, respectively, in response to increases in interstitial glucose from 5 to 20 mM, although these neurons are still not thoroughly characterized, and there are doubts about their physiological significance. However, it is important to consider that the interstitial brain glucose concentration is approximately 30% of the concentrations found in the blood. Thus, when the peripheral plasma glucose concentration is 7.6 mM, the interstitial VMH glucose is only 2.5 mM [67]. Decreasing plasma glucose to 2–3 mM or increasing to 15 mM resulted in brain glucose levels of 0.16 mM and 4.5 mM, respectively [67, 72]. Therefore, glucose concentrations found within the majority of the brain in vivo under physiological and pathophysiological conditions are within the 0.2 to 5 mM range [73-76], and it seems that the GE and GI neurons are mainly responsible for glucose sensing, since it is unclear whether brain glucose levels ever exceed 5 mM in the presence of an intact blood brain barrier. However, it should be noted that hyperglycemia impairs the integrity of the blood brain barrier [77], raising the question of whether HGE and HGI neurons could have a physiological significance in hyperglycemia-associated pathology. Nevertheless, it seems that glucose sensing neurons could be functioning to protect the brain against a severe energy deficit.

The components responsible for glucose sensing in GE neurons seem to be shared with those present in pancreatic beta-cells: GLUT2, as well as glucokinase. Furthermore, GE uses the ATP-sensitive potassium (KATP) channel to sense glucose, as occurs in beta-cells. However, while KATP channels are expressed in all GE neurons, only approximately half of VMH GE neurons express glucokinase, and approximately 30% express GLUT2 [78].

Multiple subtypes of GE neurons may exist that use alternate glucose sensing strategies. Thus, Claret et al. have shown that transgenic mice lacking the $\alpha2$ subunit of AMPK, an important cellular fuel gauge, also lack GE neurons in ARC [79]. However, other authors [80] have shown that the acute pharmacological activation or inhibition of AMPK had no effect on glucose sensing in VMH GE neurons.

GI neurons have similar components to GE and, therefore, to beta-cells in glucose sensing, such as glucokinase [78, 81], as well as GLUT2 and GLUT4. However, the signal transduction pathway, whereby changes in intracellular ATP alter the activity of GI neurons, is completely different. In this case, the activation of $\alpha2$AMPK by glucose mediates the activation of VMH GI neurons, as described by Murphy et al. [82]. Hypothalamic $\alpha2$AMPK is a key kinase involved in the energy balance and is a target for a number of hormones and a transmitter that regulates the energy balance [83-88]. The pharmacological activation of hypothalamic AMPK increases food intake [89]. It is not therefore surprising that decreased glucose activates AMPK in GI neurons.

4. AMPK, together with mTOR and its downstream target S6K1, integrate nutrient and hormonal signals to maintain energy homeostasis

AMPK is a nutrient and energy sensor. AMPK senses cellular energy availability by detecting the AMP/ATP ratio. AMPK is activated in low energy states and promotes ATP-generating catabolic pathways and inhibits anabolic reactions [90-92].

AMPK is a heterotrimeric complex that contains a catalytic α-subunit ($\alpha1$ or $\alpha2$) and two regulatory subunits, β ($\beta1$, $\beta2$) and γ ($\gamma1$, $\gamma2$, $\gamma3$). The α-subunit contains a kinase domain. The β-subunit contains the regions that permit interaction with other α and γ subunits and a carbohydrate-binding domain that facilitates binding to glycogen. The γ subunit contains four tandem repeats, which are four binding sites for adenosine derivates denominated as CBS motifs (cystathionine β-synthase) [92, 93].

Different isoforms and the alternative splicing of some mRNAs encoding these subunits give rise to a wide range of heterotrimeric combinations. The expression of the catalytic subunits ($\alpha1$ and $\alpha2$) is also different. The $\alpha2$ subunit expression has been found in pancreatic beta-cells, neurons, skeletal muscle and the heart. The liver has 50% of each AMPKα isoform ($\alpha1$ and $\alpha2$), while adipose tissue expresses higher levels of the AMPK$\alpha1$ isoform [93].

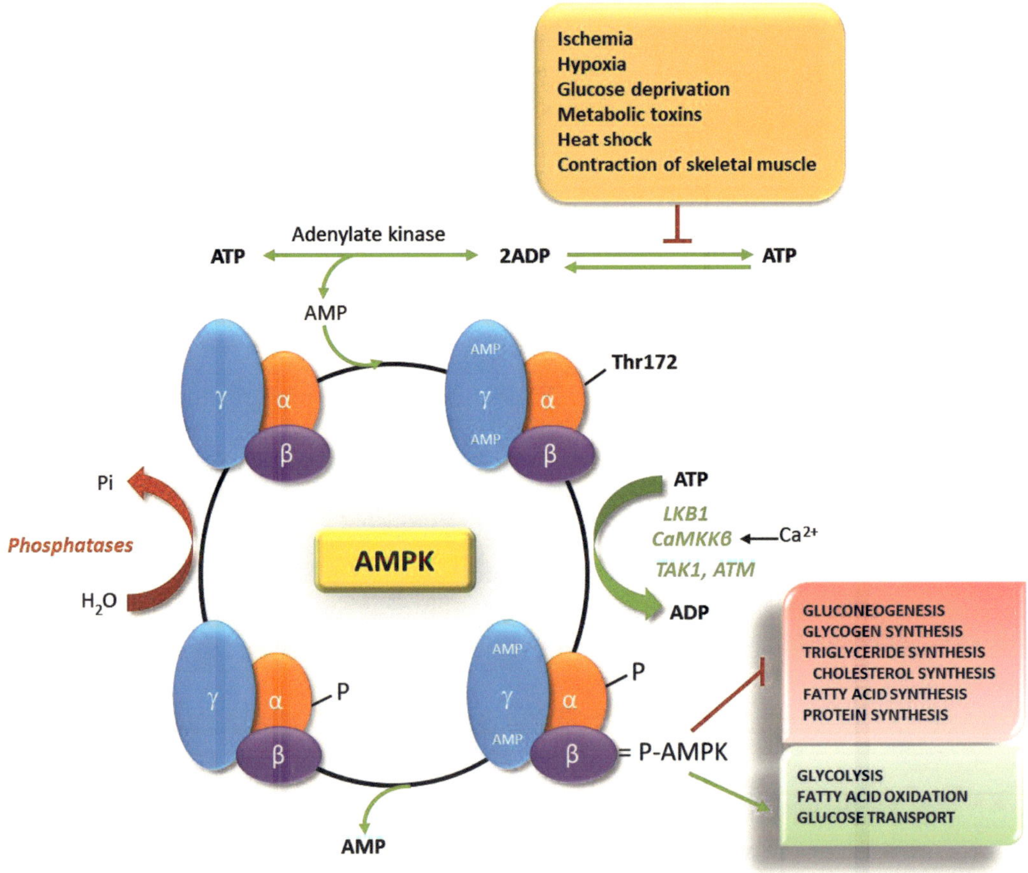

Figure 3. Schematic representation of AMPK's subunits and its activation process. AMPK detects changes in the cellular energy state that occur in response to nutrient variations or metabolic stress caused by changes in the AMP/ATP ratio. The activation of AMPK triggers key enzymes of glucose metabolism and fatty acids. The long-term effect of AMPK activation is the transcriptional control of the main elements involved in these metabolic pathways.

AMPK serine/threonine kinase activity is stimulated by the phosphorylation of the α-subunit on the Thr residue (Thr172). This activation process is regulated by several upstream kinases. The two main kinases in mammals are liver kinase B1 (LKB1), identified as a tumour-suppressor, and the Ca^{2+}/calmodulin-dependent protein kinase (mainly CaMKKβ) [92, 93]. AMPK activity is also allosterically regulated by AMP binding to the γ subunit (Figure 3). Recent studies have found that AMP or ADP binding to the γ regulatory subunit protect the activated phosphorylated form of AMPK [94, 95]. AMP, ADP and ATP bind the γ subunit with similar affinity [94]. AMPK can be activated by increases in AMP and ADP according to changes in the cellular levels of adenosine derivatives. LKB1 phosphorylates AMPK in almost all tissues, while CaMKKβ plays an important role in neurons and T lymphocytes. Other studies have suggested that a member of the MAPKKK family, TAK1 (transforming growth factor β-activated kinase) could be an important AMPK upstream kinase in cardiac cells [96], and ATM (ataxia telangiectasia mutated) may also regulate the phosphorylation of Thr172 [97]. The level of Thr172 phosphorylation depends also on the activity of protein phosphatases [98, 99]. The effect of an increase in AMP inhibits phosphatase activity, and considering that LKB1 is constitutively active [100], the response after a rise in AMP increases the phosphorylation of Thr172 and the activation of AMPK.

AMPK can detect changes in cellular energy state that occur in response to nutrient variations. Any cellular or metabolic stress that reduces ATP production (e.g., heat shock, hypoxia, ischemia, glucose deprivation) or accelerates ATP consumption (e.g., contraction of skeletal muscle) will increase the ADP/ATP ratio, which will be amplified by the action of adenylate kinase, resulting in increased AMP/ATP with the consequent activation of AMPK (Figure 3). Once activated, AMPK first directly affects the activity of key enzymes of glucose metabolism and fatty acids, and second, proceeds to the long-term regulation of the transcriptional control of the main elements involved in these metabolic pathways. The net result of the activation of AMPK will restore the energy balance, inhibiting the anabolic pathways responsible for the synthesis of macromolecules, such as proteins and glycogen, and also of the following lipids: fatty acids, triglycerides and cholesterol, while activating the catabolic pathways, such as the oxidation of fatty acids, glucose uptake and glycolysis [101] (Figure 3).

The mTOR is a serine/threonine kinase that responds to nutrients and hormonal signals [102-104]. mTOR forms two distinct complexes with different sensitivities to rapamycin: mTORC1 and mTORC2. Both complexes contain mTOR, GβL (G-protein β-protein subunit-like), mLST8 (mammalian lethal with SEC13 protein) and deptor (DEP domain containing mTOR interacting protein) [103, 105, 106]. This complex, along with raptor (rapamycin-sensitive adaptor protein of mTOR) and PRAS40 (proline-rich Akt substrate of 40 kDa) forms mTORC1, which is rapamycin and nutrient sensitive. However, mTORC2 comprises mTOR, GβL/mLST8 and deptor together with rictor (rapamycin-insensitive companion of mTOR), mSin 1 (mammalian stress-activated MAPK-interacting protein 1) and protor 1/2 (protein observed with rictor ½), which is insensitive to acute rapamycin (Figure 4)

mTORC1 regulates metabolism and cell growth in response to several environmental signals. The presence of amino acids, growth factors and mitogens stimulates mTORC1, which promotes anabolic processes. The mTORC1 activity phosphorylates multiple substrates, with S6K1 and the initiation factor 4E binding proteins (4E-BPs) being the best characterized [106-108]. The activation of mTORC1 induces the dissociation of 4E-BP from the eukaryotic translation initiation factor 4E (eIF4E), facilitating mRNA translation [109], and the activation of S6K1 promotes protein synthesis. Moreover, the mTORC2 function is less well known. It is known that mTORC2 phosphorylates Akt and appears to regulate mainly cell proliferation and cell survival [110] (Figure 4)

The effect growth factors have on mTORC1 is mediated through phosphatidylinositol-3,4,5-triphosphate kinase (PI3K) activation, the subsequent activation of phosphoinositide-dependent kinase (PDK1) and Akt. Once activated, Akt phosphorylates tuberous sclerosis complex 2 (TSC2), suppressing the inhibitory effect of the TSC1-TSC2 complex in mTORC1.

TSC2 functions as a GTPase-activating protein of Ras homolog enriched in brain (Rheb), which is an mTORC1 activator. Mitogens activating the Ras/MAPK cascade also activate mTORC1. ERK phosphorylates TSC2, inhibiting the TSC1/TSC2 complex and inducing mTORC1 activity [111]. Raptor is additionally phosphorylated by ERK [112] (Figure 4)

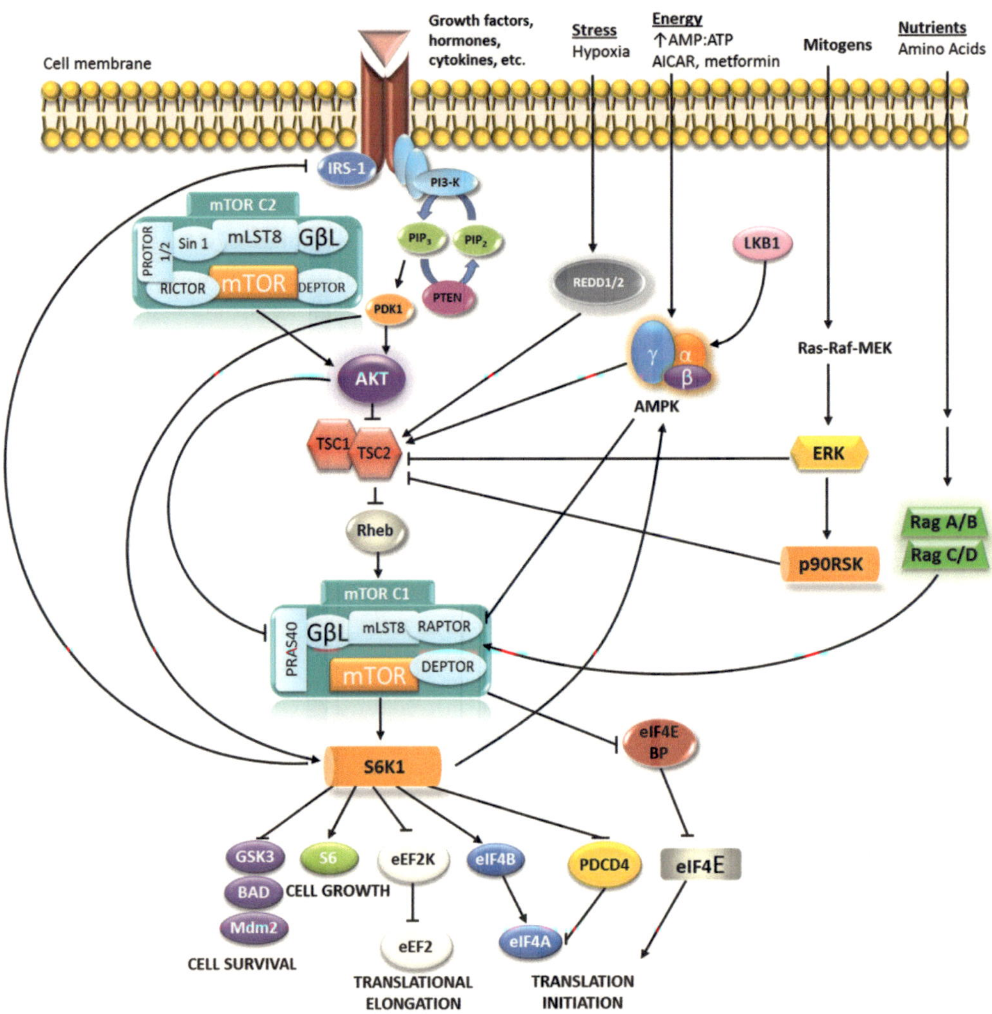

Figure 4. Network of proteins involved in the AMPK/mTOR/S6K1 signalling pathway

mTORC1 is also stimulated by amino acids, especially leucine. This activation pathway is independent of PI3K. The amino-acid regulation of mTOR needs rag GTPases and Rheb. The detailed mechanism of activation is unknown. It has been suggested that rag GTPases may control the localization of mTOR to specific vesicular membranes containing Rheb-GTP [113].

mTORC1 activity is inhibited in conditions of energy depletion coordinated with AMPK activity. An increase in AMP/ATP ratio activates AMPK, which phosphorylates the TSC2, and this modification induces the concomitant inhibition of mTORC1 mediated by the TSC1-TSC2 complex [114]. Furthermore, AMPK phosphorylates raptor in mTORC1, which downregulates this complex [115].

In addition, energy depletion inhibits mTORC1 by a mechanism that is independent of AMPK activation. This effect is mediated by eliminating the GTP loading of Rheb [116].

4.1. Expression and regulation of these sensors in the VMH and LH

Studies in recent years have established a direct relationship between metabolic sensor activity in the hypothalamus and the regulation of food intake, body weight and energy homeostasis.

AMPK is broadly expressed throughout the brain. The $\alpha 2$ catalytic subunit is present with a high distribution in neurons and activated astrocytes [117]. Hypothalamic AMPK has been assumed to play a role in the central regulation of food intake and energy balance, whereby fasting increases and re-feeding decreases AMPK activity in various hypothalamic nuclei. Alterations of hypothalamic AMPK activity specifically affected $\alpha 2$AMPK and did not change $\alpha 1$AMPK [88].

The hypothalamic AMPK role has been studied in vivo by the expression of AMPK mutants: dominant negative AMPK (DN-AMPK) or constitutively active AMPK (CA-AMPK). The expression of CA-AMPK in the medial hypothalamus by adenoviruses increased food intake and body weight, whereas the expression of DN-AMPK inhibited them [88]. These alterations change the hypothalamic neuropeptide expression: the expression of CA-AMPK enhances the effect of fasting, increasing the expression of NPY and AgRP in the ARC and the melanin-concentrating hormone in the lateral hypothalamus, whereas the hypothalamic expression of DN-AMPK decreases the expression of orexigenic neuropeptides NPY and AgRP in ARC [88, 118].

mTORC1 is another metabolic sensor that plays an important role in the regulation of feeding behaviour and body weight in the hypothalamus [119, 120]. mTOR and its downstream target S6K1 are widely distributed in the rat brain. The activated forms of mTOR and S6K1 are localized mainly in the paraventricular and arcuate nuclei [119], being co-localized in a high percentage of orexigenic neurons that express AgRP/NPY and also in around half the anorexigenic neurons that express POMC/CART in the arcuate nuclei [119].

mTORC1 activation in the rat hypothalamus decreases food intake and body weight. Similar results were found by introducing constitutively active S6K1 mediated by adenovirus into the mediobasal hypothalamus of the rat brain. By contrast, the injection of dominant-negative S6K1 leads to an increase in food intake and body weight [121].

4.1.1. Nutrient regulation

Food intake leads to periods of fasting and feeding that are associated with substantial changes in the level of available nutrients (e.g., glucose and amino acids) and accompanied by hormonal changes. Several studies describe the effect of glucose on both metabolic sensors, AMPK and mTOR, in hypothalamic areas. During fasting, the decrease in glucose concentration activates AMPK. This period is also characterized by low levels of glucose and amino acids, and the mTOR complex is kept inactive. The increase in glucose levels after food intake decreases the activity of AMPK and, conversely, the activity of the mTOR/S6K1 pathway is stimulated by higher levels of glucose and amino acids.

Thus, Kim et al. reported that decreasing intracellular glucose through the supply of 2-deoxyglucose increases hypothalamic AMPK activity and food intake. By contrast, hyperglycaemia decreases hypothalamic AMPK activity [122]. It was also observed that AMPK activity is inhibited in arcuate, ventromedial, dorsomedial, paraventricular nuclei and the LH by high glucose and re-feeding. [88]. Increases in α2-AMPK activities in arcuate-ventromedial and paraventricular nuclei are also detected during insulin-induced hypoglycaemic in rats [123]. However, fasted rats recorded a decrease in the number of hypothalamic cells expressing mTOR and S6K1 activated forms specifically in the arcuate nucleus, with these changes responding to the availability of nutrients [119]. Similar findings were subsequently confirmed, also showing that the constitutive activation of S6K in the mediobasal hypothalamic area protects against the harmful effects of a high-fat diet [121].

It has also been established that AMPK and mTOR are involved in the anorexigenic effect induced by high protein diets. Thus, a high protein diet and the intracerebroventricular administration of leucine decreased AMPK phosphorylation in the rat hypothalamus [120]. The activation of hypothalamic mTORC1 is additionally produced by a high protein diet and the intracerebroventricular administration of amino acids or leucine [119, 124].

4.1.2. Gut hormone regulation and signals from energy stores

The effects of glucose, amino acids and other nutrients are reinforced by the effects of intestinal peptides, as stated above. They are able to regulate food intake, energetic homeostasis and body weight. The gastrointestinal tract responds to gut contents by secreting hormones, which can serve to inform the CNS of nutrient status. Thus, circulating ghrelin, the only intestinal peptide with orexigenic properties, is high in the period before a meal, and the level declines an hour after eating [125]. Ghrelin stimulates food intake in lean and obese humans [126]. In contrast, anorexigenic intestinal peptides as peptide YY (PYY), pancreatic polypeptide (PP), GLP-1, oxyntomodulin and cholecystokinin are low during the fasting period, and their level increases after a meal, and some of them are released proportionally to the amount of calories ingested (Reviewed in [127]).

Other signals that inform the state of energy stores, such as leptin and insulin levels, are important modulators of feeding behaviour. Insulin regulates the storage of nutrients and also informs the brain about the energy balance [128]. Leptin is produced by adipose tissue and informs the brain about the energy storage status [128].

We now know that the function of at least some of these peptides may be mediated by the modulation of hypothalamic metabolic sensors. Thus, it has been reported that hypothalamic AMPK activity is also regulated by several orexigenic and anorexigenic signals. Ghrelin, the intestinal peptide with orexigenic properties, activates AMPK and stimulates food intake [87, 89]. By contrast, anorexigenic peptides such as leptin decrease AMPK activity in the ARC and PVN [88, 89, 129]. However, leptin treatment increased mTOR and S6K1 hypothalamic activity [130].

It has recently been suggested that ghrelin activates AMPK in presynaptic neurons, inducing an increase in activity in NPY/AgRP neurons promoting sustained food intake, and this signal stops after leptin is released by adipose tissue, signalling to stimulate POMC neurons inhibiting feeding and also to inhibit the AMPK in the presynaptic neurons, inactivating the release of NPY/AgRP [131].

Inoki et al. previously reported that the activation of AMPK induces the inhibition of mTOR activity [114]. It has recently been posited that S6K phosphorylates $\alpha 2$ AMPK. This process is necessary for the leptin effects on hypothalamic AMPK activity [132].

These findings indicate that hypothalamic AMPK and mTOR respond to changes in glucose and other nutrients in opposite ways, and their effects on the regulation of food intake may overlap.

5. Modulation of AMPK and S6K by GLP-1/exendin-4 in these hypothalamic areas

As indicated before, GLP-1 is able to induce several effects contributing to the control of feeding behaviour. It inhibited gastric acid secretion and emptying, stimulated postprandial insulin secretion and inhibited glucagon release. GLP-1 treatment to type 2 diabetic subjects normalized the fasting levels of blood glucose and decreased postprandial glucose levels. We have also reported that GLP-1 reduces glucose metabolism in the human hypothalamus and brain stem [133].

In general, the brain activity of AMPK is activated by fasting and is inhibited by re-feeding [88, 122, 123], but the effect of glucose on AMPK also regulates *Ampk* expression in VMH [134]. Thus, fasting increased *Ampk* mRNA expression in the hypothalamus of rats, and the ICV administration of GLP-1 reduced that effect [135].

The glucose effect on AMPK might be region-specific in hypothalamic areas that have opposite effects over the control of feeding behaviour. We have also reported, using rat hypothalamic slices, that high glucose levels decrease the expression of *Ampk-$\alpha 2$* mRNA, specifically in the LH, but not in the VMH [83]. The decrease in *AMPK$\alpha 2$* expression in response to high glucose levels was reversed by the presence of GLP-1 [83]. Sanz et al. have also reported a different response to glucose in the VMH and LH [136, 137]. The distinctive response in the LH compared to the VMH may be explained by the different role these two areas have in the control of food intake.

Results obtained from in vivo studies conducted on lean and obese Zucker rats showed that the effects fasting and re-feeding have on the activity of AMPK and S6K in the areas involved in the control of feeding are modulated by exendin-4 treatment [83].

It has been previously reported that the anorexigenic effects produced by the intraperitoneal administration of exendin-4 led to a reduction in food intake and increased the period between meals [138]. Additionally, the peripheral administration of exendin-4 and liraglutide regulates food intake by activating the GLP-1 receptors expressed on both vagal afferents and CNS [139]. Recent studies conducted within our group [83] have focused on clarifying the coordinated effects of fasting, re-feeding and exendin-4 administration on the activity of AMPK and S6K in the VMH and LH. The results of these studies show that fasting increases hypothalamic AMPK activity in both areas in lean Zucker rats. However, the subcutaneous administration of exendin-4 over the last hour reversed this effect, whereas exendin-4 activated AMPK in animals re-fed for two hours when AMPK activity was markedly inhibited. The activation degree of AMPK after four hours of re-feeding differed in both areas. Thus, the activation level of AMPK in the VMH was similar to fasted rats. However, AMPK activity in the LH was still low, and exendin-4 treatment decreased AMPK activity in the VMH, whereas no significant effect was detected in the LH (Figure 5).

Anorexic peptides also regulate the mTOR/S6K1 pathway in hypothalamic areas. Insulin and leptin increases the activated forms of S6K [119]. The administration of exendin-4 also regulates S6K activity and the effect is dependent on the activation status of S6K, as occurred with AMPK. We thus found that S6K activation peaked in animals re-fed for four hours. However, the administration of exendin-4 strongly stimulated S6K activity in animals re-fed for two hours. In contrast, exendin-4 decreased S6K activity in the VMH of lean rats re-fed for four hours [83] (Figure 5).

The use of rat organotypic hypothalamic slices confirmed that AMPK activity at low glucose concentrations was stimulated, and S6K activity was maintained with minimal activation [83]. GLP-1 treatment reversed the effect of glucose on AMPK and did not modify S6K activity in the VMH and LH. High levels of glucose stimulated S6K activity in both nuclei, and the presence of GLP-1 reversed such activation. Similar results were found using hypothalamic GT1-7 and neuroblastoma N2A cell lines [83]. The metabolic sensors in these cells respond to glucose as described above, and GLP-1 treatment reversed the glucose effects [83].

The effect of GLP-1 on AMPK activity was also reported in other brain areas. Thus, GLP-1R activation in hindbrain suppressed food intake, and that effect is accompanied by the suppression of AMPK activity [140].

The complexities of the regulation of hypothalamic AMPK activity have previously been described for some hormones. Thus, the cocaine-and amphetamine-regulated transcript (CART) has been reported to have an anorexic effect after intracerebroventricular administration [141], while CART injected directly into the paraventricular or arcuate nucleus of fasted rats increases food intake [142]. Likewise, differences in the effect of regulatory peptides on AMPK as a function of nutritional status have been previously described. Ghrelin or cannabinoids have ad libitum effects [143], whereas leptin [88] and adiponectin [144] only have an effect after variable periods of fasting or re-feeding.

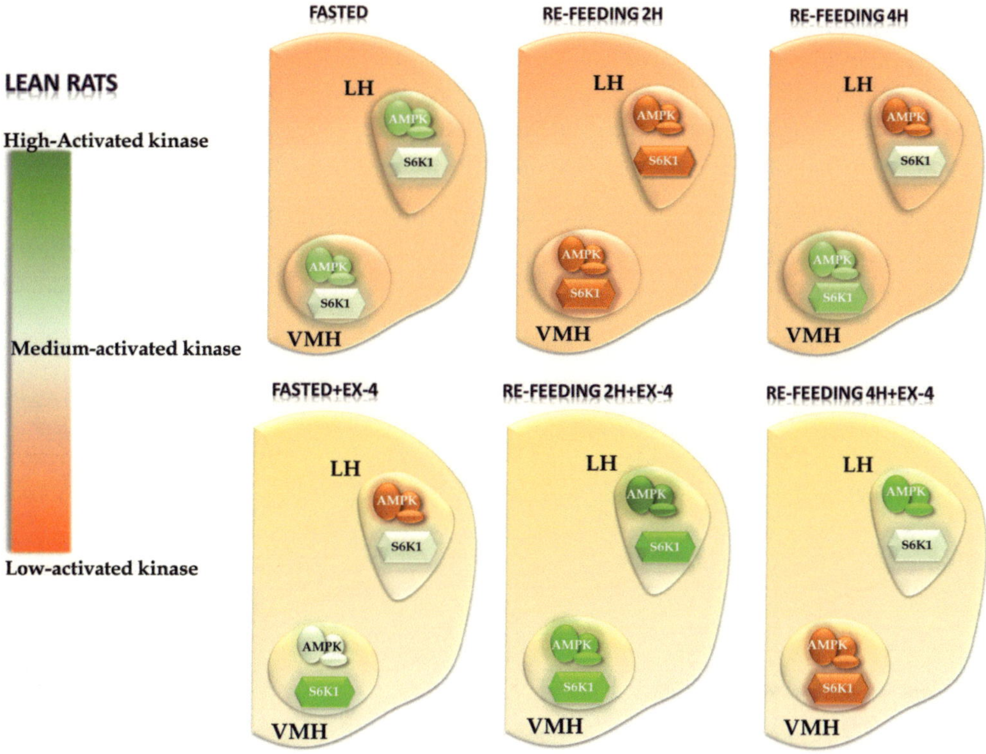

Figure 5. Effects of exendin-4 administration in fasted or re-fed lean rats on the activity of AMPK and S6K. Lean Zucker rats were fasted or re-fed for two or four hours. In some cases, the GLP-1 analogue exendin-4 (100 nM) was administrated. The activation states of AMPK and S6K were determined by quantifying phospho-specific forms in VMH and LH areas.

6. GLP-1/exendin-4 as a compensator of the disturbances in AMPK and S6K activities occurring in obesity

In obesity, the elevated levels of nutrients and hormonal modifications alter the activity of hypothalamic metabolic sensors. Thus, diet-induced obesity reduced hypothalamic AMPK activity [145]. The GLP-1 receptor agonist exendin-4 is one of the agents used in the treatment of type 2 diabetes [146] and is a long-acting receptor agonist of GLP-1 that also produces weight loss [147-149].

The obese Zucker (fa/fa) rat provides a well-established animal model of insulin resistance and genetic obesity and, in comparison with lean Zucker rats, manifests hyperinsulinemia and hyperlipidemia. We have previously noted that the peripheral long-term subcutaneous administration of exendin-4 decreased food intake and induced weight loss in both obese and lean control Zucker rats [15].

Zucker rats have been used to analyze the exendin-4 effect on the activity of AMPK and S6K in the VMH and LH areas [83]. The results obtained showed that AMPK activity was lower in the obese than in the lean Zucker rats in both areas. Interestingly, the effect of exendin-4 administration on fasted obese Zucker rats was different compared to the lean rats. The absence of exendin-4 effect in obese rats maintains AMPK activity at a level of activation similar to the lean animals after the administration of exendin-4 [83] (Figure 5).

These results suggest that GLP-1/exendin-4 might compensate for the alterations in AMPK, activity produced either by oscillations in glucose levels or by pathologies such as obesity or episodes of hyperinsulinemia (Figure 5, 6).

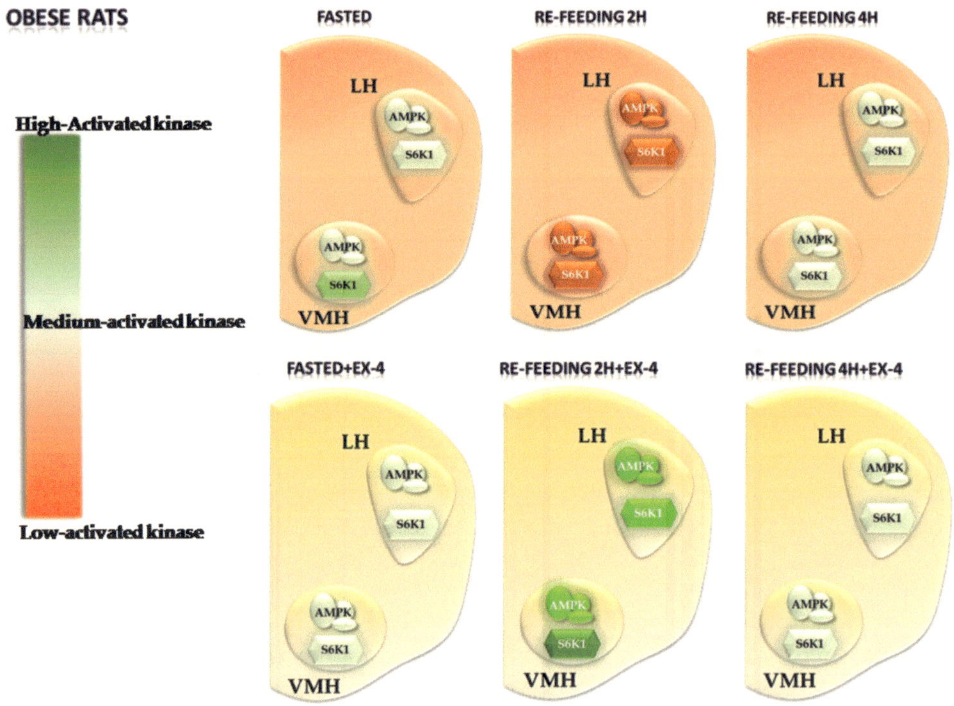

Figure 6. Effects of exendin-4 administration in fasted or re-fed obese rats on the activity of AMPK and S6K. Lean Zucker rats were fasted or re-fed for two or four hours. In some cases, the GLP-1 analogue exendin-4 (100 nM) was administrated. The activation states of AMPK and S6K were determined by quantifying phospho-specific forms in the VMH and LH areas.

Another difference in the level of activation of AMPK between obese and lean Zucker rats was observed after re-feeding for four hours. The AMPK activity in the LH was higher in obese compared to lean animals (Figure 5, 6).

After two hours of re-feeding, exendin-4 treatment increased S6K activity in the VMH and LH in obese rats. Nevertheless, the effect of exendin-4 on S6K activity in the VMH differed between obese and lean rats. Exendin-4 administration did not modify S6K activity in the

LH of lean and obese rats after four hours of re-feeding, whereas exendin-4 reduced S6K activity in the VMH of lean Zucker rats but not in their obese counterparts [83].

The prolonged activation of hypothalamic S6K inhibits insulin signalling and contributes to hepatic insulin resistance [150], suggesting that hypothalamic S6K activation would be involved in the pathogenesis of diet-induced hepatic insulin resistance. Our data indicate that S6K activity in the presence of exendin-4 could be decreased when this protein is maximally activated. This suggests that exendin-4 treatment in diabetic subjects could also improve hepatic insulin resistance.

7. Conclusions

We have reported here some of the many actions of GLP-1, such as, its role as an incretin hormone and controlling food intake. Accordingly, we have reviewed the importance of hypothalamic areas in the control of food intake, such as, for example, the ventromedial and lateral hypothalamus. In parallel, the function of AMPK and the mTOR/S6K pathway has been studied in those areas. Likewise, we have explored the coordinated response of hypothalamic AMPK and S6K to alterations in nutritional status and energy storage. Our results have revealed both the activation of AMPK and S6K in the VMH and LH in response to changes in glucose concentration or nutritional state, and that GLP-1/exendin-4 acts by counteracting the activation/inactivation of these kinases and contributing to the balance of proper AMPK and S6K activation. It therefore seems that GLP-1/exendin-4 might be acting in the VMH and LH, interacting with the AMPK/S6K signalling pathways, and modulating the activation status of AMPK and S6K in response to nutrient fluctuations. Likewise, GLP-1/exendin-4 would contribute to the normalization of the altered levels of these kinases in pathophysiological states such as obesity, for example.

Author details

Veronica Hurtado[1,2,3], Isabel Roncero[1,2,3], Enrique Blazquez[1,2,3], Elvira Alvarez[1,2,3] and Carmen Sanz[1,2,3,4]

1 Department of Biochemistry and Molecular Biology. Faculty of Medicine. University Complutense of Madrid, Spain

2 Instituto de Investigación Sanitaria del Hospital Clínico San Carlos (IdISSC), Spain

3 The Center for Biomedical Research in Diabetes and Associated Metabolic Disorders (CIBERDEM), Spain

4 Department of Cellular Biology. Faculty of Medicine. University Complutense of Madrid, Spain

References

[1] Mojsov S, Heinrich G, Wilson IB, Ravazzola M, Orci L, Habener JF. Preproglucagon gene expression in pancreas and intestine diversifies at the level of post-translational processing. J Biol Chem1986 Sep 5;261(25):11880-9.

[2] Orskov C, Holst JJ, Poulsen SS, Kirkegaard P. Pancreatic and intestinal processing of proglucagon in man. Diabetologia1987 Nov;30(11):874-81.

[3] Goke R, Trautmann ME, Haus E, Richter G, Fehmann HC, Arnold R, et al. Signal transmission after GLP-1(7-36)amide binding in RINm5F cells. Am J Physiol1989 Sep; 257(3 Pt 1):G397-401.

[4] Uttenthal LO, Blazquez E. Characterization of high-affinity receptors for truncated glucagon-like peptide-1 in rat gastric glands. FEBS Lett1990 Mar 12;262(1):139-41.

[5] Valverde I, Merida E, Delgado E, Trapote MA, Villanueva-Penacarrillo ML. Presence and characterization of glucagon-like peptide-1(7-36) amide receptors in solubilized membranes of rat adipose tissue. Endocrinology1993 Jan;132(1):75-9.

[6] Richter G, Goke R, Goke B, Schmidt H, Arnold R. Characterization of glucagon-like peptide-I(7-36)amide receptors of rat lung membranes by covalent cross-linking. FEBS Lett1991 Mar 25;280(2):247-50.

[7] Shimizu I, Hirota M, Ohboshi C, Shima K. Identification and localization of glucagon-like peptide-1 and its receptor in rat brain. Endocrinology1987 Sep;121(3): 1076-82.

[8] Kanse SM, Kreymann, B., Ghatei, M.A., Shima, K. Identification and localization of glucagon-like peptide-1(7-36) amide binding sites in the rat brain and lung. FEBS Lett1987;241:209-12.

[9] Uttenthal LO, Toledano A, Blazquez E. Autoradiographic localization of receptors for glucagon-like peptide-1 (7-36) amide in rat brain. Neuropeptides1992 Mar;21(3): 143-6.

[10] Calvo JC, Yusta B, Mora F, Blazquez E. Structural characterization by affinity cross-linking of glucagon-like peptide-1(7-36)amide receptor in rat brain. J Neurochem1995 Jan;64(1):299-306.

[11] Calvo JC, Gisolfi CV, Blazquez E, Mora F. Glucagon-like peptide-1(7-36)amide induces the release of aspartic acid and glutamine by the ventromedial hypothalamus of the conscious rat. Brain Res Bull1995;38(5):435-9.

[12] Mora F, Exposito I, Sanz B, Blazquez E. Selective release of glutamine and glutamic acid produced by perfusion of GLP-1 (7-36) amide in the basal ganglia of the conscious rat. Brain Res Bull1992 Sep-Oct;29(3-4):359-61.

[13] Turton MD, O'Shea D, Gunn I, Beak SA, Edwards CM, Meeran K, et al. A role for glucagon-like peptide-1 in the central regulation of feeding. Nature1996 Jan 4;379(6560):69-72.

[14] Navarro M, Rodriquez de Fonseca F, Alvarez E, Chowen JA, Zueco JA, Gomez R, et al. Colocalization of glucagon-like peptide-1 (GLP-1) receptors, glucose transporter GLUT-2, and glucokinase mRNAs in rat hypothalamic cells: evidence for a role of GLP-1 receptor agonists as an inhibitory signal for food and water intake. J Neurochem1996 Nov;67(5):1982-91.

[15] Rodriquez de Fonseca F, Navarro M, Alvarez E, Roncero I, Chowen JA, Maestre O, et al. Peripheral versus central effects of glucagon-like peptide-1 receptor agonists on satiety and body weight loss in Zucker obese rats. Metabolism2000 Jun;49(6):709-17.

[16] Alvarez E, Roncero I, Chowen JA, Vazquez P, Blazquez E. Evidence that glucokinase regulatory protein is expressed and interacts with glucokinase in rat brain. J Neurochem2002 Jan;80(1):45-53.

[17] Alvarez E, Roncero I, Chowen JA, Thorens B, Blazquez E. Expression of the glucagon-like peptide-1 receptor gene in rat brain. J Neurochem1996 Mar;66(3):920-7.

[18] Roncero I, Alvarez E, Chowen JA, Sanz C, Rabano A, Vazquez P, et al. Expression of glucose transporter isoform GLUT-2 and glucokinase genes in human brain. J Neurochem2004 Mar;88(5):1203-10.

[19] Roncero I, Alvarez E, Vazquez P, Blazquez E. Functional glucokinase isoforms are expressed in rat brain. J Neurochem2000 May;74(5):1848-57.

[20] Ban K, Noyan-Ashraf MH, Hoefer J, Bolz SS, Drucker DJ, Husain M. Cardioprotective and vasodilatory actions of glucagon-like peptide 1 receptor are mediated through both glucagon-like peptide 1 receptor-dependent and -independent pathways. Circulation2008 May 6;117(18):2340-50.

[21] Li Y, Duffy KB, Ottinger MA, Ray B, Bailey JA, Holloway HW, et al. GLP-1 receptor stimulation reduces amyloid-beta peptide accumulation and cytotoxicity in cellular and animal models of Alzheimer's disease. J Alzheimers Dis2010;19(4):1205-19.

[22] Barragan JM, Rodriguez RE, Blazquez E. Changes in arterial blood pressure and heart rate induced by glucagon-like peptide-1-(7-36) amide in rats. Am J Physiol1994 Mar;266(3 Pt 1):E459-66.

[23] Barragan JM, Rodriguez RE, Eng J, Blazquez E. Interactions of exendin-(9-39) with the effects of glucagon-like peptide-1-(7-36) amide and of exendin-4 on arterial blood pressure and heart rate in rats. Regul Pept1996 Nov 14;67(1):63-8.

[24] Bulotta A, Hui H, Anastasi E, Bertolotto C, Boros LG, Di Mario U, et al. Cultured pancreatic ductal cells undergo cell cycle re-distribution and beta-cell-like differentiation in response to glucagon-like peptide-1. J Mol Endocrinol2002 Dec;29(3):347-60.

[25] De Leon DD, Deng S, Madani R, Ahima RS, Drucker DJ, Stoffers DA. Role of endogenous glucagon-like peptide-1 in islet regeneration after partial pancreatectomy. Diabetes2003 Feb;52(2):365-71.

[26] Chia CW, Egan JM. Incretin-based therapies in type 2 diabetes mellitus. J Clin Endocrinol Metab2008 Oct;93(10):3703-16.

[27] Moore B. On the treatment of Diabetus mellitus by acid extract of Duodenal Mucous Membrane. Biochem J1906;1(1):28-38.

[28] Zunz E, La Barre J.. Contributions a l'etude des variations physiologiques de la secretion interne du pancreas. relations entre les secretions externe et interne du pancreas. relations entre les secretions externe et interne du pancreas.. Arch Int Physiol Biochim 1929;31:20-44.

[29] Elrick H, Stimmler L, Hlad CJ, Jr., Arai Y. Plasma Insulin Response to Oral and Intravenous Glucose Administration. J Clin Endocrinol Metab1964 Oct;24:1076-82.

[30] Unger RH, Eisentraut AM. Entero-insular axis. Arch Intern Med1969 Mar;123(3): 261-6.

[31] Creutzfeldt W. The incretin concept today. Diabetologia1979 Feb;16(2):75-85.

[32] Mudaliar S, Henry RR. The incretin hormones: from scientific discovery to practical therapeutics. Diabetologia2012 Jul;55(7):1865-8.

[33] Nauck M, Stockmann F, Ebert R, Creutzfeldt W. Reduced incretin effect in type 2 (non-insulin-dependent) diabetes. Diabetologia1986 Jan;29(1):46-52.

[34] Kreymann B, Williams G, Ghatei MA, Bloom SR. Glucagon-like peptide-1 7-36: a physiological incretin in man. Lancet1987 Dec 5;2(8571):1300-4.

[35] Nauck MA, Heimesaat MM, Orskov C, Holst JJ, Ebert R, Creutzfeldt W. Preserved incretin activity of glucagon-like peptide 1 (7-36 amide) but not of synthetic human gastric inhibitory polypeptide in patients with type-2 diabetes mellitus. J Clin Invest1993 Jan;91(1):301-7.

[36] Nauck MA, Kleine N, Orskov C, Holst JJ, Willms B, Creutzfeldt W. Normalization of fasting hyperglycaemia by exogenous glucagon-like peptide 1 (7-36 amide) in type 2 (non-insulin-dependent) diabetic patients. Diabetologia1993 Aug;36(8):741-4.

[37] Drucker DJ, Nauck MA. The incretin system: glucagon-like peptide-1 receptor agonists and dipeptidyl peptidase-4 inhibitors in type 2 diabetes. Lancet2006 Nov 11;368(9548):1696-705.

[38] Vara E, Arias-Diaz J, Garcia C, Balibrea JL, Blazquez E. Glucagon-like peptide-1(7-36) amide stimulates surfactant secretion in human type II pneumocytes. Am J Respir Crit Care Med2001 Mar;163(4):840-6.

[39] Batterham RL, Cowley MA, Small CJ, Herzog H, Cohen MA, Dakin CL, et al. Gut hormone PYY(3-36) physiologically inhibits food intake. Nature2002 Aug 8;418(6898):650-4.

[40] Tang-Christensen M, Larsen PJ, Thulesen J, Romer J, Vrang N. The proglucagon-derived peptide, glucagon-like peptide-2, is a neurotransmitter involved in the regulation of food intake. Nat Med2000 Jul;6(7):802-7.

[41] Schwartz MW, Woods SC, Porte D, Jr., Seeley RJ, Baskin DG. Central nervous system control of food intake. Nature2000 Apr 6;404(6778):661-71.

[42] Gutzwiller JP, Goke B, Drewe J, Hildebrand P, Ketterer S, Handschin D, et al. Glucagon-like peptide-1: a potent regulator of food intake in humans. Gut1999 Jan;44(1): 81-6.

[43] Orskov C, Poulsen SS, Moller M, Holst JJ. Glucagon-like peptide I receptors in the subfornical organ and the area postrema are accessible to circulating glucagon-like peptide I. Diabetes1996 Jun;45(6):832-5.

[44] Lind RW, Thunhorst RL, Johnson AK. The subfornical organ and the integration of multiple factors in thirst. Physiol Behav1984 Jan;32(1):69-74.

[45] Zueco JA, Esquifino AI, Chowen JA, Alvarez E, Castrillon PO, Blazquez E. Coexpression of glucagon-like peptide-1 (GLP-1) receptor, vasopressin, and oxytocin mRNAs in neurons of the rat hypothalamic supraoptic and paraventricular nuclei: effect of GLP-1(7-36)amide on vasopressin and oxytocin release. J Neurochem1999 Jan;72(1): 10-6.

[46] Holst JJ, Orskov, C. Glucagon an other proglucagon-derived peptides.. In: Walsh JH DG, editor. New York. : Raven; 1994.

[47] Schjoldager BT, Mortensen PE, Christiansen J, Orskov C, Holst JJ. GLP-1 (glucagon-like peptide 1) and truncated GLP-1, fragments of human proglucagon, inhibit gastric acid secretion in humans. Dig Dis Sci1989 May;34(5):703-8.

[48] Gutniak M, Orskov C, Holst JJ, Ahren B, Efendic S. Antidiabetogenic effect of glucagon-like peptide-1 (7-36)amide in normal subjects and patients with diabetes mellitus. N Engl J Med1992 May 14;326(20):1316-22.

[49] Berridge KC. 'Liking' and 'wanting' food rewards: brain substrates and roles in eating disorders. Physiol Behav2009 Jul 14;97(5):537-50.

[50] Chaudhri OB, Salem V, Murphy KG, Bloom SR. Gastrointestinal satiety signals. Annu Rev Physiol2008;70:239-55.

[51] Hetherington A, Ranson S. Hypothalamic lesions and adiposity in the rat. Anat Rec1940;78:149-72.

[52] Anand BK, Chhina GS, Sharma KN, Dua S, Singh B. Activity of Single Neurons in the Hypothalamic Feeding Centers: Effect of Glucose. Am J Physiol1964 Nov; 207:1146-54.

[53] Stellar E. The physiology of motivation. Psychol Rev1954 Jan;61(1):5-22.

[54] Kalra SP, Dube MG, Pu S, Xu B, Horvath TL, Kalra PS. Interacting appetite-regulating pathways in the hypothalamic regulation of body weight. Endocr Rev1999 Feb; 20(1):68-100.

[55] Elmquist JK. Hypothalamic pathways underlying the endocrine, autonomic, and behavioral effects of leptin. Physiol Behav2001 Nov-Dec;74(4-5):703-8.

[56] Adage T, Scheurink AJ, de Boer SF, de Vries K, Konsman JP, Kuipers F, et al. Hypothalamic, metabolic, and behavioral responses to pharmacological inhibition of CNS melanocortin signaling in rats. J Neurosci2001 May 15;21(10):3639-45.

[57] de Lecea L, Kilduff TS, Peyron C, Gao X, Foye PE, Danielson PE, et al. The hypocretins: hypothalamus-specific peptides with neuroexcitatory activity. Proc Natl Acad Sci U S A1998 Jan 6;95(1):322-7.

[58] Sakurai T, Amemiya A, Ishii M, Matsuzaki I, Chemelli RM, Tanaka H, et al. Orexins and orexin receptors: a family of hypothalamic neuropeptides and G protein-coupled receptors that regulate feeding behavior. Cell1998 Feb 20;92(4):573-85.

[59] Qu D, Ludwig DS, Gammeltoft S, Piper M, Pelleymounter MA, Cullen MJ, et al. A role for melanin-concentrating hormone in the central regulation of feeding behaviour. Nature1996 Mar 21;380(6571):243-7.

[60] Song Z, Levin BE, McArdle JJ, Bakhos N, Routh VH. Convergence of pre- and postsynaptic influences on glucosensing neurons in the ventromedial hypothalamic nucleus. Diabetes2001 Dec;50(12):2673-81.

[61] Shiraishi T. Noradrenergic neurons modulate lateral hypothalamic chemical and electrical stimulation-induced feeding by sated rats. Brain Res Bull1991 Sep-Oct; 27(3-4):347-51.

[62] Mizuno Y, Oomura Y. Glucose responding neurons in the nucleus tractus solitarius of the rat: in vitro study. Brain Res1984 Jul 30;307(1-2):109-16.

[63] Nakano Y, Oomura Y, Lenard L, Nishino H, Aou S, Yamamoto T, et al. Feeding-related activity of glucose- and morphine-sensitive neurons in the monkey amygdala. Brain Res1986 Dec 3;399(1):167-72.

[64] Raybould HE. Sensing of glucose in the gastrointestinal tract. Auton Neurosci2007 Apr 30;133(1):86-90.

[65] Koyama Y, Coker RH, Stone EE, Lacy DB, Jabbour K, Williams PE, et al. Evidence that carotid bodies play an important role in glucoregulation in vivo. Diabetes2000 Sep;49(9):1434-42.

[66] Matveyenko AV, Donovan CM. Metabolic sensors mediate hypoglycemic detection at the portal vein. Diabetes2006 May;55(5):1276-82.

[67] Silver IA, Erecinska M. Extracellular glucose concentration in mammalian brain: continuous monitoring of changes during increased neuronal activity and upon limitation in oxygen supply in normo-, hypo-, and hyperglycemic animals. J Neurosci1994 Aug;14(8):5068-76.

[68] Borg WP, Sherwin RS, During MJ, Borg MA, Shulman GI. Local ventromedial hypothalamus glucopenia triggers counterregulatory hormone release. Diabetes1995 Feb; 44(2):180-4.

[69] Dunn-Meynell AA, Sanders NM, Compton D, Becker TC, Eiki J, Zhang BB, et al. Relationship among brain and blood glucose levels and spontaneous and glucoprivic feeding. J Neurosci2009 May 27;29(21):7015-22.

[70] Ashford ML, Boden PR, Treherne JM. Glucose-induced excitation of hypothalamic neurones is mediated by ATP-sensitive K+ channels. Pflugers Arch1990 Jan;415(4): 479-83.

[71] Fioramonti X, Lorsignol A, Taupignon A, Penicaud L. A new ATP-sensitive K+ channel-independent mechanism is involved in glucose-excited neurons of mouse arcuate nucleus. Diabetes2004 Nov;53(11):2767-75.

[72] Silver IA, Erecinska M. Glucose-induced intracellular ion changes in sugar-sensitive hypothalamic neurons. J Neurophysiol1998 Apr;79(4):1733-45.

[73] Wang R, Liu X, Hentges ST, Dunn-Meynell AA, Levin BE, Wang W, et al. The regulation of glucose-excited neurons in the hypothalamic arcuate nucleus by glucose and feeding-relevant peptides. Diabetes2004 Aug;53(8):1959-65.

[74] Song Z, Routh VH. Differential effects of glucose and lactate on glucosensing neurons in the ventromedial hypothalamic nucleus. Diabetes2005 Jan;54(1):15-22.

[75] Song Z, Routh VH. Recurrent hypoglycemia reduces the glucose sensitivity of glucose-inhibited neurons in the ventromedial hypothalamus nucleus. Am J Physiol Regul Integr Comp Physiol2006 Nov;291(5):R1283-7.

[76] Murphy BA, Fioramonti X, Jochnowitz N, Fakira K, Gagen K, Contie S, et al. Fasting enhances the response of arcuate neuropeptide Y-glucose-inhibited neurons to decreased extracellular glucose. Am J Physiol Cell Physiol2009 Apr;296(4):C746-56.

[77] VanGilder RL, Kelly KA, Chua MD, Ptachcinski RL, Huber JD. Administration of sesamol improved blood-brain barrier function in streptozotocin-induced diabetic rats. Exp Brain Res2009 Jul;197(1):23-34.

[78] Kang L, Routh VH, Kuzhikandathil EV, Gaspers LD, Levin BE. Physiological and molecular characteristics of rat hypothalamic ventromedial nucleus glucosensing neurons. Diabetes2004 Mar;53(3):549-59.

[79] Claret M, Smith MA, Batterham RL, Selman C, Choudhury AI, Fryer LG, et al. AMPK is essential for energy homeostasis regulation and glucose sensing by POMC and AgRP neurons. J Clin Invest2007 Aug;117(8):2325-36.

[80] Cotero VE, Routh VH. Insulin blunts the response of glucose-excited neurons in the ventrolateral-ventromedial hypothalamic nucleus to decreased glucose. Am J Physiol Endocrinol Metab2009 May;296(5):E1101-9.

[81] Dunn-Meynell AA, Routh VH, Kang L, Gaspers L, Levin BE. Glucokinase is the likely mediator of glucosensing in both glucose-excited and glucose-inhibited central neurons. Diabetes2002 Jul;51(7):2056-65.

[82] Murphy BA, Fakira KA, Song Z, Beuve A, Routh VH. AMP-activated protein kinase and nitric oxide regulate the glucose sensitivity of ventromedial hypothalamic glucose-inhibited neurons. Am J Physiol Cell Physiol2009 Sep;297(3):C750-8.

[83] Hurtado-Carneiro V, Sanz C, Roncero I, Vazquez P, Blazquez E, Alvarez E. Glucagon-like peptide 1 (GLP-1) can reverse AMP-activated protein kinase (AMPK) and S6 kinase (P70S6K) activities induced by fluctuations in glucose levels in hypothalamic areas involved in feeding behaviour. Mol Neurobiol2012 Apr;45(2):348-61.

[84] Hegyi K, Fulop K, Kovacs K, Toth S, Falus A. Leptin-induced signal transduction pathways. Cell Biol Int2004;28(3):159-69.

[85] Kahn BB, Alquier T, Carling D, Hardie DG. AMP-activated protein kinase: ancient energy gauge provides clues to modern understanding of metabolism. Cell Metab2005 Jan;1(1):15-25.

[86] Kohno D, Sone H, Minokoshi Y, Yada T. Ghrelin raises (Ca2+)i via AMPK in hypothalamic arcuate nucleus NPY neurons. Biochem Biophys Res Commun2008 Feb 8;366(2):388-92.

[87] Kola B, Hubina E, Tucci SA, Kirkham TC, Garcia EA, Mitchell SE, et al. Cannabinoids and ghrelin have both central and peripheral metabolic and cardiac effects via AMP-activated protein kinase. J Biol Chem2005 Jul 1;280(26):25196-201.

[88] Minokoshi Y, Alquier T, Furukawa N, Kim YB, Lee A, Xue B, et al. AMP-kinase regulates food intake by responding to hormonal and nutrient signals in the hypothalamus. Nature2004 Apr 1;428(6982):569-74.

[89] Andersson U, Filipsson K, Abbott CR, Woods A, Smith K, Bloom SR, et al. AMP-activated protein kinase plays a role in the control of food intake. J Biol Chem2004 Mar 26;279(13):12005-8.

[90] Rutter GA, Da Silva Xavier G, Leclerc I. Roles of 5'-AMP-activated protein kinase (AMPK) in mammalian glucose homoeostasis. Biochem J2003 Oct 1;375(Pt 1):1-16.

[91] Hardie DG, Carling D, Carlson M. The AMP-activated/SNF1 protein kinase subfamily: metabolic sensors of the eukaryotic cell? Annu Rev Biochem1998;67:821-55.

[92] Hardie DG, Ross FA, Hawley SA. AMPK: a nutrient and energy sensor that maintains energy homeostasis. Nat Rev Mol Cell Biol2012 Apr;13(4):251-62.

[93] Viollet B, Athea Y, Mounier R, Guigas B, Zarrinpashneh E, Horman S, et al. AMPK: Lessons from transgenic and knockout animals. Front Biosci2009;14:19-44.

[94] Xiao B, Sanders MJ, Underwood E, Heath R, Mayer FV, Carmena D, et al. Structure of mammalian AMPK and its regulation by ADP. Nature2011 Apr 14;472(7342):230-3.

[95] Oakhill JS, Steel R, Chen ZP, Scott JW, Ling N, Tam S, et al. AMPK is a direct adenylate charge-regulated protein kinase. Science2011 Jun 17;332(6036):1433-5.

[96] Xie M, Zhang D, Dyck JR, Li Y, Zhang H, Morishima M, et al. A pivotal role for endogenous TGF-beta-activated kinase-1 in the LKB1/AMP-activated protein kinase energy-sensor pathway. Proc Natl Acad Sci U S A2006 Nov 14;103(46):17378-83.

[97] Zhou K, Bellenguez C, Spencer CC, Bennett AJ, Coleman RL, Tavendale R, et al. Common variants near ATM are associated with glycemic response to metformin in type 2 diabetes. Nat Genet2011 Feb;43(2):117-20.

[98] Garcia-Haro L, Garcia-Gimeno MA, Neumann D, Beullens M, Bollen M, Sanz P. The PP1-R6 protein phosphatase holoenzyme is involved in the glucose-induced dephosphorylation and inactivation of AMP-activated protein kinase, a key regulator of insulin secretion, in MIN6 beta cells. Faseb J2010 Dec;24(12):5080-91.

[99] Steinberg GR, Michell BJ, van Denderen BJ, Watt MJ, Carey AL, Fam BC, et al. Tumor necrosis factor alpha-induced skeletal muscle insulin resistance involves suppression of AMP-kinase signaling. Cell Metab2006 Dec;4(6):465-74.

[100] Sanders MJ, Grondin PO, Hegarty BD, Snowden MA, Carling D. Investigating the mechanism for AMP activation of the AMP-activated protein kinase cascade. Biochem J2007 Apr 1;403(1):139-48.

[101] Lim CT, Kola B, Korbonits M. AMPK as a mediator of hormonal signalling. J Mol Endocrinol2010 Feb;44(2):87-97.

[102] Foster KG, Acosta-Jaquez HA, Romeo Y, Ekim B, Soliman GA, Carriere A, et al. Regulation of mTOR complex 1 (mTORC1) by raptor Ser863 and multisite phosphorylation. J Biol Chem2010 Jan 1;285(1):80-94.

[103] Alessi DR, Pearce LR, Garcia-Martinez JM. New insights into mTOR signaling: mTORC2 and beyond. Sci Signal2009;2(67):pe27.

[104] Zoncu R, Efeyan A, Sabatini DM. mTOR: from growth signal integration to cancer, diabetes and ageing. Nat Rev Mol Cell Biol2011 Jan;12(1):21-35.

[105] Sengupta S, Peterson TR, Sabatini DM. Regulation of the mTOR complex 1 pathway by nutrients, growth factors, and stress. Mol Cell2010 Oct 22;40(2):310-22.

[106] Magnuson B, Ekim B, Fingar DC. Regulation and function of ribosomal protein S6 kinase (S6K) within mTOR signalling networks. Biochem J2012 Jan 1;441(1):1-21.

[107] Meyuhas O, Dreazen A. Ribosomal protein S6 kinase from TOP mRNAs to cell size. Prog Mol Biol Transl Sci2009;90:109-53.

[108] Fenton TR, Gout IT. Functions and regulation of the 70kDa ribosomal S6 kinases. Int J Biochem Cell Biol Jan;43(1):47-59.

[109] Ma XM, Blenis J. Molecular mechanisms of mTOR-mediated translational control. Nat Rev Mol Cell Biol2009 May;10(5):307-18.

[110] Sarbassov DD, Guertin DA, Ali SM, Sabatini DM. Phosphorylation and regulation of Akt/PKB by the rictor-mTOR complex. Science2005 Feb 18;307(5712):1098-101.

[111] Ma L, Chen Z, Erdjument-Bromage H, Tempst P, Pandolfi PP. Phosphorylation and functional inactivation of TSC2 by Erk implications for tuberous sclerosis and cancer pathogenesis. Cell2005 Apr 22;121(2):179-93.

[112] Carriere A, Romeo Y, Acosta-Jaquez HA, Moreau J, Bonneil E, Thibault P, et al. ERK1/2 phosphorylate Raptor to promote Ras-dependent activation of mTOR complex 1 (mTORC1). J Biol Chem2011 Jan 7;286(1):567-77.

[113] Flinn RJ, Yan Y, Goswami S, Parker PJ, Backer JM. The late endosome is essential for mTORC1 signaling. Mol Biol Cell2010 Mar 1;21(5):833-41.

[114] Inoki K, Zhu T, Guan KL. TSC2 mediates cellular energy response to control cell growth and survival. Cell2003 Nov 26;115(5):577-90.

[115] Gwinn DM, Shackelford DB, Egan DF, Mihaylova MM, Mery A, Vasquez DS, et al. AMPK phosphorylation of raptor mediates a metabolic checkpoint. Mol Cell2008 Apr 25;30(2):214-26.

[116] Zheng M, Wang YH, Wu XN, Wu SQ, Lu BJ, Dong MQ, et al. Inactivation of Rheb by PRAK-mediated phosphorylation is essential for energy-depletion-induced suppression of mTORC1. Nat Cell Biol2011 Mar;13(3):263-72.

[117] Turnley AM, Stapleton D, Mann RJ, Witters LA, Kemp BE, Bartlett PF. Cellular distribution and developmental expression of AMP-activated protein kinase isoforms in mouse central nervous system. J Neurochem1999 Apr;72(4):1707-16.

[118] Minokoshi Y, Shiuchi T, Lee S, Suzuki A, Okamoto S. Role of hypothalamic AMP-kinase in food intake regulation. Nutrition2008 Sep;24(9):786-90.

[119] Cota D, Proulx K, Smith KA, Kozma SC, Thomas G, Woods SC, et al. Hypothalamic mTOR signaling regulates food intake. Science2006 May 12;312(5775):927-30.

[120] Ropelle ER, Pauli JR, Fernandes MF, Rocco SA, Marin RM, Morari J, et al. A central role for neuronal AMP-activated protein kinase (AMPK) and mammalian target of

rapamycin (mTOR) in high-protein diet-induced weight loss. Diabetes2008 Mar; 57(3):594-605.

[121] Blouet C, Ono H, Schwartz GJ. Mediobasal hypothalamic p70 S6 kinase 1 modulates the control of energy homeostasis. Cell Metab2008 Dec;8(6):459-67.

[122] Kim MS, Park JY, Namkoong C, Jang PG, Ryu JW, Song HS, et al. Anti-obesity effects of alpha-lipoic acid mediated by suppression of hypothalamic AMP-activated protein kinase. Nat Med2004 Jul;10(7):727-33.

[123] Han SM, Namkoong C, Jang PG, Park IS, Hong SW, Katakami H, et al. Hypothalamic AMP-activated protein kinase mediates counter-regulatory responses to hypoglycaemia in rats. Diabetologia2005 Oct;48(10):2170-8.

[124] Lynch CJ, Gern B, Lloyd C, Hutson SM, Eicher R, Vary TC. Leucine in food mediates some of the postprandial rise in plasma leptin concentrations. Am J Physiol Endocrinol Metab2006 Sep;291(3):E621-30.

[125] Cummings DE, Purnell JQ, Frayo RS, Schmidova K, Wisse BE, Weigle DS. A preprandial rise in plasma ghrelin levels suggests a role in meal initiation in humans. Diabetes2001 Aug;50(8):1714-9.

[126] Wren AM, Seal LJ, Cohen MA, Brynes AE, Frost GS, Murphy KG, et al. Ghrelin enhances appetite and increases food intake in humans. J Clin Endocrinol Metab2001 Dec;86(12):5992.

[127] Hameed S, Dhillo WS, Bloom SR. Gut hormones and appetite control. Oral Dis2009 Jan;15(1):18-26.

[128] Benoit SC, Clegg DJ, Seeley RJ, Woods SC. Insulin and leptin as adiposity signals. Recent Prog Horm Res2004;59:267-85.

[129] Mountjoy PD, Bailey SJ, Rutter GA. Inhibition by glucose or leptin of hypothalamic neurons expressing neuropeptide Y requires changes in AMP-activated protein kinase activity. Diabetologia2007 Jan;50(1):168-77.

[130] Cota D, Matter EK, Woods SC, Seeley RJ. The role of hypothalamic mammalian target of rapamycin complex 1 signaling in diet-induced obesity. J Neurosci2008 Jul 9;28(28):7202-8.

[131] Yang Y, Atasoy D, Su HH, Sternson SM. Hunger states switch a flip-flop memory circuit via a synaptic AMPK-dependent positive feedback loop. Cell2011 Sep 16;146(6): 992-1003.

[132] Dagon Y, Hur E, Zheng B, Wellenstein K, Cantley LC, Kahn BB. p70S6 Kinase Phosphorylates AMPK on Serine 491 to Mediate Leptin's Effect on Food Intake. Cell Metab2012 Jul 3;16(1):104-12.

[133] Alvarez E, Martinez MD, Roncero I, Chowen JA, Garcia-Cuartero B, Gispert JD, et al. The expression of GLP-1 receptor mRNA and protein allows the effect of GLP-1 on

glucose metabolism in the human hypothalamus and brainstem. J Neurochem2005 Feb;92(4):798-806.

[134] McCrimmon RJ, Fan X, Cheng H, McNay E, Chan O, Shaw M, et al. Activation of AMP-activated protein kinase within the ventromedial hypothalamus amplifies counterregulatory hormone responses in rats with defective counterregulation. Diabetes2006 Jun;55(6):1755-60.

[135] Seo S, Ju S, Chung H, Lee D, Park S. Acute effects of glucagon-like peptide-1 on hypothalamic neuropeptide and AMP activated kinase expression in fasted rats. Endocr J2008 Oct;55(5):867-74.

[136] Sanz C, Roncero I, Vazquez P, Navas MA, Blazquez E. Effects of glucose and insulin on glucokinase activity in rat hypothalamus. J Endocrinol2007 May;193(2):259-67.

[137] Sanz C, Vazquez P, Navas MA, Alvarez E, Blazquez E. Leptin but not neuropeptide Y up-regulated glucagon-like peptide 1 receptor expression in GT1-7 cells and rat hypothalamic slices. Metabolism2008 Jan;57(1):40-8.

[138] Williams DL, Baskin DG, Schwartz MW. Evidence that intestinal glucagon-like peptide-1 plays a physiological role in satiety. Endocrinology2009 Apr;150(4):1680-7.

[139] Kanoski SE, Fortin SM, Arnold M, Grill HJ, Hayes MR. Peripheral and central GLP-1 receptor populations mediate the anorectic effects of peripherally administered GLP-1 receptor agonists, liraglutide and exendin-4. Endocrinology2011 Aug;152(8): 3103-12.

[140] Hayes MR, Leichner TM, Zhao S, Lee GS, Chowansky A, Zimmer D, et al. Intracellular signals mediating the food intake-suppressive effects of hindbrain glucagon-like peptide-1 receptor activation. Cell Metab2011 Mar 2;13(3):320-30.

[141] Kristensen P, Judge ME, Thim L, Ribel U, Christjansen KN, Wulff BS, et al. Hypothalamic CART is a new anorectic peptide regulated by leptin. Nature1998 May 7;393(6680):72-6.

[142] Abbott CR, Rossi M, Wren AM, Murphy KG, Kennedy AR, Stanley SA, et al. Evidence of an orexigenic role for cocaine- and amphetamine-regulated transcript after administration into discrete hypothalamic nuclei. Endocrinology2001 Aug;142(8): 3457-63.

[143] McCrimmon RJ, Shaw M, Fan X, Cheng H, Ding Y, Vella MC, et al. Key role for AMP-activated protein kinase in the ventromedial hypothalamus in regulating counterregulatory hormone responses to acute hypoglycemia. Diabetes2008 Feb;57(2): 444-50.

[144] Kubota N, Yano W, Kubota T, Yamauchi T, Itoh S, Kumagai H, et al. Adiponectin stimulates AMP-activated protein kinase in the hypothalamus and increases food intake. Cell Metab2007 Jul;6(1):55-68.

[145] Martin TL, Alquier T, Asakura K, Furukawa N, Preitner F, Kahn BB. Diet-induced obesity alters AMP kinase activity in hypothalamus and skeletal muscle. J Biol Chem2006 Jul 14;281(28):18933-41.

[146] Niswender K. Diabetes and obesity: therapeutic targeting and risk reduction - a complex interplay. Diabetes Obes Metab2010 Apr;12(4):267-87.

[147] Blonde L, Klein EJ, Han J, Zhang B, Mac SM, Poon TH, et al. Interim analysis of the effects of exenatide treatment on A1C, weight and cardiovascular risk factors over 82 weeks in 314 overweight patients with type 2 diabetes. Diabetes Obes Metab2006 Jul; 8(4):436-47.

[148] Buse JB, Rosenstock J, Sesti G, Schmidt WE, Montanya E, Brett JH, et al. Liraglutide once a day versus exenatide twice a day for type 2 diabetes: a 26-week randomised, parallel-group, multinational, open-label trial (LEAD-6). Lancet2009 Jul 4;374(9683): 39-47.

[149] Montanya E, Sesti G. A review of efficacy and safety data regarding the use of liraglutide, a once-daily human glucagon-like peptide 1 analogue, in the treatment of type 2 diabetes mellitus. Clin Ther2009 Nov;31(11):2472-88.

[150] Ono H, Pocai A, Wang Y, Sakoda H, Asano T, Backer JM, et al. Activation of hypothalamic S6 kinase mediates diet-induced hepatic insulin resistance in rats. J Clin Invest2008 Aug;118(8):2959-68.

Chapter 8

The Insulin-Like Growth Factor System in the Human Pathology

Emrah Yerlikaya and Fulya Akin

Additional information is available at the end of the chapter

http://dx.doi.org/10.5772/55213

1. Introduction

1.1. Physiology

Insulin-like growth factors are single chain polypeptides. There are two principle IGFs referred to as IGF-I and IGF-II. IGF-1 is a polypeptide hormone with a molecular weight of 7.6-kDa structurally similar to insulin. In 1957, it is identified by Salmon and Daughaday. Because of the its ability to stimulate the sulfation of the cartilage proteoglycans, it was regarded as a sulphation factor [1]. The IGF-1 gene is on the long arm of chromosome 12q23–23. IGF-1 gene contains 6 exons [2, 3]. The alternate extension peptide at carboxy terminal, encoded by exons 5 and 6 determines the subforms of IGF-1: IGF-1B and IGF-1A. The most abundant isoform of the IGF-1 (153 aminoacid) is IGF-1A [4, 5]. IGF1B peptide (195 amino acids) is a less abundant IGF1 isoform. IGF-2 is also a peptide with 67 amino acids and molecular weight of 7.4-kDa. IGF-2 is encoded by a gene on the short arm of chromosome 11 at position 15.5. This gene consists of nine exons [6]. In the plasma, 99% of IGFs are bound to a family of binding cysteine-rich proteins. There are six binding proteins (IGFBP-1 to IGFBP-6) [7]. They act as carriers for IGFs in the circulation, regulate the bioavailability of IGFs to spesific tissues and modulates the biological activities of IGF proteins. Six IGF-binding proteins (IGFBPs) can inhibit or enhance the actions of IGFs [8]. Potentiation of IGF activity by some of the IGFBPs, described for IGFBP-1 and IGFBP-3, is also documented for IGFBP-5. Each of IGFBPs is the product of a seperate gene. These genes share a common structural organization in which four conserved exons are located within genes ranging from 5 kb (IGFBP-1) to more than 30 kb (IGFBP-2 and IGFBP-5) [9]. IGFBPs contain N terminal and C terminal domains which are similar in aminoacid sequence. Post-translational modifications of IGFBP, including glycosylation, phosphorylation and proteolysis modify the affinities of the binding proteins to IGF. IGFs mediate their action on target cells by three receptors that bind IGFs with differing affinities. These receptors are type 1 IGF receptor, type 2 IGF receptor and Insulin receptors. The type 1 IGF receptor (IGF-1R), structurally homologous to the insulin receptor, exhibits four transmembrane spanning subunits and an intracellular tyrosine kinase domain [10]. The IGF-1R and IR are both synthesized as a precursor that is glycosylated on the extracellular regions, dimerized and proteolytically processed to yield separate α and β chains [11]. IGF-1R binds insulin, IGF-1, or IGF-2. IGF1R binds to IGF1 with greater affinity than IGF-2. IGF-1R affinity for insulin is lower than for IGF-1. Type 2 IGF receptor is structurally and functionally different from the IGF-1R. The receptor is a 250-kDa protein with a large extracellular domain, which binds M6P, lysosomal enzymes, and IGF-2 [12]. IGF-2R binds to IGF-2 with high affinity whereas IGF-1 binding is weak and insulin does not bind at all [13]. Binding of IGF-1 and IGF-2 to the cognate IGF-1R stimulates the intrinsic tyrosine kinase activity of this receptor [14]. Upon IGF binding, the tyrosine kinase activity of IGF-1 receptor leads to the phosphorylation of several substrates, including the insulin receptor substrate family of proteins (such as Insulin receptor substrate 1 (IRS-1), SHC (Src homology 2 domain containing) transforming protein 1 (Shc) and some others. Once phosphorylated, these docking proteins activate downstream intracellular signaling through the Phosphatidylinositol 3-kinase (PI3K) or Growth factor receptor-bound protein 2 (GRB2)/ Son of sevenless homolog (SOS)/ v-Ha-ras Harvey rat sarcoma viral oncogene homolog (H-Ras) pathways that ultimately leads to cellular proliferation [15,16].

Ligand binding to IGF-1R activates the tyrosine kinase higher concentration of the anti-apoptotic proteins bcl-2 and bcl-Xl, a lower level of the apoptotic proteins bax and bcl-xs activates phosphatidylinositol 3-kinase (P13-K), and activates protein kinase B (PKB/Akt) that also prevent apoptosis. Activation of PI 3-kinase generates inositol triphosphate activation of protein tyrosine kinase-B activate mTOR, p70/S6 kinase and GSK-3β results in protein glucose uptake, glycogen synthesis. Most IGF-1 is secreted by the liver and is transported to other tissues, acting as an endocrine hormone. IGF-1 is also secreted by other tissues, including cartilagenous cells, and acts locally as a paracrine hormone. In response to GH, IGF-1 synthesis is increased in connective tissues. Growth hormone released from the anterior lobe of the pituitary binds to receptors on the surface of liver cells which stimulates the synthesis and release of IGF-1 from them. STAT5B is a transcription factor mediating effect of GH on liver. Low IGF-1 and IGFBP-3 levels in cirrhosis occurs due to decreased hepatic synthesis [17, 18]. IGFBP-3 that binds 95% of circulating IGFs is also produced by the endothelial lining and Kupffer cells in the liver.

2. Factors affecting IGF system

IGF-1 peaks during puberty. Advanced age is associated with a progressive decrease in serum IGF-1 because GH secretion declines; 14% per decade of life [19, 20]. During lifetime, GH production is reduced nearly 30-fold. This decrement in IGF-1 is attributable to increased somatostatinergic tone and a generalized reduction in the pulses of GH-releasing hormones and GH-releasing peptides [21]. Although GH may be responsible for the decrement it is not the only factor responsible for the increment in childhood. Serum estradiol concentrations correlate with IGF-1 in both men and women [22]. Stimulated and spontaneous GH secretion is higher in young women than in postmenopausal women or young men, with the difference strongly correlated with circulating estradiol levels [23, 24, 25]. Use of oral estrogen resulted in a significant reduction in IGF1 levels but no effect of transdermal estrogen was shown in patients with hypopitutiarism [26]. Transdermally delivered estrogen stimulates IGF-1 production. When delivered orally, estrogen reduces IGF-1 [27]. IGF-1 mRNA expressed by endometrium. Progesterons increases IGF-1 expression İn the endometrial stroma. There is circumstantial evidence to suggest a positive association between circulating levels of testosterone and IGF-1. Administration of testosterone to younger men with hypogonadism and boys with isolated gonadotropin-releasing hormone deficiency increases serum IGF-1 [28]. Endogenous testosterone levels correlate with IGF-1 in hypopituitary women with unsubstituted growth hormone deficiency [29]. Serum dehydroepiandrosterone concentrations decline with age, and absolute concentrations in postmenopausal women correlate with serum IGF-1 [30]. Thyroxine is also another hormone affecting IGF-1 levels. In patients with T4 deficiency due to primary and central hypothyroidism IGF-1 and ALS are low at baseline. In most of these T4-treated patients, T4 therapy increased IGF-1 and ALS concentrations [31]. The major effect of thyroid hormones on IGF-1 and IGFBP-3 in vivo has been considered to occur by increased expression and secretion of growth hormone by the pituitary gland [32]. IGFBP-3 also increases with thyroxine replacement in primary hypothyroidism [33]. One key function of IGF-1 is the stimulation of anabolic processes and body growth. Protein and energy content of the diet influence plasma IGF-1 concentrations [34]. IGF-1 is reduced in conditions of energy restriction, such as short-term fasting [35] and malnutrition [36]. Zinc deficiency is a common component of protein-calorie malnutrition. IGF-1 synthesis can be impaired by zinc deficiency. A reduction in circulating IGF-1 concentrations has been proposed as a potential mechanism for growth retardation induced by zinc deficiency [37]. Significant elevation in the IGF-1 level after zinc supplementation occurs [38]. Similarly, nutritional deprivation results in a major decrease in IGF-1 mRNA that can be restored with refeeding. In the population of healthy well-nourished men, greater dietary intakes of protein, zinc, red meat, and fish and seafood were associated with higher IGF-1 concentrations [39]. The anabolic effect of PTH may be mediated by local growth factors. PTH has been shown to stimulate IGF-1 production at the transcriptional and polypeptide levels [40]. Low IGF-1 and IGFBP-3 levels occurs in liver cirrhosis due to decreased synthesis and low IGF-1 levels may be involved in the development of cirrhotic complications including malnutrition, insulin resistance, impaired immunity, and osteoporosis [41].

Any factors affecting IGFBP concentrations in blood and extracellular fluids also affects the IGF levels and its avaibility to tissues. Binding of IGF-1 to ALS and IGFBPs form ternary complexes. Acid Labile Subunit (ALS) is a liver-derived protein that exists in a ternary complex with IGFBP-3 also with IGFBP-5. Formation of the ternary complexes restricts the IGFs to the circulation prolongs their half-lives and allows them to be stored at high concentration in plasma. ALS is a single-copy gene, and was mapped to bands A2-A3 of mouse chromosome 17 and to the short arm of human chromosome 16 at p13 3 [42, 43]. ALS has no affinity for free

IGF-1 or IGF-2 and very low affinity for uncomplexed IGFBP-3. Main binding protein of IGFs is IGFBP-3 and its synthesis is mainly determined by growth hormone. IGFBP-3 is the most abundant form of the IGFBPs. IGFBP-3 concentrations decreases in patientes with growth hormone deficiency and increaes by GH secretion. Testesterone administration adminstration increases IGFBP-3 levels in serum. IGFBP-3 level is also affected by thyroid hormone levels. Low IGFBP-3 levels were found in hypothyroid patients and IGFBP-3 levels are increased by thyroxine replacement in hypothyroid patients. The IGFBP-1 that is present in the circulation is also synthesized in the liver. At concentrations higher than IGF-1, IGFBP-1 inhibit DNA synthesis, glucose transportation [44]. Postprandial increase in serum insulin concentrations results in a four- to five-fold decrease in IGFBP-1 [45]. Intrauterine growth retardation correlates with high levels of serum IGF binding protein-1 (IGFBP-1). Overexpression of IGFBP-1 may affect body growth and skeletal formation as well as biomineralization. IGFBP-1 overexpression may also reduce carbohydrate resources necessary for growth and survival [46]. IGFBP-1 play roles in the endometrial and ovarian physiology. The IGFBP-2 that is present in the circulation originates from hepatocytes, GH is a main determinant of IGFBP-2 levels in circulation. IGF-1 is a potent stimulant of IGFBP-2 concentrations in serum. IGFBP-2 gene transcription is increased in starved rodents and plasma concentrations are increased in fasted humans [47]. IGFBP-2 has mostly inhibitory effects. IGF-1 stimulated collagen synthesis is inhibited by IGFBP-2.

The serum concentrations of intact IGFBP-4 are quite low. IGFBP-4 level is increased with low bone turnover and low parathyroid hormone levels. Sunlight exposure, vitamin D or its active metabolites also may regulate serum IGFBP-4. It may play a role in bone metabolism. IGFBP-5 circulates as incomplete fragments, intact IGFBP-5 is at very low levels. Its concentration are also regulated with GH ang IGF-1. IGFBP-6 inhibits the effects of IGF-2 in several tissues and cell types. IGFBP-6 differs from the other IGFBPs, it has a markedly higher affinity for IGF-2 than for IGF-1, whereas the other IGFBPs bind the two IGFs with similar affinities and IGFBP-2 has a slight IGF-2 binding preference [48, 49, 50].

However, IGF bioactivity in tissues is not determined by the circulating levels of IGFs, IGFBPS, ALS. Proteases that digest IGFBPs are also important in determining the acions of IGFs at tissue level. In addition IGFBPs have their own separate roles in the extravascular tissue compartment.

3. IGFs and bone

Osteoblasts and preosteoblasts secrete IGF-1. Several bone trophic factors, estrogens, PTH stimulate the synthesis of the IGF-1 while glucocorticoids, FGF, PDGF, TGF-B decreases IGF1 expression.

IGF-1 released from the bone matrix during bone remodeling stimulates osteoblastic differentiation of recruited mesenchymal stem cells by activation of mammalian target of rapamycin (mTOR), thus maintaining proper bone microarchitecture and mass. It is well known that both BMD and serum concentration of IGF-1 decrease with age, in age-related osteoporosis in humans, it is found that bone marrow IGF-1 concentrations were 40% lower in individuals with osteoporosis than in individuals without osteoporosis [51]. As compared to healthy controls, total bone mass was found lower in men with GH deficiency and The total BMD was found positively related to plasma IGF-1 and median of GH values [52]. GH deficiency in adulthood is associated with reduced BMD. IGF-1 may be an early marker for low bone mass [53]. Short term treatment with recombinant human IGF-1 in healthy postmenopausal women resulted in increases in bone turnover markers [54]. However, certain effects of the long-term treatment with IGF-1 is unknown.

4. IGFs and growth

Linear bone growth at the epiphyseal plate occurs by a process that is similar to endochondral ossification. The epiphyseal plate between the epiphysis and the metaphysis grows by mitosis. This process continues throughout childhood and the adolescent years until the cartilage growth slows and finally stops. GH may act directly at the growth plate to amplify the production of chondrocytes from germinal zone precursors and then to induce local IGF-1 synthesis, which is thought to stimulate the clonal expansion of chondrocyte columns in an autocrine/paracrine manner [55, 56]. IGF-2 mRNA expression is higher in the proliferative and resting zones than the hypertrophic zone. IGF-1 and GH receptors are expressed throughout the growth plate. Molecular studies revealed that the causes of GH resistance are deletions[57] or mutations [58] in the GH receptor gene, resulting in the failure to generate IGF-1 and a reduction in the synthesis of several other substances,including IGFBP-3.

The expression of IGF-I, IGF-II, IGFBP-3, and ALS is tightly controlled by GH. STAT5B is a transcription factor mediating effect of GH on liver. Six cases of homozygous mutations of the signal transducer and activator of transcription STAT5B gene have also been described [59]. These mutations result in a type of dwarfism characterised by high serum GH values. Studies revealed that these patients cannot generate IGF-1. Several cases have been reported of mutations of the gene for the ALS, which encodes a protein which forms part of the ternary complex that transports IGF-1 in serum [60, 61]. These cases have markedly low serum IGF-1 concentrations and modest growth failure. Syndrome of GH resistance (insensitivity) was named by Elders et al as Laron dwarfism, a name subsequently changed to Laron syndrome [62]. Long term treatment of patients with LS promotes growth and, if treatment is started at an early age, there is a considerable potential for achieving height normalisation [63]. The recently available recombinant human insulin-like growth factor I has shown promise as a promoter of growth in children with Laron syndrome. Main adverse effects with IGF-1 treatment is hypoglycemia. Other adverse effects of IGF-1 treatment appear to be related to hyperstimulation of lymphoid tissue growth: tonsillar growth, snoring, sleep apnea, recurrent ear infections, thymic hypertrophy, and splenic enlargement [64, 65, 66, 67]. Injection site hypertrophy has been observed, but is generally amenable to proper rotation of injection sites. Arthralgias and myalgias have been reported in as many as 20% of recipients in uncontrolled studies, but are usually transient. Benign intracranial hypertension has been reported in ~4% of recipients. Although this number appears somewhat larger than that observed with GH treatment, it is usually transient, disappearing following temporary cessation of treatment. Craniofacial growth, sometimes with coarsening of features, has been described in a number of patients [64, 65, 66, 67].

5. IGFs and cancer

The IGF-1R can regulate cell-cycle progression through control of several cycle checkpoints. It can facilitate G0-G1 transition through activation of p70S6K, leading to phosphorylation of the S6 ribosomal protein and an increased ribosomal pool necessary for entry into the cycle [68]. It can promote G1-S transition by increasing cyclin D1 and CDK4 gene expression, leading to retinoblastoma protein phosphorylation, release of the transcription factor E2F, and synthesis of cyclin E [69, 70]. Alterations in cyclin D1 expression to play a role in tumor formation. IGF's are also important for the development and progression of angiogenesis in tumors. Tumor-induced neovascularization is one of the pathologic mechanisms lying underlying cancer metastasis. IGF-1 and IGF-2 can induce angiogenesis by stimulating the migration and morphological differentiation of endothelial cells [71, 72]. Hypoxia is a major trigger for tumor-dependent angiogenesis. IGF-1 and IGF-2 can induce the expression of hypoxia-inducible factor 1α and this can lead to the formation of the HIF-1/arylhydrocarbon receptor nuclear translocator complex which is involved in transcriptional regulation of hypoxia response element-containing genes such as VEGF [73], a major tumor-derived angiogenic factor. The IGF system can cooperate with other tyrosine kinase receptors such as the EGFR in the induction of angiogenesis [74].

Accumulating evidence has suggested that GH and IGF-1 may be important components of the pathophysiologic mechanisms that underlie the growth of neoplasms, including colorectal carcinoma [75, 76, 77, 78]. Many epidemiology studies have indicated that high levels of IGF - I or altered levels of its binding proteins, or both, are associated with an increased risk of the most common cancers, including cancers of the lung [79], colon and rectum [80], prostate, and breast [81].

Patients with acromegaly, who have elevated levels of circulating GH and IGF-1, may be at increased risk of developing colorectal adenoma and carcinoma [82, 83].

Two prospective epidemiologic studies [84, 85] have shown that higher plasma IGF-1 and lower plasma IGFBP-3 concentrations are associated with an increased risk of colorectal adenoma and cancer among both men and women. These observations suggest that the ratio of circulating IGF-1/IGFBP-3 may be a marker of circulating and tissue IGF-1 bioavailability. Cancer can cause proteolysis of insulin-like growth factor binding protein-3 and affect concentrations of IGFBP-2. These changes in IGF system can affect distribution and clearance of IGFs, thus bioavaibility of IGFs to spesific tissues. In vitro studies on human colon cancer cells, which showed that IGF-1 promoted cell proliferation, IGF-1 receptors were frequently overexpressed on colon cancer cells and IGF-1R blockade with a monoclonal antibody inhibited cell proliferation [85]. A larger case-control study from Sweden reported a similar positive association between IGF-1 level and prostate cancer risk [86]. In the Physicians' Health

Study, a prospective epidemiological study, the associations between IGF-1 and IGFBP-3 levels and subsequent prostate cancer risk among 152 patients and 152 age-matched controls were investigated. There was a significant linear trend between IGF-1 and prostate cancer risk [87]. Strong association between IGF-1 and IGFBP-3 levels and the risk of advanced prostate cancer but no association with early stage disease was found. Measurement of IGF-1 and IGFBP-3 levels may predict the risk of advanced stage prostate cancer years before the cancer is actually diagnosed and may be helpful in aiding decision making about treatment [88]. No trend in the relative risk of prostate cancer with increasing IGF-1 was found in another study; rather, the highest incidence of prostate cancer was in the lowest quartile of IGF-1, and the incidence in the other quartiles of IGF-1 was slightly lower but not statistically significantly different from incidence rates in the lowest quartile [89]. A multiethnic study was performed to determine the associations between prediagnostic levels of IGF-1 and IGFBP-3 and risk of prostate cancer. In this study no association was observed for levels of IGF-1 or IGF-to-IGFBP-3 ratio and prostate cancer risk [90]. In one metaanalyze including included both retrospective and prospective studies and demonstrated that average 21% increase risk of prostate cancer per standard deviation increase in IGF-1. A stronger association of IGF-1 was found in more aggressive and advanced cancers in comparison to nonaggressive and localized ones [91]. Considerable evidence has accumulated that suggests that the IGF system is involved in the pathophysiology of prostate cancer. GH is believed to be the pituitary factor responsible for mammary ductal morphogenesis [92, 93]. It has been reported that IGF-1 or amino-terminally truncated IGF-1, des(1–3) IGF-1, mimic the action of GH on mammary development in hypophysectomized gonadectomized rats [94, 95]. IGF-1 mRNA is localized to stromal fibroblasts surrounding normal breast epithelium while high levels of IGF-2 mRNA are found in fibroblasts adjacent to malignant epithelium [96, 97]. Malignant breast epithelial cells can induce expression of IGF-2 in the stroma in vitro [98]. IGF-1R has been found on the surface of malignant breast epithelial cells [99] and IGFs provide radioprotection and resistance of breast cancer cells to chemotherapeutic agents [100, 101]. Some epidemiologic studies have associated high circulating levels of IGF-1 with increased risk of breast cancer among premenopausal women. In a meta-analysis, circulating levels of IGF-1 were not significantly higher in breast cancer patients than in controls for all women and for the postmenopausal group but were significantly higher for the premenopausal group [102]. Literature on the relationship between breast cancer risk and circulating concentrations of IGF-1 and IGFBP-3 showed an increased risk for premenopausal women with increasing levels of IGF-1 and IGFBP-3. More prospective studies are needed to clarify the association between IGF-1 and IGFBP-3 and breast cancer.

Overexpression of IGF-2 mRNA and peptide has been described in human pheochromocytomas [103, 104]. Despite to this finding, very little tumoral IGF-2 is released into the circulation, unlike catecholamines [104]. IGF-1 also seems to be secreted by pheochromocytoma cells in an autocrine or paracrine manner. In rat pheochromocytoma PC12 cells IGF-1R has been shown to be important for the stimulation of cell replication [105]. Significant overexpression of the IGF-1R in human pheochromocytomas was found. [106]. IGF-1 was 10 times more potent in stimulating DNA synthesis than IGF-2, suggesting that these effects are mediated by the IGF-1R [107, 108]. In Wilms' tumor, a childhood kidney neoplasm expresses IGF-2 mRNA and protein [109]. Wilms' tumors contain receptors that recognize and respond to exogenous IGF

[110]. Deletions or point mutations of the Wilms tumor suppressor gene-1 (WT-1) on chromosome 11p13 are associated with Wilms' tumors. WT1 binds to multiple sites in the promoter region of the IGF-2 gene, and that it acts as a potent repressor of IGF-2 transcription [111]. A molecular basis for the overexpression of IGF-2 in Wilms' tumor may have autocrine effects in tumor progression.

IGF-1R is expressed in pancreatic cancer cell lines and human pancreatic cancers and also IGF-1 is markedly overexpressed in these cancers [112]. The anti-IGF-1R antibody inhibited the action of IGF-1 on cell proliferation. Moderately strong IGF-2R immunoreactivity was present in the cytoplasm of islet cells and mild cytoplasmic immunoreactivity was evident occasionally in ductal and acinar cells. In the pancreatic cancers, regions of strong IGF-2R immunoreactivity were present in the duct-like cancer cells within the tumor mass often exhibiting nuclear localization [113].

IGF-2R may contribute to the pathobiology of pancreatic cancer. Insulin-like growth factor 2 mRNA binding protein 3 (IGF2BP-3) was found to be selectively overexpressed in pancreatic ductal adenocarcinoma tissues but not in benign pancreatic tissues. The highest rate of expression was seen in poorly differentiated cancers. Overall survival was found to be significantly shorter in patients with IGF2BP-3 expressing tumors [114]. Enhanced expression of IGF-1 and IGF-2 mRNA transcripts has been demonstrated in gliomas, meniningiomas, and other tumours [115]. Patients with malignant CNS tumours showed increased IGFBP-2 concentrations in CSF. Patients with CNS tumours and microscopically detectable malignant cells in their CSF had the highest IGFBP-2 values [116]. The IGFs have important roles in the normal ovary and exert intra-ovarian control in the replication and differentiation processes of folliculogenesis. [117, 118]. The IGFs, their receptors and IGFBPs were identified in ovarian tumours. IGFBP-2 levels are high in the sera of patients with epithelial ovarian cancer and they may be useful as a possible tumour marker [119, 120]. Primary ovarian epithelial cell lines derived from previously untreated ovarian cancers expressed all major components of the IGF system and were able to demonstrate functional responses to exogenous IGFs [121]. Expression of the IGF-2 gene was more than 300-fold higher in ovarian cancers compared with normal ovarian surface epithelium samples. High IGF-2 expression was associated with advanced stage disease at diagnosis, high-grade cancers and sub-optimal surgical cytoreduction. Relative IGF-2 expression was regarded as an independent predictor of poor survival [122]. IGF-1 mRNA expression and peptide concentrations were also analyzed in epithelial ovarian cancer. High levels of free IGF-1 peptide were associated with elevated risk of disease progression. Women with high IGF-1 mRNA and peptide were found to be at greater risk for disease progression compared to those with low in both [123].

6. IGFs and hypoglycemia

Hypoglyaemia from malignant tumours is rare. This is the only paraneoplastic syndrome caused by the IGF2 overproduction. This phenomenon, referred to as non islet cell tumour hypoglycaemia (NICTH). Hypoglycaemia secondary to mesenchymal tumours account for

64% of the cases with hepatomas, adrenal carcinomas, and gastrointestinal malignancies accounting for others [124, 125]. Endogenous IGFs which circulate in adults fail to exert their immense potential hypoglycaemic activity because they are largely trapped within the vascular space due to their sequestration in a high molecular weight protein complex. IGF-2 leads to an increased peripheral glucose uptake in different tissues as well as inhibition of hepatic gluconeogenesis and lipolysis [126]. IGF-2 has also been shown to have high affinity binding with the insulin receptor. The insulin receptor exon 11+ (IR-B) isoform is the form best known for the classic metabolic responses induced upon insulin binding and this isoform has low affinity for the IGFs. IGF-2 binds with high affinity to the insulin receptor exon 11− (IR-A) isoform of the IR. Activation of IR-A leads to mitogenic responses similar to those described for the IGF-1R [127]. IGF-2 gene can be expressed to produce proteins of various molecular weights. The most active form, with regard to binding of IGF receptors, is 7.5kDa [128]. IGF-2 gene expression regulation, post-translational processing of the 156-amino acid IGF-2 precursor is abnormal in tumors [129]. Larger forms lack posttranslational cleavage plays role in hypoglycemia. Incompletely processed IGF-II (Big-IGF-II) has a strongly reduced affinity for ALS. Impaired formation of the 150 kDa complex, tumour-derived 'big'-IGF-II primarily forms smaller binary complexes with IGFBPs and a greater fraction may stay in the free unbound form [130, 131, 132]. These smaller complexes have a greater capillary permeability and thus are thought to increase IGF bioavailability to the tissues, resulting in hypoglycaemia through action on the insulin receptors and IGF1R [133]. Patients whose underlying condition is one of GH resistance, especially if it is complete and at the level of the GHR, having lost the counter-regulatory effects of GH, are susceptible to hypoglycemia with the IGF-1 treatment [134]. Administration of IGF-I with meals may overcome with this problem.

7. IGFs and diabetes

Reduced IGF-1 levels have been proposed to have a role in diabetes [135]. In animal studies deletion of IGF-1 gene expression in liver caused increased GH secretion and reduced insülin sensitivity. A positive association between low IGF-1 levels and glucose intolerance/ diabetes in a sample of 615 subjects aged 45-65 years was found [136]. In contrast, recently Rajpatak et al did not find an independent association between IGF-1 and diabetes among 922 subjects aged >/=65 yrs from the Cardiovascular Health Study [137]. In a study was to evaluate the association between IGF-1 level and insulin resistance, both low and high normal IGF-1 levels are found to be related to insulin resistance [138]. A study in 7,665 subjects showed that low and high baseline IGF-1 serum concentrations were both related to a higher risk of developing type 2 diabetes within 5 years [139]. This U-shaped association seems to be likely in face of a higher prevalence of metabolic syndrome or type 2 diabetes in patients with GH deficiency [140]. A state of low IGF-1 levels, as well as with acromegaly [141], a disease characterized by high IGF-1 levels, although endogenous GH secretion may confound short-term glucose homeostasis in these patients. IGF-1 administration reduces the GH hypersecretion of adolescents and adults with type 1 diabetes [142, 143]. IGF-1 administration increases systemic IGF-1 levels, resulting in reduced GH secretion and improves insulin sensitivity in adults with type 1 diabetes [144]. Also in patients with types 2 diabetes, glycemic control improves with IGF-1 treatment [145]. In one study, subcutaneous administration of of recombinant human IGF-1 (for 6 weeks) significantly lowered blood glucose. Glycosylated hemoglobin, which was 10.4% pretreatment, declined to 8.1% at the end of therapy and this improvement in glycemic control was accompanied by a change in body composition with a 2.1% loss in body fat without change in total body weight [146]. Paracrine or autocrine effects of IGF-1 may paly a role in the pathogenesis of diabetic complications. Hyperglycemia and IGF-1 stimulate the endothelial cell migration, and tubular formation is induced by a combination of IGF-1 and hyperglycemia [147]. Animal models have provided direct evidence that IGF-1 contributes to the development of retinopathy induced by retinal ischemia. Active capillary proliferation has been documented after implantation of intracorneal pellets containing IGF-1 [148]. The progression of retinopathy is slowed in diabetic patients with hypopituitarism who have low serum IGF-1 levels [149, 150]. Patients with more rapid progression of their retinopathy had the highest levels of IGF-1 in the vitreous [151]. However, Data concerning the relationship between serum IGF-1 levels and diabetic retinopathy is contradictory. Some studies have shown no association between serum IGF-I levels and the development or progression of diabetic retinopathy. In patients with diabetic retinopathy IGF-1 reducing treatment strategies with either somatostatins or pegvisomant have been tried. Glomerular hypertrophy is thought to be one of the key early changes in the development of diabetic nephropathy. IGF-I has been associated with renal/glomerular hypertrophy and compensatory renal growth. Epithelial, mesangial, and endothelial cells derived from the kidney respond to IGF-1 binding with increased protein synthesis, migration, and proliferation. Both GH and IGF-I increase renal plasma flow and glomerular filtration rate. Microalbuminuric patients display higher levels of urinary IGF-1, urinary GH, and plasma IGF-1 than normoalbuminuric diabetic subjects [152]. Patients with microalbuminuria had higher levels of urinary IGFBP-3 even when compared to patients without microalbuminuria matched for metabolic control [152, 153, 154]. Hyperglycemic conditions limit the protective role of IGF-I against podocyte apoptosis. IGFBP-3 can facilitate podocyte apoptosis. Podocyte structural changes also contribute to the pathogenesis of albuminuria in diabetes. IGF-1 binding to its type 1 receptors stimulates mesengial cell proliferation [155]. Mesengial cell proliferation is one of the factors that contributes diabetic nephropathy.

Higher IGF-1 bioavailability may protect against the onset of ischemic heart disease [156, 157]. Potential beneficial actions of IGF-1 in cardiovascular physiology include increased nitric oxide synthesis and K+ channel opening [158,159] and this may explain the impaired small-vessel function associated with low IGF-1 levels in patients with cardiovascular syndrome X [159]. Higher IGF-1 bioavailability may offer improved metabolic control and prevent vascular complications in type 2 diabetic patients. In contrast to this finding, posttranslational phosphorylation of IGFBP-1 increases its affinity for IGF-1 and modify IGF bioavailability. Low circulating levels of hpIGFBP-1 are found to be closely correlated with macrovascular disease and hypertension in type 2 diabetes [160]. further studies are needed to better understand the true value of the IGF-1/IGFBP axis in macrovascular complications of diabetes.

Author details

Emrah Yerlikaya* and Fulya Akin

Pamukkale University Division of Endocrinology and Metabolism, Denizli, Turkey

References

[1] Salmon W, Daughaday W. Journal of Laboratory and Clinical Medicine 1957;49 (6): 825–36.

[2] Brissenden JE, Ullrich A, Francke U. Human chromosomal mapping of genes for insulin-like growth factors 1 and 2 and epidermal growth factor. Nature 1984;310:781–4.

[3] Rotwein P. Structure, evolution, expression and regulation of insulin-like growth factors I and II. Growth Factors 1991;5:3–18.

[4] Sussenbach JS, Steenbergh PH, Holthuizen P. Structure and expression of the human insulin-like growth factor genes. Growth Regulation 1992;2:1–9.

[5] Jansen E, Steenbergh PH, van Schaik FM, Sussenbach JS. The human IGF-1 gene contains two cell type-specifically regulated promoters. Biochemical and Biophysical Research Communications 1992;187:1219–1226.

[6] Baxter RC. Insulin-like growth factor (IGF)-binding proteins: interactions with IGFs and intrinsic bioactivities. American Journal of Physiology-Endo 2000; 278:967-E976

[7] Hwa V, Oh Y, Rosenfeld RG. The insulin-like growth factor binding protein (IGFBP) superfamily. Endocrine Reviews 1999;20: 761–87.

[8] Yu H, Rohan T. Role of the insulin-like growth factor family in cancer development and progression. Journal of the National Cancer Institute. 2000; 92:1472-89.

[9] Baxter RC. Molecular aspects of insulin-like growth factor binding proteins. Molecular and Cellular Endocrinology1997;1:123–159.

[10] Morgan, DO, Jarnagin K. and Roth RA. Purification and characterization of the receptor for insulin-like growth factor 1. Biochemistry 1986; 25:5560-5564.

[11] Adams TE, Epa VC, Garrett TP, Ward CW. Structure and function of the type 1 insulin-like growth factor receptor. Cellular and Molecular Life Sciences 2000; 57:1050–1093.

[12] Kornfeld S. Structure and function of the mannose-6-phosphate/insulin like growth factor II receptors. Annu Rev Biochem 1992; 61 : 307-30.

[13] Tong PY, Tollefsen SE, Kornfeld S. The cation-independent mannose 6-phosphate receptor binds insulin-like growth factor 2. Journal of Biological Chemistry 1988;263:2585–8.

[14] Vincent AM, Feldman EL. Control of cell survival by IGF signaling pathways. Growth hormone & IGF research 2002;12(4):193-7.

[15] [15]. Kuemmerle JF. IGF-1 elicits growth of human intestinal smooth muscle cells by activation of PI3K, PDK-1, and p70S6 kinase. American journal of physiology. 2003;284(3):G411-22

[16] Galvan V, Logvinova A, Sperandio S, Ichijo H, Bredesen DE. Type 1 insulin-like growth factor receptor signaling inhibits apoptosis signal-regulating kinase 1 (ASK1). The Journal of biological chemistry 2003;278(15):13325-32.

[17] Donaghy A, Ross R, Gimson A, et al. Growth hormone, insulinlike growth factor-1, and insulinlike growth factor binding proteins 1 and 3 in chronic liver disease. Hepatology 1995; 21(3):680-8.

[18] Wu YL, Ye J, Zhang S, et al. Clinical significance of serum IGF-1, IGF-2 and IGFBP-3 in liver cirrhosis. World Journal of Gastroenterology 2004; 10(18):2740-3.

[19] Veldhuis JD, Iranmanesh A, Weltman A. Elements in the pathophysiology of diminished GH secretion in aging humans. Endocrine 1997;7:41–8.

[20] Toogood AA, O'Neil PA, Shalet SA. Beyond the somatopause: GHD in adults over age 60. Journal of Clinical Endocrinology & Metabolism 1996;81:460–3.

[21] Hoffman AR, Lieberman SA, Butterfield G, Thompson J, Hintz RRL, Ceda GP, Marcus R. Functional consequences of the somatopause and its treatment. Endocrine 1997;7:73–6.

[22] Greendale GA, Delstein S, Barrett Connor E. Endogenous sex steroids and bone mineral density in older men and women. Journal of Bone and Mineral Research 1997;12:1833–43.

[23] Ho KY, Evans WS, Blizzard RM, Veldhuis JD, Merriam GR, Samojlik E, Furlanetto R, Rogol AD, Kaiser DL, Thorner MO. Effects of sex and age on the 24-hour profile of growth hormone secretion in man: importance of endogenous estradiol concentrations. Journal of Clinical Endocrinology & Metabolism 1987; 64:51–58.

[24] Thompson RG, Rodriguez A, Kowarski A, Blizzard RM. Growth hormone: metabolic clearance rates, integrated concentrations, and production rates in normal adults and the effect of prednisone. Journal of Clinical Investigation 1972; 51:3193–3199.

[25] Van den Berg G, Veldhuis JD, Frolich M, Roelfsema F. An amplitude-specific divergence in the pulsatile mode of growth hormone (GH) secretion underlies the gender difference in mean GH concentrations in men and premenopausal women. Journal of Clinical Endocrinology & Metabolism 1996; 81:2460–2467.

[26] Isotton AL, Wender MC, Casagrande A, Rollin G, Czepielewski MA. Effects of oral and transdermal estrogen on IGF1, IGFBP3, IGFBP1, serum lipids, and glucose in patients with hypopituitarism during GH treatment: a randomized study. European Journal of Endocrinology 2012 ;166(2):207-13.

[27] Greendale GA, Delstein S, Barrett Connor E. Endogenous sex steroids and bone mineral density in older men and women. Journal of Bone and Mineral Research 1997;12:1833–43.

[28] Hobbs CJ, Plymate SR, Rosén CJ, Adler RA: Testosterone administration increases insulinlike growth factor I levels in normal men. Journal of Clinical Endocrinology & Metabolism 1993; 77: 776–779.

[29] Fisker S, Jørgensen JOL, Vahl N, Ørskov H, Christiansen JS. Impact of gender and androgen status on IGF-1 levels in normal and GH deficient adults. European Journal of Endocrinology 1999; 141:601–608.

[30] DePugola G, Lespite L, Grizzulli VA. IGF-1 and DHEA-S in obese females. International Journal of Obesity an Related Metabolic Disorders 1993;11:481–3.

[31] Schmid C, Zwimpfer C, Brändle M, Krayenbühl PA, Zapf J, Wiesli P. Effect of thyroxine replacement on serum IGF-1, IGFBP-3 and the acid-labile subunit in patients with hypothyroidism and hypopituitarism Clinical Endocrinology 2006: 65;706–711

[32] Nanto-Salonen K & Muller HL, Hoffman AR, Vu TH & Rosenfeld RG. Mechanisms of thyroid hormone action on the insulin-like growth factor system: all thyroid hormone effects are not growth hormone mediated. Endocrinology 1993; 132:781–788.

[33] Schmid C, Brandle M, Zwimpfer C, Zapf J & Wiesli P. Effect of thyroxine replacement on creatinine, insulin-like growth factor 1, acid-labile subunit, and vascular endothelial growth factor. Clinical Chemistry 2004; 50:228–231.

[34] Isley WL, Underwood LE, Clemmons DR. Changes in plasma somatomedin-C in response to diets with variable protein and energy content. Journal of Parenteral and Enteral Nutrition 1984; 8: 407-411.

[35] Clemmons DR, Klibanski A, Underwood LE et al. Reduction of plasma immunoreactive somatomedin-C during fasting in humans. Journal of Clinical Endocrinology & Metabolism 1981; 53: 1247-1250.

[36] Untermann TG, Vazquez RM, Slas AJ, Martyn PA, Phillips LS. Nutrition and somatomedin. XIII. Usefulness of somatomedin-C in nutritional assessment. Am J Med 1985; 78: 228-234.

[37] Prasad A. Zinc and growth. Journal of the American College of Nutrition 1996; 15: 341–42.

[38] Nakamura T, Nishiyama S, Suginohara YF, Matsuda I, Higashi A. Mild to moderate zinc deficiency in short children. Journal of Pediatrics 1993; 123: 65–9.

[39] Larsson SC, Wolk K, Brismar K, and Wolk A. Association of diet with serum insulin-like growth factor 1 in middle-aged and elderly men American Journal of Clinical Nutrition 2005; 81(5):1163-1167.

[40] Schmid C, Schläpfer I, Peter M, Böni-Schnetzler M, Schwander J, Zapf J, Froesch ER. Growth hormone and parathyroid hormone stimulate IGFBP-3 in rat osteoblasts. American Journal of Physiology. 1994; 267: 226-33

[41] Aleem E, Elshayeb A, Elhabachi N, Mansour AR, Gowily A, Hela A. Serum IGFBP-3 is a more effective predictor than IGF-1 and IGF-2 for the development of hepatocellular carcinoma in patients with chronic HCV infection. Oncology Letters 2012; 3:704-712

[42] Boisclair YR, Seto D, Hsieh S, Hurst KR & Ooi GT. Organization and chromosomal localization of the gene encoding the mouse acid labile subunit of the insulin-like growth factor binding complex. Proceedings of the National Academy of Sciences 1996;93:10028–10033.

[43] Suwanichkul A, Boisclair YR, Olney RC, Durham SK & Powell DR. Conservation of a growth hormone-responsive promoter element in the human and mouse acid-labile subunit genes. Endocrinology 2000; 141 833–838.

[44] Burch WW, Correa J, Shively JE, Powell DR. The 25-kilodalton insulin-like growth factor (IGF)-binding protein inhibits both basal and IGF-1 mediated growth in chick embroyonic pelvic cartilage in vitro. Journal of Clinical Endocrinology & Metabolism 1990; 70:173

[45] Busby WH, Snyder DK, Clemmons DR. Radioimmunoassay of a 26,000-dalton plasma insulin-like growth factor-binding protein: control by nutritional variables. Journal of Clinical Endocrinology & Metabolism. 1988 Dec;67(6):1225-30.

[46] Lagha NB , Seurin D, Bouc YL, Binoux, M, Berdal A , Menuelle P and Babajko S. Insulin-Like Growth Factor Binding Protein (IGFBP-1) Involvement in Intrauterine Growth Retardation: Study on IGFBP-1 Overexpressing Transgenic Mice. Endocrinology 2006;147(10): 4730-4737.

[47] Clemmons DR, Busby WH, Snyder DK. Variables con- trolling the secretion of insulin-like growth factor binding protein-2 in normal human subjects. Journal of Clinical Endocrinology & Metabolism 1991, 73, 727-733.

[48] Roghani M, Hossenlopp P, Lepage P, Balland A & Binoux M. Isolation from human cerebrospinal fluid of a new insulin-like growth factor-binding protein with a selective affinity for IGF-2. FEBS Letters 1989;255 253–258.

[49] Bach LA. Insulin-like growth factor binding protein-6: The 'forgotten' binding protein? Hormone and Metabolic Research 1999; 31:226–234.

[50] Bach LA, Hsieh S, Sakano K, Fujiwara H, Perdue JF & Rechler MM. Binding of mutants of human insulin-like growth factor 2 to insulin-like growth factor binding proteins 1–6. Journal of Biological Chemistry 1993; 268 9246–9254.

[51] Xian L, Matrix IGF-1 maintains bone mass by activation of mTOR in mesenchymal stem cells. Nature Medicine 2012: 18;1095–1101.

[52] Johansson AG, Burman P, Westermark K, Ljunghall S. The bone mineral density in acquired growth hormone deficiency correlates with circulating levels of insulin-like growth factor I. Journal of Internal Medicine 1992; 232(5):447-52.

[53] Liu J, Zhao H, Ning G, Zhang YCL, Sun L, Xu YZM, Chen J. IGF-1 as an early marker for low bone mass or osteoporosis in premenopausal and postmenopausal women Journal of Bone and Mineral Metabolism 2008;26:159–164.

[54] Ghiron LJ, Thompson JL, Holloway L, Hintz RL, Butterfield GE, Hoffman AR, Marcus R. Effects of recombinant insulin-like growth factor-I and growth hormone on bone turnover in elderly women. Journal of Bone and Mineral Research 1995; 10:1844–1852.

[55] Nilsson O, Marino R, De Luca F, Phillip M, Baron J. Endocrine regulation of the growth plate. Horm Res. 2005;64(4):157-65

[56] Ohlsson C, Bengtsson BA, Isaksson OG, Andreassen TT, Slootweg MC. Growth hormone and bone. Endocr Rev. 1998; 19(1):55-79.

[57] Godowski PJ, Leung DW, Meacham LR, et al. Characterization of the human growth hormone receptor gene and demonstration of a partial gene deletion in 2 patients with Laron type dwarfism. Proceedings of the National Academy of Sciences 1989;86:8083–7.

[58] Amselem S, Duquesnoy P, Attree O, et al. Laron dwarfism and mutations of the growth hormone-receptor gene. New England Journal of Medicine 1989;321:989–95.

[59] Rosenfeld RG, Belgorsky A, Camacho-Hubner C, Savage MO, Wit JM & Hwa V. Defects in growth hormone receptor signaling as causes of short stature. Trends in Endocrinology 2007; 18 134–141.

[60] Domene HM, Bengolea SV, Martinez AS, Ropelato MG, Pennisi P, Scaglia P, Heinrich JJ & Jasper HG. Deficiency of the circulating insulin-like growth factor system associated with inactivation of the acid-labile subunit. New England Journal of Medicine 2004; 350:570–577.

[61] Hwa V, Haeusler G, Pratt KL, Little B, Frisch H, Koller D & Rosenfeld RG. Total absence of functional acid labile subunit, resulting in severe insulin-like growth factor deficiency and moderate growth failure. Journal of Clinical Endocrinology and Metabolism 2006; 91:1826–1831.

[62] Laron Z, Parks JS, eds. Lessons from Laron syndrome (LS) 1966–1992. A model of GH and IGF-1 action and interaction. Pediatric and Adolescent Endocrinology 1993;24:1–367.

[63] Ranke MB, Savage MO, Chatelain PG, et al. Long-term treatment of growth hormone insensitivity syndrome with IGF-1. Hormone Research 1999;51:128–34.

[64] Guevara-Aguirre J, Rosenbloom AL, Vasconez O, Martinez V, Gargosky SE, Allen L & Rosenfeld RG. Two-year treatment of growth hormone (GH) receptor deficiency with recombinant insulin-like growth factor I in 22 children: comparison of two dosage levels and to GH-treated GH deficiency. Journal of Clinical Endocrinology and Metabolism 1997; 82:629–633.

[65] Ranke MB, Savage MO, Chatelain PG, Preece MA, Rosenfeld RG & Wilton P. Long-term treatment of growth hormone insensitivity syndrome with IGF-1. Results of the European Multicentre Study. Hormone Research 1999; 51:128–134.

[66] Backeljauw PF & Underwood LE. Therapy for 6.5–7.5 years with recombinant insulin-like growth factor I in children with growth hormone insensitivity syndrome: a Clinical Research Center Study. Journal of Clinical Endocrinology and Metabolism 2001; 86:1504–1510.

[67] Chernausek SD, Backeljauw PF, Frane J, Kuntze J & Underwood LE. Long-term treatment with recombinant IGF-1 in children with severe IGF-1 deficiency due to growth hormone insensitivity. Journal of Clinical Endocrinology and Metabolism 2007; 92 902–910.

[68] Dupont J, Pierre A, Froment P, Moreau C. The insulin-like growth factor axis in cell cycle progression. Hormone and Metabolic Research 2003; 35:740–750

[69] Rosenthal SM, Cheng ZQ. Opposing early and late effects of insulin-like growth factor I on differentiation and the cell cycle regulatory retinoblastoma protein in skeletal myoblasts. Proceedings of the National Academy of Sciences 1995; 92:10307–10311

[70] Dupont J, Karas M, LeRoith D. The potentiation of estrogen on insulin-like growth factor I action in MCF-7 human breast cancer cells includes cell cycle components. Journal of Biological Chemistry 2000; 275:35893–35901.

[71] Shigematsu S, Yamauchi K, Nakajima K, Iijima S, Aizawa T, Hashizume K. IGF-1 regulates migration and angiogenesis of human endothelial cells. Endocrine Journal 1999; 46: 59–S62

[72] Lee OH, Bae SK, Bae MH, Lee YM, Moon EJ, Cha HJ, Kwon YG, KimKW. Identification of angiogenic properties of insulin-like growth factor II in in vitro angiogenesis models. British Journal of Cancer 2000; 82: 385–391

[73] Zelzer E, Levy Y, Kahana C, Shilo BZ, Rubinstein M, Cohen B. Insulin induces transcription of target genes through the hypoxia inducible factor HIF-1α/ARNT. EMBO Journal 17:5085–5094.

http://dx.doi.org/10.5772/55213

[74] Samani AA, Yakar S, LeRoith D and Brodt P. The Role of the IGF system in cancer growth and metastasis: Overview and recent insights Endocrine Reviews 2007;28(1): 20–47

[75] LeRoith D, Baserga R, Helman L, Roberts CT Jr. Insulin-like growth factors and cancer. Annals of Internal Medicine 1995; 122:54–9.

[76] Baserga R. The insulin growth factor I receptor: a key to tumour growth? Cancer Research 1995; 55:249–52.

[77] Singh P, Rubin R. Insulin-like growth factors and binding proteins in colon cancer. Gastroenterology 1993;105:1218–37.

[78] Tricoli JV, Rall LB, Karakousis CP, Herrara L, Petrelli NJ, Bell GI, et al. Enhanced levels of insulin-like growth factor mRNA in human colon carcinomas and liposarcomas. Cancer Research 1986;46:6169–73.

[79] Karamouzis MV, Papavassiliou AG. The IGF -1 network in lung carcinoma therapeutics. Trends in Molecular Medicine 2006; 12:595–602.

[80] Durai R, Davies M, Yang W, et al. Biology of insulin-like growth factor binding protein-4 and its role in cancer. International Journal of Oncology 2006; 28:1317–25.

[81] Renehan AG, Zwahlen M, Minder C, O'Dwyer ST, Shalet SM, Egger M. Insulin-like growth factor (IGF)- I, IGF binding protein- 3, and cancer risk: systematic review and meta-regression analysis. Lancet 2004;363:1346–53.

[82] Jenkins PJ, Besser GM, Fairclough PD. Colorectal neoplasia in acromegaly. Gut 1999; 44:585–7.

[83] Orme SM, McNally RJ, Cartwright RA, Belchetz PE. Mortality and cancer incidence in acromegaly: a retropsective cohort study. United Kingdom Acromegaly Study Group. Journal of Clinical Endocrinology & Metabolism 1998; 83:2730–4.

[84] Giovannucci E, Pollak MN, Platz EA, Willett WC, Stampfer MJ, Majeed N, et al. A prospective study of plasma insulin-like growth factor-1 and binding protein-3 and the risk of colorectal neoplasia in women. Cancer Epidemiology, Biomarkers & Prevention 2000; 9:345–49.

[85] Ma J, Pollak MN, Giovannucci E, Chan JM, Tao Y, Hennekens C, et al. Prospective study of colorectal cancer risk in men and plasma levels of insulin-like growth factor (IGF)-1 and IGF binding protein-3. Journal of the National Cancer Institute 1999 ; 91:620–5.

[86] Wolk A, Mantzoros CS, Andersson SO, Bergström H, Signorello LB, Lagiou P, et al. Insulin-like growth factor 1 and prostate cancer risk: a population-based, case-control study. Journal of the National Cancer Institute 1998; 90(12):911-5.

[87] Chan JM, Stampfer MJ, Giovannucci E, Gann PH, Ma J, Wilkinson P, Hennekens CH, Pollak M. Plasma insulin-like growth factor-I and prostate cancer risk: a prospective study. Science. 1998; 279(5350):563-6.

[88] Chan JM et al. Insulin-like growth factor-1 (IGF-1) and IGF binding protein-3 as predictors of advanced-stage prostate cancer. Journal of the National Cancer Institute. 2002; 94:1099-1106.

[89] [89]. Schaefer C, Gary D. Friedman, Charles P. Quesenberry Jr. IGF-1 and Prostate Cancer. Science 1998; 282:199

[90] BorugianMJ, Spinelli JJ, Sun Z, Kolonel LN, Girvan IO, Pollak MD, Whittemore AS, Wu AH and Gallagher RP. Prostate Cancer Risk in Relation to Insulin-like Growth Factor (IGF)-I and IGF-Binding Protein-3: A Prospective Multiethnic Study. Cancer Epidemiology, Biomarkers & Prevention 2008; 17:252-254.

[91] Rowlands MA, David Gunnell D, Ross Haris R, Vatten LJ, Holly JMP and Martin RM. Circulating insulin-like growth factor (IGF) peptides and prostate cancer risk: a systematic review and meta-analysis. International Journal of Cancer 2009; 124(10): 2416–2429.

[92] Kleinberg DL, Ruan W, Catanese V, Newman CB & Feldman M. Non-lactogenic effects of growth hormone on growth and insulin-like growth factor-1 messenger ribonucleic acid of rat mammary gland. Endocrinology 1990; 126:3274–3276.

[93] Feldman M, Ruan W, Cunningham BC, Wells JA & Kleinberg DL. Evidence that the growth hormone receptor mediates differentiation and development of the mammary gland. Endocrinology 1993; 133:1602–1608.

[94] Ruan W, Newman CB & Kleinberg DL. Intact and amino-terminally shortened forms of insulin-like growth factor 1 induce mammary gland differentiation and development. Proceedings of the National Academy of Sciences 1992; 89:0872–10876.

[95] Ruan W, Catanese V, Wieczorek R, Feldman M & Kleinberg DL. Estradiol enhances the stimulatory effect of insulin-like growth factor- 1 (IGF-1) on mammary development and growth hormone-induced IGF-1 messenger ribonucleic acid. Endocrinology 1995; 136:1296–1302.

[96] Pekonen F, Partanen S, Makinen T & Rutanen EM. Receptors for epidermal growth factor and insulin-like growth factor 1 and their relation to steroid receptors in human breast cancer. Cancer Research 1988; 48:1343–1347.

[97] Toropainen EM, Lipponen PK & Syrjanen KJ. Expression of insulin-like growth factor 2 in female breast cancer as related to established prognostic factors and long-term prognosis. AntiCancer Research 1995; 15:2669–2674.

[98] Singer C, Rasmussen A, Smith HS, Lippman ME, Lynch HT, Cullen KJ. Malignant breast epithelium selects for insulin-like growth factor-2 expression in breast stroma: evidence for paracrine function. Cancer Research 1995; 55:2448–2454.

[99] Pollak MN, Perdue JF, Margolese RG, Baer K, Richard M. Presence of somatomedin receptors on primary human breast and colon carcinomas. Cancer Letters 1987; 38:223–230.

[100] Dunn SE, Hardman RA, Kari FW, Barrett JC. Insulin-like growth factor 1 alters drug sensitivity of HBL100 human breast cancer cells by inhibition of apoptosis induced by diverse anticancer drugs. Cancer Research 1997; 57:2687–2693.

[101] Gooch JL, Van Den Berg CL, Yee D. Insulin-like growth factor-1 rescues breast cancer cells from chemotherapy induced cell death – proliferative and anti-apoptotic effects. Breast Cancer Research and Treatment 1999; 56:1–10.

[102] [102]. Shi R, Yu H, McLarty J, Glass J. IGF-1 and breast cancer: a meta-analysis. International Journal of Cancer. 2004; 111(3):418-23.

[103] 103] Haselbacher GK, Irminger JC, Zapf J, Ziegler WH, Humbel RE. Insulin-like growth factor 2 in human adrenal pheochromocytomas and Wilms tumors: expression at the mRNA and protein level. Proceedings of the National Academy of Sciences 1987; 84 1104–1106.

[104] Gelato MC, Vassalotti J. Insulin-like growth factor-2: possible local growth factor in pheochromocytoma. Journal of Clinical Endocrinology and Metabolism. 1990; 71(5): 1168-74.

[105] Dahmer MK, Hart PM, Perlman RL. Studies on the effect of insulin-like growth factor 1 on catecholamine secretion from chromaffin cells. Journal of Neurochemistry 1990; 54 931–936.

[106] Christian Fottner C, Timo Minnemann T, Sarah Kalmbach S and Matthias M Weber MM. Overexpression of the insulin-like growth factor I receptor in human pheochromocytomas. Journal of Molecular Endocrinology 2006 Apr;36(2):279-87.

[107] Dahmer MK, Perlman RL. Insulin and insulin-like growth factors stimulate desoxyribonucleic acid synthesis in PC12 pheochromocytoma cells. Endocrinology 1988; 122 2109–2113.

[108] Nielsen FC, Gammeltoft S. Insulin-like growth factors are mitogens for rat pheochromocytoma PC 12 cells. Biochemical and Biophysical Research Communications 1988; 154:1018–1023.

[109] Ren-Qiu Q, Schmitt S, Ruelicke T, Stallmach T and Schoenle EJ. Autocrine regulation of growth by insulin like growth Factor-2 mediated by type 1 IGF-Receptor in Wilms tumor cells. Pediatric Research 1996 ;39:160–165.

[110] Gansler T, Allen KD, Burant CF, Inabnett T, Scott A, Buse MG, Sens DA, Garvin AJ. Detection of type 1 insulinlike growth factor (IGF) receptors in Wilms' tumors. American Journal of Pathology. 1988 ;130(3):431-5.

[111] Drummond IA, Madden SL, Rohwer-Nutter P, Bell GI, Sukhatme VP, Rauscher FJ. Repression of the insulin-like growth factor II gene by the Wilms tumor suppressor WT1. Science. 1992; 257(5070):674-8.

[112] Hakam A, Fang Q, Karl R, Coppola D. Coexpression of IGF-1R and c-Src proteins in human pancreatic ductal adenocarcinoma. Digestive Diseases and Sciences. 2003;48(10):1972-8.

[113] Ishiwata T, Bergmann U, Kornmann M, Lopez M, Beger HG and Korc M. Altered expression of insulin like growth factor-2 receptor in human pancreatic cancer. Pancreas 1997; 4;367-373.

[114] David F Schaeffer DF, Daniel R Owen DR et al. Insulin-like growth factor 2 mRNA binding protein 3 overexpression in pancreatic ductal adenocarcinoma correlates with poor survival BMC Cancer 2010; 10:59

[115] Russo, VC, Gluckman, PD, Feldman, EL, et al. The insulin-like growth factor system and its pleiotropic functions in brain. Endocrine Reviews 2005; 26: 916-43.

[116] Müller HL, Oh Y, Lehrnbecher T, et al. Insulin-like growth factor-binding protein-2 concentrations in cerebrospinal fluid and serum of children with malignant solid tumors or acute leukemia. Journal of Clinical Endocrinology & Metabolism 1994; 79:428–34

[117] Adashi EY, Resnick CE, D'Ercole AJ, Svoboda ME, van Wyk JJ. Insulin-like growth factors as intraovarian regulators of granulosa cell growth and function. Endocrine Reviews 1985; 6:400-420.

[118] Giordano G, Barreca A, Minuto F. Growth factors in the ovary. Journal of Endocrinological Investigations 1992; 15:689-707.

[119] Karasik A, Menczer J, Pariente C, Kanety H. Insulin-like growth factor-1 and IGF-binding protein-2 are increased in cyst fluids of epithelial ovarian cancer. Journal of Clinical Endocrinology and Metabolism1994;78:271-276.

[120] Flyvberg A, Mogenson O, Mogensen B & Nielsen OS. Elevated serum insulin-like growth factor binding protein 2 and decreased IGFBP-3 in epithelial ovarian cancer: correlation with cancer antigen 125 and tumorassociated trypsin inhibitor. Journal of Clinical Endocrinology and Metabolism 1997; 82:2308-2313.

[121] Conover CA, Hartmann LC, Bradley S, Stalboerger P, Klee GG, Kalli KR, et al. Biological characterization of human epithelial ovarian cancer cells in primary culture: the insulin-like growth factor system. Experimental Cell Research 1998; 238:439– 49.

[122] Sayer RA, Lancaster JM, Pittman J, Gray J, Whitaker R, Marks JR, Berchuck A. High insulin-like growth factor-2 gene expression is an independent predictor of poor survival for patients with advanced stage serous epithelial ovarian cancer. Gynecologic Oncology 2005; 96(2):355-61.

[123] Brokaw J, Katsaros D, Wiley A, Lu L, Su D, Sochirca O, de la Longrais IA, Mayne S, Risch H, Yu H. IGF-1 in epithelial ovarian cancer and its role in disease progression. Growth Factors. 2007; 25(5):346-54.

[124] Odell WD, Wolfsen AR. Humoral Syndromes associated with cancer. Annual Review of Medicine 1978; 29:379-406.

[125] Blackman, NR, Rosen SW, Weintraub BD. Ectopic Hormones. Advances in Internal Medicine 1978; 23: 85-113.

[126] Zachariah S, Brackenbridge A, Jones DR. Effects of IGF-2 on glucose metabolism. Endocrine Abstracts 2006;11:220

[127] Denley A, Wallace JC, Cosgrove LJ, Forbes BE. The insulin receptor isoform exon 11– (IR-A) in cancer and other diseases: a review. Hormone and Metabolic Research 2003; 35:778–785.

[128] Kiess W, Yang Y, Kessler U, et al. Insulin-like growth factor 2 and the IGF-2 mannose-6-phosphate receptor—the myth continues. Hormone Research. 1994 ;41: 66–73.

[129] Duguay SJ, Jin Y, Stein J, Duguay AN, Gardner P and Steiner DF. Post-translational processing of the insulin like growth factor-2 precursor: Analysis of O-glycosylation and endoproteolysis The Journal of Biological Chemistry 1998; 273:18443-18451.

[130] Daughaday WH, Kapadia M. Significance of abnormal serum binding of insulin-like growth factor II in the development of hypoglycemia in patients with non-islet-cell tumors. PNAS 1989; 86:6778–6782.

[131] Zapf J, Schmid C, Guler HP, Waldvogel M, Hauri C, Futo E, Hossenlopp P, Binoux M & Froesch ER. Regulation of binding proteins for insulin-like growth factors (IGF) in humans. Increased expression of IGF binding protein 2 during IGF I treatment of healthy adults and in patients with extrapancreatic tumor hypoglycemia. Journal of Clinical Investigation 1990; 86:952–961.

[132] Zapf J, Futo E, Peter M & Froesch ER Can 'big' insulin-like growth factor II in serum of tumor patients account for the development of extrapancreatic tumor hypoglycemia? Journal of Clinical Investigation 1992; 90:2574–2584.

[133] de Groot JW, Rikhof B, van Doorn J, Bilo HJ, Alleman MA, Honkoop AH, van der Graaf WT. Non-islet cell tumour-induced hypoglycaemia: a review of the literature including two new cases. Endocr Relat Cancer. 2007; 14:979-93.

[134] Rosenfeld RG, Rosenbloom AL & Guevara-Agurre J. Growth hormone (GH) insensitivity due to primary GH receptor deficiency. Endocrine Reviews 1994; 15:369–390.

[135] Clemmons DR. Role of insulin-like growth factor iin maintaining normal glucose homeostasis. Hormone Research 2004; 62(1):77-82.

[136] Sandhu MS, Heald AH, Gibson JM, Cruickshank JK, Dunger DB, Wareham NJ. Circulating concentrations of insulin-like growth factor-I and development of glucose intolerance: a prospective observational study. Lancet 200; 359(9319):1740-5.

[137] Rajpathak SN, Gunter MJ, Wylie-Rosett J, Ho GY, Kaplan RC, Muzumdar R, Rohan TE, Strickler HD. The role of insulin-like growth factor-I and its binding proteins in glucose homeostasis and type 2 diabetes. Diabetes/Metabolism Research and Reviews 2009; 25(1):3-12.

[138] Friedrich N, Thuesen B, Jørgensen T, Juul A, Spielhagen C, Wallaschofksi H and Linneberg A. The association between IGF-1 and insulin resistance: A general population study in Danish adults. Diabetes Care. 2012 Apr;35(4):768-73.

[139] Schneider HJ, Friedrich N, Klotsche J, et al. Prediction of incident diabetes mellitus by baseline IGF1 levels. European Journal of Endocrinology 2011;164:223–229.

[140] van der Klaauw AA, Biermasz NR, Feskens EJ, et al. The prevalence of the metabolic syndrome is increased in patients with GH deficiency, irrespective of long-term substitution with recombinant human GH. European Journal of Endocrinology 2007;156:455–462.

[141] Melmed S. Medical progress: acromegaly. New England Journal of Medicine 2006;355:2558–2573.

[142] Cheetham T, Jones J, Taylor AM, Holly J, Matthews DR, Dunger DB: The effects of recombinant insulin-like growth factor-I administration on growth hormone levels and insulin requirements in adolescents with type 1 diabetes mellitus. Diabetologia 1993; 36:678–681

[143] Carroll PV, Umpleby M, Ward GS, Imuere S, Alexander E, Dunger D, Sönksen PH, Russell-Jones DL: rhIGF-1 administration reduces insulin requirements, decreases growth hormone secretion, and improves the lipid profile in adults with IDDM. Diabetes 1997; 46:1453–1458.

[144] Paul V. Carroll, Emanuel R. Christ, A. Margot Umpleby, Ian Gowrie, Nicola Jackson, Susan B. Bowes, Roman Hovorka, Premila Croos, Peter H. Sönksen, and David L. Russell-Jones. IGF-1 Treatment in Adults With Type 1 Diabetes Effects on Glucose and Protein Metabolism in the Fasting State and During a Hyperinsulinemic-Euglycemic Amino Acid Clamp. Diabetes 49:789–796, 2000.

[145] Zenobi PD, Jaeggi-Groisman SE, Riesen WF, Roder ME, Froesch ER: Insulin like growth factor-1improves glucose and lipid metabolism in type II diabetes mellitus. Journal of Clinical Investigation 90:2234–2241, 1993

[146] Moses AC, Young SC, Morrow LA, O'Brien M, Clemmons DR. Recombinant human insulin-like growth factor I increases insulin sensitivity and improves glycemic control in type II diabetes. Diabetes. 1996;45(1):91-100.

[147] Shigematsu S, Yamauchi K, Nakajima K, Iijima S, Aizawa T, Hashizume K. IGF-1 regulates migration and angiogenesis of human endothelial cells. Endocrinology 1999;46:59-62.

[148] Grant MB, Mames RN, Fitzgerald C, et al. Insulin-like growth factor I acts as an angiogenic agent in rabbit cornea and retina: comparative studies with basic fibroblast growth factor. Diabetologia 1993; 36:282.

[149] Merimee TJ. A follow-up study of vascular disease in growth-hormone-deficient dwarfs with diabetes. New England Journal of Medicine 1978;298: 1217.

[150] Merimee TJ, Fineberg SE, McKusick VA, Hall J. Diabetes mellitus and sexual ateliotic dwarfism: a comparative study. Journal of Clinical Investigation 1970;49:1096.

[151] Merimee TJ, Zapf J, Froesch ER. Insulin-like growth factors. Studies in diabetics with and without retinopathy. New England Journal of Medicine 1983; 309:527.

[152] Spagnoli A, Chiarelli F, Vorwerk P, Boscherini B, Rosenfeld RG. Evaluation of the components of insulin-like growth factor (IGF)-IGF binding protein system in adolescents with type 1 diabetes and persistent microalbuminuria: relationship with increased urinary excretion of IGFBP-3 18 kD N-terminal fragment. Clinical Endocrinology 1999; 51: 587–596

[153] Verrotti A, Cieri F, Petitti MT, Morgese G, Chiarelli F. Growth hormone and IGF-1 in diabetic children with and without microalbuminuria. Diabetes, Nutrition and Metabolism 1999;12:271–276.

[154] Shinada M, Akdeniz A, Panagiotopoulos S, Jerums G, Bach LA. Proteolysis of insulin-like growth factor-binding protein-3 is increased in urine from patients with diabetic nephropathy. Journal of Clinical Endocrinology and Metabolism 2000; 85 :1163–1169.

[155] Abrass C, Raugi G, Gabourel L, Lovet DH. Insulin and insulin-like growth factor I binding to cultured rat glomerular mesangial cells. Endocrinology 1988;123:2432–2439.

[156] Juul A, Scheike T, Davidsen M, Gyllenborg J, Jorgensen T: Low serum insulin-like growth factor 1 is associated with increased risk of ischemic heart disease: a population-based case control study. Circulation 106:939–944.

[157] Conti E, Crea F, Andreotti F: IGF-1 and risk of ischemic heart disease. Circulation 2004; 110: 2260-2265.

[158] Muniyappa R, Walsh MF, Rangi JS, Zayas RM, Standley PR, Ram JL. Insulin-like growth factor 1 increases vascular smooth muscle nitric oxide production. Life Science 61:925–931, 1997.

[159] E Andreotti FE, Sestito A, Riccardi P, Menini E, Crea F, Maseri A, Lanza GA. Markedly reduced insulin-like growth factor-1 associated with insulin resistance in syndrome X patients. American Journal of Cardiology 2002; 89:973–975

[160] Heald AH, Siddals KW, Fraser W, Taylor W, Kaushal K, Morris J, Young RJ, White A, Gibson JM. Low circulating levels of insulin-like growth factor binding protein-1 are closely associated with the presence of macrovascular disease and hypertension in type 2 diabetes. Diabetes 2002 Aug;51(8):2629-36.

Chapter 9

Pediatric Nonalcoholic Fatty Liver Disease

Ebe D'Adamo, M. Loredana Marcovecchio,
Tommaso de Giorgis, Valentina Chiavaroli,
Cosimo Giannini, Francesco Chiarelli and
Angelika Mohn

Additional information is available at the end of the chapter

http://dx.doi.org/10.5772/53463

1. Introduction

Paralleling the burgeoning epidemics of childhood obesity, nonalcoholic fatty liver disease (NAFLD) is now recognized as the most common cause of chronic liver disease in children [1,2].

NAFLD is a clinic-pathological condition defined by the accumulation of intrahepatic triglyceride fat (IHTF) content in the absence of alcohol consumption [1,2].

NAFLD encompasses a wide spectrum of liver damage, ranging from asymptomatic steatosis with elevated or normal aminotransferases to steatosis with inflammation, ballooning degeneration and pericellular fibrosis (Nonalcoholic Steatohepatitis, NASH) to cirrhosis [2,3].

Although there are limited long-term data on the natural history of NAFLD in children, NASH is increasingly diagnosed in obese children [4] and it may progress to cirrhosis even in this age group [2,5]. In addition, children with NAFLD have a 13.6-fold higher risk of mortality or requiring a liver transplant as compared to age/sex matched controls [6].

During the last years there has been a growing interest in the relationship between NAFLD and the development of metabolic and cardiovascular diseases [7-9].

Several lines of evidence have shown that in obese children and adolescents excessive accumulation of IHTF is associated with important alterations in glucose, fatty acid (FA), lipoprotein metabolism and inflammation, suggesting that IHTF represents a strong risk factor for the development of the Metabolic Syndrome (MetS) and type 2 diabetes mellitus (T2D) [7-10].

Although a multifactorial pathogenesis of NAFLD has been postulated [12-14], obesity and insulin resistance represent two important players in the development of the early stages of the disease [2,14]. Interestingly, although the insulin resistance state could explain the relationship between NAFLD and the development of metabolic alterations [10,15], the presence of liver steatosis is also an important marker of multiorgan insulin resistance [16], opening a debate as to whether hepatic steatosis is a consequence or cause of insulin resistance.

Therefore, it would be of paramount importance to identify children affected by NAFLD and to better understand the pathogenesis of this condition in order to prevent the development of the associated metabolic complications early in life.

2. Definition and prevalence of NAFLD

Despite fatty liver is becoming one of the most common hepatic alterations in obese children [1,2], the prevalence of pediatric NAFLD is uncertain, mainly due to the methods used to assess fatty liver.

NAFLD is defined as an IHTF content > 5% of liver volume or weight and as a presence ≥5% of hepatocytes containing intracellular triglycerides, in the absence of alcohol consumption [17,18].

The gold standard for diagnosing NAFLD is liver biopsy [19,20]. Liver biopsy allows an accurate assessment of histopatological findings, providing information on the type of NAFLD (simple steatosis or steatohepatitis) and the various degrees of hepatic fibrosis [20]. However, the main limitation of the application of liver biopsy in the pediatric age group is due to the fact that it is an invasive procedure; thus, it is not considered as first line to screen the presence of liver disease [19,20].

Although non-invasive methods, such as computer tomography, MRI, or ultrasonography are unable to distinguish between NASH and other forms of NAFLD [19,21], they have an acceptable sensitivity and specificity for the diagnosis of increased fat accumulation in the liver [21]. Furthermore, ultrasound has been shown to have a good correlation with the histological findings of liver biopsy, particularly macrovescicular steatosis [22].

In clinical practice, combining liver function tests, such as serum aminotransferases [18], with liver ultrasound represents a useful way of identifying the presence of liver steatosis in obese children.

In spite of the method used, it is clear that the prevalence of NAFDL is increasing in children and adolescence. NAFLD affects 2.6% of normal children [23] and up to 77% of obese individuals [24,25]. Pediatric NAFLD extends beyond North America according to centers in Europe, Asia, South America and Australia [2,3]. The prevalence of fatty liver in obese children in China, Italy, Japan, and the United States has been reported to be between 10% and 77% [2,3]. Data derived from the National Health and Nutrition Examination Survey III (1988-1994) suggest that approximately 3% of adolescents present abnormal serum aminotransferase values [26]. Moreover, studies from autopsies of 742 children (ages 2–19 years) reported fatty liver prevalence at 9.6%, and in obese children this rate increased to an alarming 38% [25].

NAFLD has been also described in obese prepubertal children. In the study by Manco et al. [27] NAFLD was detected in children as young as 3 years old.

The prevalence of NAFLD is around 30% in children with a Tanner pubertal stage I, significantly lower when compared to that found in the pubertal age [28].

Alarming data come from our study population of prepubertal Caucasian obese children [29]. Out of 100 severely obese prepubertal children, liver steatosis was found in 52% and was equally distributed between the two sexes [29].

Thus, NAFLD in an emerging health problem even in very young age groups.

3. Pathogenesis and risk factors of NAFLD

Although the pathogenetic mechanism of NAFLD is not completely understood, in accordance with the "two hit hypothesis", insulin resistance and oxidative stress represent two key factors for the development and progression of NAFLD/NASH [12,17,20].

3.1. Insulin resistance and central obesity

The "two-hit" model proposes that fat accumulation in the hepatocytes is a prerequisite for a second hit that induces fibrosis and inflammation [30].

Fat accumulation in the liver is likely to result from insulin resistance and concomitant impairment of fatty acid (FA) metabolism within liver, skeletal muscle and adipose tissue [31].

Insulin resistance seems to be responsible for abnormalities in lipid storage and lipolysis in insulin-sensitive tissues, leading to an increased fatty acids flux from adipose tissue to the liver and subsequent accumulation of triglycerides in the hepatocytes [31]. In particular, steatosis develops when the rate of FA input (uptake and synthesis with subsequent esterification to triglycerides (TG)) is greater than the rate of FA output (oxidation and secretion) [11]. The amount of TG in the hepatocytes represents a complex interaction among [11,31]: hepatic FA uptake, derived from plasma free fatty acid (FFA) released from hydrolysis of adipose tissue and FFA released from hydrolysis of circulating TG; de novo FA synthesis (de novo lipogenesis [DNL]); fatty acid oxidation (FAO); FA export within very low-density lipoprotein (VLDL)-TG.

Obesity is the most important cause in the development of insulin resistance and it has been demonstrated that the critical determinant of insulin sensitivity is not the degree of obesity *per se* but the distribution of fat partitioning [32,33].

Several studies [32,33] have demonstrated that obese adolescents presenting increased intramyocellular lipid content (IMCL) [32] and visceral fat and decreased subcutaneous fat deposition are more likely to develop insulin resistance.

There is extensive evidence indicating that central obesity is associated with an impaired insulin action in obese pediatric populations. Although controversy remains regarding the contribution of visceral and subcutaneous fat to the development of insulin resistance [33], a previous study by Cruz et al. [35] showed a direct impact of visceral fat accumulation on insulin sensitivity and secretion, independently of total body adiposity, in obese children with a family history of T2D. Indeed, by stratifying a multiethnic cohort of obese adolescents into tertiles based on the proportion of visceral fat in the abdomen (visceral/subcutaneous fat ratio), insulin resistance (homeostasis model assessment) significantly increased and insulin sensitivity (Matsuda index) decreased in obese adolescents with high proportion of visceral fat and relatively low abdominal subcutaneous fat [33].

These findings suggest that obese children and adolescents at risk for developing metabolic complications are not necessarily the most severely obese, but are characterized by an unfavorable lipid partitioning profile.

3.2. Insulin resistance and fatty liver disease: Which comes first?

Despite the demonstrated relationship between IMCL, visceral fat and metabolic dysfunction, the ectopic fat deposition in the liver is emerging as the most important marker of insulin resistance in adults [15] as well as in obese pediatric population [36].

In healthy nondiabetic humans the correlation between the IHTF content and peripheral insulin resistance was much stronger than the correlation with intramyocellular lipid content, visceral fat content or subcutaneous fat content [37]. The relationship between liver steatosis and insulin resistance has been clearly demonstrated in children [36,29]. In our cross sectional study, we evaluated insulin resistance indexes between obese prepubertal children with and without liver steatosis; furthermore insulin resistance indexes were compared to values of normal weight children. Our results showed that children with NAFLD not only presented severe obesity but also an increased degree of insulin resistance when compared to the sex- and age-matched normal weight children [29].

The relationship between insulin resistance and fatty liver disease is not only related to the presence of liver steatosis, but also to the degree of fatty liver. In a multiethnic cohort of obese adolescents, Calì et al. [36] clearly showed a significant decrease in insulin sensitivity and an imbalance between anti- and pro-inflammatory markers [adiponectin and interleukin 6 (IL-6)] paralleling the severity of hepatic steatosis [36]. In particular, adiponectin, the most abundant secretory protein produced by adipose tissue, is closely related with insulin action. Plasma adiponectin concentrations are inversely associated with hepatic steatosis and metabolic complications [37,38].

Although these findings support the central role of insulin resistance in the development of fatty liver, several studies have demonstrated that the presence of liver steatosis is an important marker of multiorgan insulin resistance, independently of BMI, percent body fat, and visceral fat mass [11,15,36]. In particular, NAFLD has been found to be associated with insulin resistance in liver (impaired suppression of insulin-mediated glucose production) [39,40], skeletal muscle (reduced insulin stimulated glucose uptake) [40] and adipose tissue (decrease inhibition of lipolysis by insulin) [41] in obese children and adolescents, independently of adiposity.

Recently, Caprio et al. [16] reported that obese adolescents with high liver fat content, independent of visceral and IMCL had an impaired insulin action (as assessed by the hyperinsulinemic-euglycemic clamp) in the liver and in the muscle and early defects in β-cell function [16]. These results suggest that the liver has a central role in the complex phenotype of the insulin resistance state in obese adolescents with fatty liver.

Although it is clear that there is an important correlation between insulin resistance and hepatic steatosis, the mechanisms responsible for the interrelationships between fatty liver disease and insulin resistance are not clearly understood. In fact, it remains unclear whether hepatic steatosis is a consequence or the primary event leading to hepatic and subsequently peripheral insulin resistance.

Petersen et al. [42] showed that the lack of adipose tissue in the congenital lipodystrophy is characterized by extreme insulin resistance associated with massive hepatic fat accumulation; intervention with subcutaneous leptin administration in these patients improved whole-body insulin sensitivity mainly due to the mobilization of the excessive fatty liver content.

Models of patients with liver cirrhosis in which hepatic dysfunction is known to be the primary disturbance provide strong support that insulin resistance in peripheral tissues develops secondary to liver disease [43]. 60-80% of patients with liver cirrhosis are glucose intolerant and in 10-15% diabetes occurs relatively rapidly (over a period of 5 years). Diabetes complicating liver cirrhosis, also known as hepatogenous diabetes, and the common form of T2D are the results of a marked reduction in insulin action and a β-cell secretion defect that is not able to compensate the severity of insulin resistance [43,44]. The important role of peripheral insulin resistance in the glucose tolerance of cirrhosis has been highlighted by the observation that liver transplantation, when the dosage of immunosuppressive agents was reduce and corticosteroids withdrawn, was able to restore normal insulin sensitivity not only in the liver but also at the level of the skeletal muscle and adipose tissue and normalizes glucose tolerance in most patients with diabetes [43,44].

The mechanism by which IHTF has an important systemic consequence to adversely affect insulin sensitivity is unknown. However, it has been proposed that fatty liver might interfere with insulin degradation [45]; the resultant hyperinsulinemia may potentially be able to impair insulin action in peripheral tissues, as shown in benign insulinoma induced hyperinsulinemia [43,44,46]. This hyperinsulinemia-induced mechanism may be justified also based on the finding of the reverse experiment: when the prolonged infusion of octreotide was administered to extremely insulin-resistant cirrhotic individuals, the correlation of hyperinsulinemia was paralleled by the restoration of normal insulin sensitivity [43,47].

Although these data showed a clear possibility that intrahepatic fat accumulation plays a key role in the onset of insulin resistance and insulin resistance syndrome, longitudinal data are needed in order to clarify which abnormality comes first.

3.3. Oxidative stress

In accordance with the "two hit hypothesis", dysfunction of various oxidation pathways within the hepatocytes and subsequent overproduction of reactive oxygen species (ROS), may result in the peroxidation of accumulated lipids, inflammation, hepatocellular apoptosis and fibrogenesis [31].

Obese subjects affected by NAFLD present an impaired oxidant-antioxidant status than subjects without [12,48].

Interestingly, we recently observed [48] that obese prepubertal children affected by liver steatosis had impaired levels of receptors for advanced glycation endproducts (RAGEs), which has been demonstrated to be correlated with the progression of several metabolic and cardiovascular diseases. In particular, obese prepubertal children with liver steatosis presented decreased RAGEs levels compared with children without liver disease, underling that oxidative stress could play a role even in the early stages of the disease [48].

3.4. Genetic and environmental factors associated with fatty liver disease

Several genetic and environmental factors are likely responsible for NAFLD and its progression from simple steatosis to NASH.

In fact, although the development of NAFLD is strongly linked to obesity and insulin resistance, there are obese individuals who do not have NAFLD, and since NAFLD can occur in normal-weight individuals with normal metabolic profile, thus multiple genetic and environmental factors should be involved in its development [49].

Initial evidence for a *genetic component* of NAFLD comes from ethnic variation in NAFLD prevalence [50]. Children from certain ethnicities are predisposed to NAFLD, primarily Hispanics, Asians and Native Americans [25,50].

Furthermore, a familial aggregation study of fatty liver in overweight children with and without NAFLD found that fatty liver is a highly heritable trait. Family members of children with biopsy-proven NAFLD and overweight children without NAFLD were evaluated by magnetic resonance imaging (MRI). Fatty liver was identified in 17% of siblings and 37% of parents of overweight children without NAFLD and in 59% of siblings and 78% of parents of children with NAFLD [51].

Interestingly, Romeo et al. [52] conducted the first genome-wide association scan conducted in a large multiethnic population. The authors demonstrated that the patatin-like phospholipase domain containing protein 3 (also known as adiponutrin) gene was strongly associated with IHTF content in adults [52].

These findings have been recently supported by Santoro et al. [53]. By genotyping the *PNLPA3* SNP in a multiethnic group of 85 obese youths, the authors found that the *PNPLA3* rs738409 SNP gene confers susceptibility to hepatic steatosis.

Nutrition and physical activity are important *environmental factors* that determine risk in NAFLD.

Excess food intake and lack of exercise contribute to weight gain, which has been shown to contribute to the progression of liver fibrosis in patients with NAFLD [54]. Specific dietary factors may also play either protective or antagonistic roles in the development and progression of NAFLD. An increased consumption of meat and soft drinks and low consumption of fish were found to be associated with NAFLD cases compared with controls [49]. Furthermore, low intakes of polyunsaturated fatty acid (PUFA) and high intakes of saturated fat and cholesterol were also shown to be associated with NAFLD [49]. Other studies have shown higher-carbohydrate and lower-fat diets to be associated with more progressive disease [49,55]. Notably, very recent animal data have shown that in both mice [49,56] and non-human primates [49] exposure to a maternal high-fat diet leads to a disturbing development and progression of NAFLD in the offspring.

It has been proposed that increase consumption of fructose in soft drinks and fruit drinks may have a role in the pathogenesis of NAFLD [2]. In one study, children with biopsy-proven NAFLD were shown to have significantly elevated plasma TG levels and oxidative stress levels after consumption of fructose as compared with glucose [57]. However, children without NAFLD were found to have no differences in TG or oxidative stress levels following the consumption of glucose compared with fructose [2].

Small intestinal bacterial overgrowth may be an additional environmental factor involved in NAFLD pathogenesis, and dietary supplements such as probiotics could have a beneficial effect [49]. Evidences from animal studies have shown that small intestinal bacterial overgrowth increases gut permeability leading to portal endotoxaemia and increased circulating inflammatory cytokines, both of which have been implicated in the progression of NAFLD [58,59].

4. NAFLD, metabolic and cardiovascular complications in obese children and adolescents

4.1. NAFLD and metabolic complications

NAFLD is nowadays considered the hepatic manifestation of the MetS in adults as well as in children [60]. This is not surprising since NAFLD is closely associated with obesity, insulin resistance, and alterations in glucose and lipid metabolism [44].

The association between NAFLD and MetS has been clearly demonstrated by Burgert et al. [61,62]. In 392 obese adolescents, elevated alanine aminotransferases (ALT) (>35 U/L) levels were found in 14% of participants, with a predominance of White/Hispanic. After adjusting for potential confounders, rising ALT levels were associated with deterioration in insulin sensitivity and glucose tolerance, as well as increasing FFA and TG levels. Furthermore, increased hepatic fat accumulation was found in 32% of obese adolescents and was associated with decreased insulin sensitivity and increased lipid levels and visceral fat [61]. These results demonstrate that in obese children and adolescents, hepatic fat accumulation is associated with insulin resistance, dyslipidemia and altered glucose metabolism.

In addition, the Korean National Health and Nutrition Examination Survey found participants aged 10 – 19 years with three or more risk factors for MetS had an odds ratio that of 6.2 (95 % CI 2.3 – 16.8) for an elevated serum ALT, which they used as an indicator of fatty liver [62]. Furthermore, a case – control study of overweight children with biopsy-proven NAFLD and age-, sex-, and obesity-matched controls found that children with NAFLD were significantly more likely to have MetS than obese controls without evidence of fatty liver disease [9].

More recently, in a large histology-based study conducted in children with NAFLD [63], MetS was diagnosed in 25.6 % of the subjects, with central obesity and hypertension being the most common of the MetS features observed. In addition, a diagnosis of MetS was predictive of steatosis severity, NASH, hepatocellular ballooning and NAFLD pattern [63].

In a recent study by our group [64], we assessed the role of liver steatosis in defining MetS in prepubertal children. The prevalence of the MetS was around 14% and increased to 20% when liver steatosis was included as an additional diagnostic criterion. These findings underline not only the relevance of the MetS even among prepubertal children but also emphasize the potential importance of testing for fatty liver as a component of the MetS already in this age group [64] (figure 1).

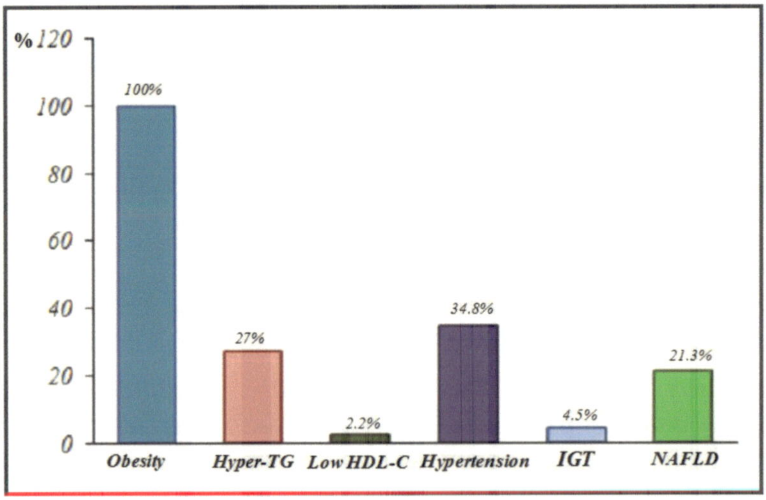

Figure 1. Prevalence of components of the MetS among obese prepubertal children [64].(TG, triglycerides; HDL-C, high density lipoprotein cholesterol; IGT, impaired glucose tolerance; NAFLD, non alcoholic fatty liver disease)

NAFLD in youth may be considered not only a strong risk factor for MetS, but also for T2D [36]. In a cohort of 118 obese adolescents [36] stratifyied according to tertiles of hepatic fat content (as assessed by fat gradient MRI), independently of obesity, the severity of fatty liver was associated with the presence of prediabetes [impaired glucose tolerance (IGT) and impaired fasting glucose (IFG)/IGT]. In fact, paralleling the severity of hepatic steatosis, there was a significant decrease in insulin sensitivity and impairment in β-cell function, as indicated by the fall in the disposition index (DI). Furthermore, paralleling the severity of fatty liver, there was a significant increase in the prevalence of MetS, suggesting that hepatic steatosis may probably be a predictive factor of MetS in children [36].

The important role of intrahepatic fat content in the development of metabolic complications in obese subject has been recently underlined by Fabbrini et al. [15]. The authors showed that in adults with high IHTF insulin action in liver, skeletal muscle and adipose tissue was impaired and hepatic VLDL-TG secretion rate was increased. In contrast, they were not able to observe these metabolic alterations in subjects with high visceral fat volume and matched for IHTF. Therefore, the authors demonstrated that IHTF and not visceral fat is a better marker of metabolic derangements associated with obesity [15,16].

4.2. NAFLD and cardiovascular disease

Recent evidences suggests that individuals with NAFLD are also at high risk for coronary heart disease [3,43]. In adults, elevated serum ALT have been associated with increased risk of cardiovascular and all cause mortality (in addition to liver mortality) [3,65].

A study in Turkish children [66] showed that carotid artery intima-media thickness is significantly higher in obese children with fatty liver than in obese children without fatty liver or normal weight control.

In addition, Pacifico et al. [67] reported that carotid artery intima-media thickness was highest in obese children with echogenic liver and severity of liver fat was an independent predictor of intima-media thickness after adjustment for known cardiovascular factors.

However, given the lack of long-term longitudinal cohort studies in pediatric fatty liver disease, the relationship between the natural history of the disease and the actual risk for future cardiac events is unclear.

5. Conclusions

The prevalence of fatty liver disease is increasing in obese children and adolescence.

Although the exact pathogenetic mechanism is still unclear, there is an urgent need to screen obese children for this pathology. A misdiagnosis of fatty liver could represent a serious risk factor for the development of its associated metabolic and cardiovascular complications during childhood and for exacerbated metabolic abnormalities later in life.

Author details

Ebe D'Adamo[1,2*], M. Loredana Marcovecchio[1,2], Tommaso de Giorgis[1,2],
Valentina Chiavaroli[1,2], Cosimo Giannini[1,2], Francesco Chiarelli[1,2] and Angelika Mohn[1,2]

*Address all correspondence to: ebe.dadamo@yahoo.com

1 Department of Pediatrics, University of Chieti, Chieti, Italy

2 Center of Excellence on Aging, "G. D'Annunzio" University Foundation, University of Chieti, Italy

References

[1] Roberts EA. Pediatric nonalcoholic fatty liver disease (NAFLD): A "growing" problem? J Hepatol 2007;46:1133-1142.

[2] Barshop NJ, Francis CS, Schwimmer JB, Lavine JE. Nonalcoholic fatty liver disease as a comorbidity of childhood obesity. Ped Health 2009;3:271-81.

[3] Loomba R, Sirlin CB, Schwimmer JB, Lavine JE. Advances in Pediatric Nonalcoholic Fatty Liver Disease. Hepatology 2009;50:1282-1293.

[4] Hesham A-Kader H. Nonalcoholic fatty liver disease in children living in the obeseogenic society. World J Pediatr 2009;5:245-254.

[5] Molleston JP, White F, Teckman J, Fitzgerald JF. Obese children with steatohepatitis can develop cirrhosis in childhood. Am J Gastroenterol 2002;97:2460-2.

[6] Feldstein AE, Charatcharoenwitthaya P, Treeprasertsuk S, Benson JT, Enders FB, Angulo P. The natural history of nonalcoholic fatty liver disease in children: a follow-up study for up to 20 years. Hepatology 2008;48(S1):335A.

[7] Pacifico L, Nobili V, Anania C, Verdecchia P, Chiesa C. Pediatric nonalcoholic fatty liver disease, metabolic syndrome and cardiovascular risk. World J Gastroenterol 2011; 14;17:3082-91.

[8] Alisi A, Feldstein AE, Villani A, Raponi M, Nobili V. Pediatric nonalcoholic fatty liver disease: a multidisciplinary approach. Nat Rev Gastroenterol Hepatol 2012;9:152-61.

[9] Ryan MC, Wilson AM, Slavin J, Best JD, Jenkins AJ, Desmond PV. Associations between liver histology and severity of the metabolic syndrome in subjects with nonalcoholic fatty liver disease. Diabetes Care 2005;28:1222-1224.

[10] Fabbrini E, deHaseth D, Deivanayagam S, Mohammed BS, Vitola BE, Klein S. Alterations in fatty acid kinetics in obese adolescents with increased intrahepatic triglyceride content. Obesity (Silver Spring) 2009;17:25-29.

[11] D'Adamo E, Northrup V, Weiss R, Santoro N, Pierpont B, Savoye M, O'Malley G, Caprio S. Ethnic differences in lipoprotein subclasses in obese adolescents: importance of liver and intraabdominal fat accretion. Am J Clin Nutr 2010:92:500-8.

[12] Browning JD, Horton JD. Molecular mediators of hepatic steatosis and liver injury. J Clin Invest. 2004;114:147-52.

[13] Sinatra FR. Nonalcoholic fatty liver disease in pediatric patients. JPEN J Parenter Enteral Nutr 2012;36:43S-8S.

[14] Brunt EM. Pathology of nonalcoholic fatty liver disease. Nat Rev Gastroenterol Hepatol 2010;7:195-203.

[15] Fabbrini E, Magkos F, Mohammed BS, Pietka T, Abumrad NA, Patterson BW, Okunade A et al. Intrahepatic fat, not visceral fat, is linked with metabolic complications of obesity. Proc Natl Acad Sci U S A 2009;106:15430-15435.

[16] D'Adamo E, Cali AMG, Weiss R, Santoro N, Pierpont B, Northrup V, Caprio S. Central Role of Fatty Liver in the Pathogenesis of Insulin Resistance in Obese Adolescents. Diabetes Care 2012;33:1817–1822.

[17] Manco M. Metabolic syndrome in childhood from impaired carbohydrate metabolism to nonalcoholic fatty liver disease. J Am Coll Nutr 2011;30(5):295-303.

[18] Angulo P. Nonalcoholic fatty liver disease. N Engl J Med 2002; 346: 1221-1231.

[19] Pais R, Lupşor M, Poantă L, Silaghi A, Rusu ML, Badea R, Dumitraşcu DL. Liver Biopsy versus Noninvasive Methods – Fibroscan and Fibrotest in the Diagnosis of Non-alcoholic Fatty Liver Disease: A Review of the Literature. Rom J Intern Med. 2009;47(4):331-40.

[20] Janczyk W, Socha P. Non-alcoholic fatty liver disease in children. Clin Res Hepatol Gastroenterol 2012;36:297-300.

[21] Joseph AE, Saverymuttu SH, Al-Sam S, Cook MG, Maxwell JD. Comparison of liver histology with ultrasonography in assessing diffuse parechymal liver disease. Clin Radiol 1991: 43:26-31.

[22] Tominaga K, Kurata JH, Chen YK, Fujimoto E, Miyagawa S, Abe I, Kusano Y. Prevalence of fatty liver in Japanese children and relationship to obesity. An epidemiological ultrasonographic survey. Dig Dis Sci 1995;40:2002-2009.

[23] Agawal N, Sharma BC. Insulin resistance and clinical aspects of non-alcoholic steatohepatitis (NASH). Hepatol Res 2005;33:92-96.

[24] Franzese A, Vajro P, Argenziano A, Puzziello A, Iannucci MP, Saviano MC, Brunetti F, Rubino A. Liver involvement in obese children. Ultrasonography and liver en-

zymes levels at diagnosis and during follow-up in an Italian population. Dig Dis Sci 1997;42:1428-1432.

[25] Schwimmer JB, Deutsch R, Kahen T, Lavine JE, Stanley C, Behling C. Prevalence of fatty liver in children and adolescents. Pediatrics 2006;118:1388-1393.

[26] Strauss RS, Barlow SE, Dietz WH. Prevalence of abnormal serum amino transferase values in overweight and obese adolescents. J Pediatr Gastroenterol Nutr 2000;136:727-733.

[27] Manco M, Bedogni G, Marcellini M, Devito R, Ciampalini P, Sartorelli MR, Comparcola D, Piemonte F, Nobili V. Waist circumference correlates with liver fibrosis in children with non-alcoholic steatohepatitis. Gut 2008;57(9):1283-7.

[28] Fishbein MH, Miner M, Mogren C, Chalekson J. The spectrum of fatty liver in obese children and the relationship of serum aminotransferases to severity of steatosis. J Pediatr Gastoenterol Nutr 2003;36:54-61.

[29] D'Adamo E, Impicciatore M, Capanna R, Loredana Marcovecchio M, Masuccio FG, Chiarelli F, Mohn AA. Liver steatosis in obese prepubertal children: a possible role of insulin resistance. Obesity (Silver Spring) 2008;16:677-683.

[30] Day CP, James OFW. Steatohepatitis: a tale of two "hits". Gastroenterology 1998;114:842-845.

[31] Tiniakos DG, Vos BM, Brunt EM. Nonalcoholic Fatty Liver Disease: Pathology and Pathogenesis. Annu Rev Patholo Mech Dis 2010:5:145-171.

[32] Weiss R, Dufour S, Taksali SE, Tamborlane WV, Petersen KF, Bonadonna RC, Boselli L, Barbetta G, Allen K, Rife F, Savoye M, Dziura J, Sherwin R, Shulman GI, Caprio S. Prediabetes in obese youth: a syndrome of impaired glucose tolerance, severe insulin resistance, and altered myocellular and abdominal fat partitioning. Lancet 2003;362:951-957.

[33] Taksali SE, Caprio S, Dziura J, Dufour S, Calí AM, Goodman TR, Papademetris X, Burgert TS, Pierpont BM, Savoye M, Shaw M, Seyal AA, Weiss R. High visceral and low abdominal subcutaneous fat stores in the obese adolescent. Diabetes 2008;57:367-371.

[34] Weiss R, Dufour S, Groszmann A, Petersen K, Dziura J, Taksali SE, Shulman G, Caprio S. Low adiponectin levels in adolescent obesity: a marker of increased intramyocellular lipid accumulation. J Clin Endocrinol Metab 2003;88:2014-2018.

[35] Cruz ML, Bergman RN, Goran MI. Unique effect of visceral fat on insulin sensitivity in obese Hispanic children with a family history of type 2 diabetes. Diabetes Care 2002;25:1631-1636.

[36] Cali A, De Oliveira AM, Kim H, et al. Glucose Dysregulation and Hepatic Steatosis in Obese Adolescents: Is There a Link? Hepatology 2009;49:1896-1903.

[37] Hwang JH, Stein DT, Barzilai N, Cui MH, Tonelli J, Kishore P, Hawkins M. Increased intrahepatic triglyceride is associated with peripheral insulin resistance: in vivo MR imaging and spectroscopy studies. Am J Physiol Endocrinol Metab 2007;293:1663-1669.

[38] Matsuwaka Y. Adiponectin: a key player I obesity related disorders. Curr Pharm Des 2010;16:1896-1901.

[39] Deivanayagam S, Mohammed BS, Vitola BE, Naguib GH, Keshen TH, Kirk EP, Klein S. Nonalcoholic fatty liver disease is associated with hepatic and skeletal muscle insulin resistance in overweight adolescents. Am J Clin Nutr 2008;88:257-262.

[40] Perseghin G, Bonfanti R, Magni S, Lattuada G, De Cobelli F, Canu T, Esposito A, et al. Insulin resistance and whole body energy homeostasis in obese adolescents with fatty liver disease. Am J Physiol Endocrinol Metab 2006;291:697-703.

[41] Seppälä-Lindroos A, Vehkavaara S, Häkkinen AM, Goto T, Westerbacka J, Sovijärvi A, Halavaara J, Yki-Järvinen H. Fat accumulation in the liver is associated with defects in insulin suppression of glucose production and serum free fatty acids independent of obesity in normal men. J Clin Endocrinol Metab 2002;87:3023-3028.

[42] Petersen KF, Oral EA, Dufour S, Befroy D, Ariyan C, Yu C, Cline GW, DePaoli AM, Taylor SI, Gorden P, Shulman GI. Leptin reverses insulin resistance and hepatic steatosis in patients with severe lipodystrophy. J Clin Invest 2002;109:1345-1350.

[43] Perseghin G. Viewpoints on the way to a consensus session: where does insulin resistance start? The liver. Diabetes Care 2009;32 Suppl 2:S164-167.

[44] Perseghin G, Mazzaferro V, Sereni LP, Regalia E, Benedini S, Bazzigaluppi E, Pulvirenti A, Leão AA, Calori G, Romito R, Baratti D, Luzi L. Contribution of reduced insulin sensitivity and secretion to the pathogenesis of hepatogenous diabetes: effect of liver transplantation. Hepatology 2000;31:694-703.

[45] Kotronen A, Yki-Järvinen H. Fatty Liver: A Novel Component of the Metabolic Syndrome. Arterioscler Thromb Vasc Biol 2008;28:27-38.

[46] Battezzati A, Terruzzi I, Perseghin G, Bianchi E, Di Carlo V, Pozza G, Luzi L. Defective insulin action on protein and glucose metabolism during chronic hyperinsulinemia in subjects with benign insulinoma. Diabetes 1995;44:837-844.

[47] Petrides AS, Stanley T, Matthews DE, Vogt C, Bush AJ, Lambeth H. Insulin resistance in cirrhosis: prolonged reduction of hyperinsulinemia normalizes insulin sensitivity. Hepatology 1998;28:141-149.

[48] de Giorgis T, D'Adamo E, Giannini C, Chiavaroli V, Scarinci A, Verrotti A, Chiarelli F, Mohn A. Could receptors for advanced glycation end products be considered cardiovascular risk markers in obese children? Antioxid Redox Signal 2012: 15;17:187-91.

[49] Moore JB. Non-alcoholic fatty liver disease: the hepatic consequence of obesity and the metabolic syndrome. Proc Nutr Soc 2010; 69: 211-220.

[50] Louthan MV, Theriot JA, Zimmerman E, Stutts JT, McClain CJ. Decreased prevalence of nonalcoholic fatty liver disease in black obese children. J Pediatr Gastroenterol Nutr 2005;41:426-429.

[51] Schwimmer JB, Celedon MA, Lavine JE, Salem R, Campbell N, Schork NJ, Shiehmorteza M, Yokoo T, Chavez A, Middleton MS, Sirlin CB.Heritability of nonalcoholic fatty liver disease. Gastroenterology 2009;136:1585-1592.

[52] Romeo S, Kozlitina J, Xing C, Pertsemlidis A, Cox D, Pennacchio LA, Boerwinkle E, Cohen JC, Hobbs HH. Genetic variation in PNPLA3 confers susceptibility to nonalcoholic fatty liver disease. Nat Genet 2008;40, 1461-1465.

[53] Santoro N, Kursawe R, D'Adamo E, Dykas DJ, Zhang CK, Bale AE, Calí AM, Narayan D, Shaw MM, Pierpont B, Savoye M, Lartaud D, Eldrich S, Cushman SW, Zhao H, Shulman GI, Caprio S.A Common Variant in the Patatin-Like Phopholipase 3 Gene (PNPLA3) is Associated with Fatty Liver Disease in Obese Children and Adolescents. Hepatology 2010;52:1281-1290.

[54] Ekstedt M, Franzén LE, Mathiesen UL, Thorelius L, Holmqvist M, Bodemar G, Kechagias S.Long-term follow-up of patients with NAFLD and elevated liver enzymes. Hepatology 2006;44,865-873.

[55] Solga S, Alkhuraishe AR, Clark JM, Torbenson M, Greenwald A, Diehl AM, Magnuson T.Dietary composition and nonalcoholic fatty liver disease. Dig Dis Sci 2004;49:1578-1583.

[56] Bruce KD, Cagampang FR, Argenton M, Zhang J, Ethirajan PL, Burdge GC, Bateman AC, Clough GF, Poston L, Hanson MA, McConnell JM, Byrne CD.Maternal high-fat feeding primes steatohepatitis in adult mice offspring, involving mitochondrial dysfunction and altered lipogenesis gene expression. Hepatology 2009;50,1796-1808.

[57] Vos M, McClain CJ, Jones D. Fructose is associated with increased oxidative stress and elevated plasma triglycerides in children with nonalcoholic fatty liver disease. Hepatology 2008;48 (S1):820A.

[58] Brun P, Castagliuolo I, Di Leo V, Buda A, Pinzani M, Palù G, Martines D. Increased intestinal permeability in obese mice: new evidence in the pathogenesis of nonalcoholic steatohepatitis. Am J Physiol Gastrointest Liver Physiol 2007;292:518-525.

[59] Wigg AJ, Roberts-Thomson IC, Dymock RB, McCarthy PJ, Grose RH, Cummins AG.The role of small intestinal bacterial overgrowth, intestinal permeability, endotoxaemia, and tumour necrosis factor alpha in the pathogenesis of non-alcoholic steatohepatitis. Gut 2001;48,206-211.

[60] D'Adamo E, Santoro N, Caprio S. Metabolic Syndrome in Pediatrics: Old Concepts Revised, New Concepts Discussed. Endocrinol Metab Clin N Am 2009;38:549-563.

http://dx.doi.org/10.5772/53463

[61] Burgert TS, Taksali SE, Dziura J, Goodman TR, Yeckel CW, Papademetris X, Constable RT, Weiss R, Tamborlane WV, Savoye M, Seyal AA, Caprio S.Alanine aminotransferase levels and fatty liver in childhood obesity: associations with insulin resistance, adiponectin, and visceral fat. J Clin Endocrinol Metab 2006;91:4287-4294.

[62] Kang H, Greenson JK, Omo JT, Chao C, Peterman D, Anderson L, Foess-Wood L, Sherbondy MA, Conjeevaram HS.Metabolic syndrome is associated with greater histologic severity, higher carbohydrate, and lower fat diet in patients with NAFLD. Am J Gastroenterol 2006;101:2247-2253.

[63] Patton HM, Yates K, Unalp-Arida A, et al. Association Between Metabolic Syndrome and Liver Histology Among Children With Nonalcoholic Fatty Liver Disease. Am J Gastroenterol 2010; 105:2093-2102.

[64] D'Adamo E, Marcovecchio ML, Giannini C, Capanna R, Impicciatore M, Chiarelli F, Mohn A.The possible role of liver steatosis in defining metabolic syndrome in prepubertal children. Metabolism 2010;59:671-676.

[65] Lee TH, Kim WR, Benson JT, Therneau TM, Melton LJ 3rd.Serum aminotransferase activity and mortality risk in a United States community. Hepatology 2008; 47: 277-283.

[66] Demircioğlu F, Koçyiğit A, Arslan N, Cakmakçi H, Hizli S, Sedat AT. Intima-media thickness of carotid artery and susceptibility to atherosclerosis in obese children with nonalcoholic fatty liver disease. J Pediatr Gastroenterol Nutr 2008;47:423-427.

[67] Pacifico L, Cantisani V, Ricci P, Osborn JF, Schiavo E, Anania C, Ferrara E, Dvisic G, Chiesa C.Nonalcoholic fatty liver disease and carotid atheroscelrosis in children. Pediatr Res 2008; 63:423-427.

Chapter 10

Anabolic/Androgenic Steroids in Skeletal Muscle and Cardiovascular Diseases

Carla Basualto-Alarcón, Rodrigo Maass,
Enrique Jaimovich and Manuel Estrada

Additional information is available at the end of the chapter

http://dx.doi.org/10.5772/53080

1. Introduction

Testosterone exerts significant effect on muscle cells, and abnormalities of plasma concentrations can cause both skeletal muscle and cardiovascular diseases. Low levels are known to be associated with hypogonadism and have recently been linked to sarcopenia and metabolic syndrome; high levels are associated with hypertrophy. However, most evidence of the link between testosterone and metabolic actions is observational. Studies targeted to establish the mechanisms for such effects at the cell level and their correlation with *in vivo* models will broaden our understanding of the role played by these male steroid hormones in the pathophysiology of muscular and metabolic diseases.

1.1. Physiology of the androgens

Anabolic/androgenic steroid hormones are part of the male reproductive endocrine axis. Androgens are the male sex hormones responsible for development of the male reproductive system. Testosterone is the main androgen circulating in the blood and it is secreted from the testes, while other androgens, such as androstenedione and dehydroepiandrostenedione (DHEA) come mainly from the adrenal gland. In some tissues the androgen actions require that testosterone can be converted to dihydrotestosterone by action of 5α-reductase, and in other tissues, including adipose tissue, testosterone can also be converted into estradiol by aromatization of the androgen ring.

Endocrine actions of testosterone are under control of the hypothalamus-pituitary-gonad axis. The hypothalamus secretes gonadotropin-releasing hormone (GnRH), which stimulates the secretion of luteinizing hormone (LH) from the anterior pituitary (adenohypophysis). In the Leydig cells of the testes, the binding of LH to its receptor activates the uptake of circulating cholesterol, the steroid precursor for biosynthesis of all androgens. In the last step of testosterone biosynthesis, androstenedione is converted to testosterone, which is the main secreted component (95% of circulating androgens). In some cases testosterone acts directly on the cells of the target organ, but in others the active hormone is formed within the cells of the target organ by reduction of testosterone at position 5 of the steroid ring to yield the more active dihydrotestosterone. Androgens are responsible for primary and secondary sexual characteristics in men and also for the development of skeletal muscle mass and strength, erythropoiesis, and bone density, amongst other functions.

The divergent effects that androgens have between the sexes can be explained by differences in concentration, metabolism, and receptor expression. Male sex hormones are also known to fluctuate along the day and throughout life. Testosterone levels are usually low in males before puberty. However, after puberty, the testosterone level increases and reaches its peak around the age of 20–25 in men. As aging occurs, testosterone levels decline.

From total circulating levels of testosterone, only the free fraction of testosterone, the part dissolved in the plasma, is biologically active. In blood, free circulating testosterone is around a 2%, while the rest of the hormone is bound in different proportions to sex hormone binding globulin (SHBG) and albumin. However, the bio-available bound testosterone can be released on demand, as the albumin binding is weak. Thus, a higher apparent concentration of free testosterone is available to act in specific tissues.

The androgens have a variety of peripheral actions. They are anabolic throughout the body. That is, they stimulate protein synthesis. It is for this reason that the male body composition is generally larger and more muscular than the female. Androgen axis alterations are due mainly to deficiency or excess of testosterone, and the final effect will depend on whether the imbalance occurs before or after puberty. Before puberty, it can lead to delayed activation or never reached puberty (hypogonadism). If in excess, the hormone will have the opposite effect promoting early puberty accompanied by growth problems characterized by bone epiphysis alterations. Testosterone deficiency during embryonic development will condition a feminization of the external genitalia in men. After puberty, given the role of the male sex hormone on spermatogenesis, testosterone deficiency can induce infertility. Exogenously induced elevated testosterone concentrations cause hypertrophy in several tissues, with the effects on skeletal and cardiac muscle being critical.

In men, plasma testosterone concentrations range from 300 to 1000 ng/dL, whereas in women circulating levels of testosterone are about 10% of those observed in men [2, 3]. The body composition of men is regulated by testosterone concentrations [4, 5]. Pharmacological suppression of endogenous testosterone levels in healthy young subjects increased fat mass and decreased fat free mass and protein synthesis in muscle, suggesting a direct effect of androgens on body metabolism of lipids and proteins [6]. Healthy young subjects suppressed of endogenous testosterone levels and supplemented with different testosterone doses (from 25 mg to 600 mg testosterone enanthate/week) for 20 weeks increased the volume of the quadriceps muscle in a dose dependent manner, as determined by nuclear magnetic resonance. At the histological level, this increase was explained by an increase in the area of type I and II muscle fibers [7]. In bone tissue, testosterone deficiency is associated with decreased bone density with increasing tissue turnover markers. Thus, hormone replacement therapy in patients with hypogonadism has been established as effective to increase bone density [5]. Although testosterone and its derivatives are well known for their androgenic properties and anabolic effects, so far the effects of androgens on muscle remain incompletely understood.

1.2. Androgen mechanisms of action

Androgens exert most of their effects through direct binding to specific intracellular receptors acting as transcriptional activators [8]. Intracellular androgen receptors have been described in skeletal and cardiac muscle cells in addition to other tissues [9, 10]. The intracellular receptor mediates the "classic" genomic response to testosterone and is characterized as a 110-kDa protein with domains for androgen binding, nuclear localization, DNA binding, and transactivation. The conserved domain structure has 3 major functional regions, an NH-terminal transactivation domain, a centrally located DNA binding domain (DBD), and a COOH-terminal hormone-binding domain (HBD). The COOH-terminus contains an additional activation domain and a hinge region connecting the HBD and the DBD. Upon ligand binding, the nuclear receptors translocate to the nucleus, where they dimerize and bind to regulatory DNA sequences on target genes to either activate or repress transcription [11]. These effects are slow, with a latency period before onset, but they are also long lasting, remaining active for several hours after hormone stimulation. Several co-regulatory proteins that bind and regulate the activity of receptors have been identified. These include both co-activators that positively regulate transcriptional effects of intracellular receptors after ligand binding and co-repressors that negatively regulate receptor activity. In addition to this transcriptional or genomic mode of action, increasing evidence suggests that androgens can exert rapid, non-genomic effects. The time course of these responses is not compatible with the classic genomic mechanism for the action of steroids, since they have a rapid onset without an apparent latency period. Common to these early effects is a fast increase in intracellular Ca^{2+} and activation of Ca^{2+}-dependent pathways and second messenger cascades [12, 13]. Second messenger induction by non-genomic steroid action is insensitive to inhibitors of either transcription or translation. Little is known about these non-genomic effects in cardiac and skeletal muscle cells other than the generation of different patterns of Ca^{2+} signals and also the activation of complementary Ca^{2+}-dependent pathways involved in these responses. An interesting hypothesis is that these second messenger cascades may ultimately serve to modulate the transcriptional activity of the intracellular androgen receptor and its associated global response [14-16].

2. Musculoskeletal conditions related to androgens

Emerging syndromes and new approaches to classic diseases are now being linked to androgens. The androgen-associated diseases that will be discussed in this section include hypogonadism of the elderly (late onset hypogonadism [LOH]), sarcopenia, and the "metabolic syndrome." The interrelation between these diseases and decreased androgen levels is complex in the sense that these diseases are not only androgen dependent but that many other factors intervene in their development. Figure 1 shows the relationship between each of these diseases with the others, demonstrating that they are not "pure" androgen-dependent syndromes. With exception of LOH, which has implicit the concept of low androgen levels, neither sarcopenia nor metabolic syndrome are solely androgen-dependent diseases. It is important to bear this characteristic in mind when considering sarcopenia and metabolic syndrome, as there are numerous causes that may be behind the same clinical presentation. Further, the role of each of the hypothesized components may be very different from one patient to the other. The fourth disease that will be discussed here is Kennedy's disease, a hereditary X-linked neurodegenerative disease that affects mainly the androgen receptor function. In this sense, the pathophysiology of this disease is somewhat different from the 3 previously considered syndromes.

We will review the current definition of each syndrome, the epidemiology, the pathophysiology, and the effects that testosterone supplementation has demonstrated upon the evolution of the disease. After presenting these syndromes, we will highlight the differences observed among clinical studies in relation to age of populations analyzed, type of study, and expected outcome. This issue is important because it may affect the obtained results and therefore the subsequent conclusions.

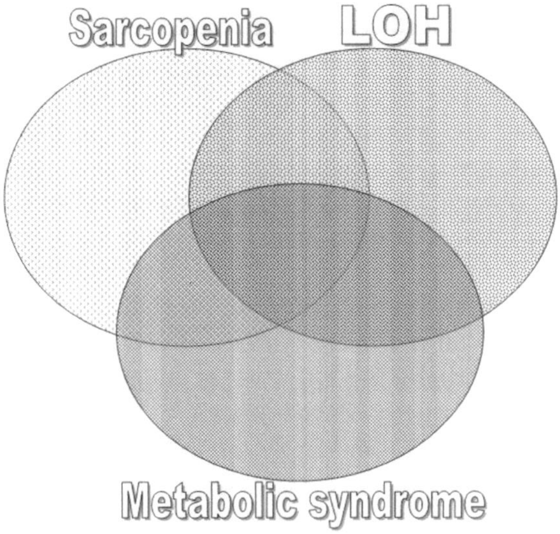

Figure 1. Clinical expression of 3 syndromes, their relationships, and androgen dependence. Each syndrome has components of "pure" disease. Thus, certain components particular to metabolic syndrome are expressed without muscle mass compromise (sarcopenia) or androgen levels decrease (LOH), although frequently, in association with the common dependence of these diseases upon advanced age, the clinical picture will associate the presence of more than 1 of these syndromes (i.e., metabolic syndrome plus sarcopenia). In another scenario, the expression of a disease, for example, sarcopenia may have decreased androgen levels among its pathophysiologic determinants.

2.1. Late onset hypogonadism (LOH)

Definition: Hypogonadism in the adult male can be considered as a syndrome, i.e., a constellation of signs and symptoms that collectively characterize a disease/disorder. Currently, there are guidelines to the diagnosis and treatment of this emerging disorder. According to these guidelines [17] the diagnosis of late onset hypogonadism (LOH) should be considered in patients who complain of specific symptoms, mainly in the areas of sexual function (decreased libido, impaired erectile function, shrinking testes), the musculoskeletal system (muscle weakness, increased adiposity, low bone mineral density), and psychological symptoms (depressed mood, decreased vitality, sleep disturbance). In these patients, a low morning serum total testosterone level, measured on 2 different occasions, will confirm the diagnosis of LOH [17, 18]. Wu et al. (2010) [19] conducted a study to establish criteria to more accurately diagnose LOH in the clinical setting. They look for the presence of characteristic symptoms that could help to reach an accurate diagnosis of LOH. After evaluating 3369 men in a cross-sectional study along with data obtained from questionnaires and a single testosterone measurement, the authors came to the conclusion that the combination of at least 3 sexual symptoms and decreased testosterone levels would make the diagnosis of LOH more accurate.

The normal reference levels for total testosterone in adult males vary from 300–1000 ng/dL. Morning levels (before 10 AM) below 250 ng/dL will make the diagnosis highly probable. A second total testosterone measurement is required to confirm the diagnosis. These tests should generally be followed by studies that help in determining the anatomical level of the endocrine failure, in order to confirm the cause of hypogonadism (primary, secondary, or mixed) [19, 20].

Epidemiology: According to the definition of Wu et al. (2010), the actual prevalence of LOH is 2.1% in a random population sample from Europe in men aged 40 to 79 years. The prevalence increased with increasing age of the participants, ranging from 0.1% in men aged 40 to 49 years to 5.1% in men 70 to 79 years of age [19]. Another study carried out in Boston, USA, used slightly different symptoms to define symptomatic hypogonadism. This study indicated an overall prevalence of symptomatic hypogonadism of 5.6%, showing an increased prevalence of 18.4% in men in their 70s [21]. A study performed in Hong Kong established a prevalence of 9.5%. As in the above-cited studies, an increase in the prevalence of hypogonadism was seen with increasing age of patients. Other conclusions that can be obtained from the epidemiological studies are that hypogonadism starts as early as the fourth decade, and that the presence of comorbid conditions (such as type 2 diabetes mellitus and cardiovascular diseases) also increases the prevalence of this syndrome [18].

Pathophysiology: Mean values of testosterone levels have declined in 75 year old men to approximately two-thirds of the values seen in young males [22]. Cross sectional and longitudinal studies have confirmed the observation that testosterone levels decline with age [18, 23-25], and that general health status plays a crucial role in arresting the fall of plasma testosterone. The time of blood sampling also affects the testosterone level, and the slope of the relationship between testosterone and aging [26, 27]. It was shown in healthy North-American men that testosterone decreased progressively at a rate that did not vary significantly with age from the third to the ninth decades. In this study, the magnitude of the decrease in total testosterone was 3.2 ng/dL per year, similar to other studies [23]. Other investigators reported a decrease of 0.8% per year in total testosterone levels (cross-sectionally) in a population of men ranging from 40–70 years [26]. Free and albumin-bound testosterone decreased at 2% per year, whereas SHBG tended to increase at 1.6% per year. These changes tend to include a shift toward inactive bound testosterone *vs* free bioavailable testosterone [24, 26].

The mechanisms behind this age-associated decline in male hormone levels are still unclear. Various alterations have been described in the elderly men that can lead to LOH. The main points where the physiology of androgens has been found to be affected by age are the testes, the hypothalamus, and the transport protein, SHBG. Primary testicular changes play an important role in age-associated testosterone decline. Leydig cells in the elderly have demonstrated a reduced secretory capacity in response to stimulation with recombinant LH [28]. This decrease has been related to a reduction in the number of Leydig cells. In addition to the decline in testicular reserve seen in the elderly, an altered neuroendocrine regulation, mainly at a hypothalamic level, has been suggested. Moderate increases of basal gonadotropin levels have been observed in response to the decline in testosterone levels, but not all studies agree with this observation [22]. The increases in GnRH as well as LH are thought to be abnormally low in response to the testosterone decline induced by the aforementioned Leydig cell alterations, implying a failure at some point in the neuroendocrine axis. It has been shown that the anterior pituitary has a preserved LH response to exogenous pulsate GnRH stimulation [28], suggesting, in line with other studies, the role played by the hypothalamus and the deficit of GnRH. Finally, increases in SHBG binding capacity have also been related to LOH. This change would result in an even greater decrease of free and bioavailable (albumin-bound) testosterone levels. The cause for this increase in SHBG binding capacity is still unknown.

In conclusion, testosterone decline in the elderly appears to have multiple causes, involving the testicular, hypothalamic, and transport levels. These alterations may be present in different proportions in different patients, making LOH a difficult syndrome both to understand and to treat.

Considerations for testosterone administration: The ability to diagnose hypogonadism with increasing accuracy does not mean that the decision of which patients to treat, how to treat them, and for how long, will be easy. Probably, because of the lack of long-term longitudinal studies that prove the safety of testosterone treatment, there is some degree of agreement not to reach supra-physiological levels with testosterone supplementation. This method of testosterone replacement therapy, in non-pharmacological doses, is presently accepted as a treatment for men diagnosed with LOH. Assuming that a correct diagnosis of hypogonadism has been made, following the above-mentioned guidelines, the choice of whom to treat should be clearer. Next, in the process of treating LOH, it is important to bear in mind the desired outcomes of androgen supplementation, i.e., whether to look only for normalization of plasma testosterone levels or also for prevention or amelioration of generally associated conditions such as osteoporosis and frailty, among others. Testosterone ad-

http://dx.doi.org/10.5772/53080

ministration to elderly men has been shown to induce beneficial effects on bone, muscle, heart, blood vessels, and mood. The problem is that many of these studies have been unable to demonstrate significant changes in endpoints such as functionality, independence, risk of fractures, etc. Furthermore, in earlier studies about testosterone supplementation, not only "pure" hypo-androgenic men were enrolled to participate, but also men with low-normal testosterone levels, which may have altered the final results. The risks associated with testosterone supplementation are an important issue influencing the decision to treat or not to treat. The development of polycythemia is a common complication of androgen therapy. It has been observed that hematocrit invariably increases with testosterone administration, and that this complication is the most frequent reason for the discontinuation of therapy [24, 29]. Concerning the cardiovascular risks, a recent study conducted in elderly patients with mobility limitations was terminated early because of an increase in the number of adverse cardiovascular events in the testosterone treated group [30]. However, a meta-analysis of randomized controlled trials that included 19 studies showed that there were no statistical differences between placebo and treated groups in relation to cardiovascular events [29]. One of the hypothesis to explain the increased cardiovascular risk is that exogenous testosterone can shift plasma lipids to a pro-atherogenic state [24], and another meta-analysis [4] that examined 29 randomized controlled trials showed a significant decrease in total cholesterol values that was more pronounced in hypogonadal men along with a reduction in HDL-cholesterol (HDL-C) that was detectable only in study populations with higher pre-treatment testosterone concentrations. This effect was dependent on the formulation of testosterone used.

Finally, one of the most recognized concerns about testosterone replacement therapy is the risk of developing prostate cancer. It has long been postulated that exogenous androgens can have a causative role in prostate cancer. On the other hand, androgen deprivation therapy has demonstrated a clear role for endogenous androgens in an already settled prostatic cancer. Therefore, the question remains open whether subclinical, "occult," prostatic lesions could develop into a neoplasia due to exogenous androgen administration. At the level of the prostate tissue, 6 months of testosterone replacement therapy in men with LOH showed no differences with placebo when considering prostate histology, tissue biomarkers, gene expression, and incidence or severity of prostate cancer [31]. Other studies that analyzed the association between testosterone treatment and prostate cancer did not find convincing evidence for this relationship [32, 33]. Nevertheless a meta-analysis [29] has shown a higher risk of detection of prostate events (incidence of prostate cancer, elevated prostatic-specific antigen, prostate biopsies) and increases in International Prostate Symptom Score (IPSS) in treated *vs* placebo groups.

In conclusion, benefits of testosterone replacement in LOH men have been established, but functional studies that demonstrate a significant improvement in large population samples are scarce and clinical studies of the risks of testosterone replacement therapy are still contradictory. Larger longitudinal, randomized placebo controlled studies are needed to draw definitive conclusions. At present, treatment is recommended for men diagnosed with LOH with appropriate monitoring of the prostate and the cardiovascular and hematological systems.

2.2. Sarcopenia

Definition: This term was proposed in 1989 by Irwin Rosenberg to describe a multifactorial syndrome that occurs with age and results in a loss of skeletal muscle mass and function [34]. The Greek word "sarx" means flesh, and "penia" means loss, suggesting with this name the principal organ and function targeted by this syndrome [35]. In 2010, a European Consensus definition and diagnosis of sarcopenia stated that sarcopenia is a syndrome characterized by progressive and generalized loss of skeletal muscle mass and strength, with the risk of adverse outcomes including physical disability, poor quality of life, and death. This working group also recommended criteria for the diagnosis of sarcopenia and highlighted the need to confirm low skeletal muscle mass to make the diagnosis [36].

Epidemiology: Janssen et al. [37] conducted a study to establish reference parameters for total and regional skeletal muscle mass in men and women between 18 and 88 years old. They studied 468 healthy men and women using magnetic resonance imaging, and confirmed previous reports indicating that there are gender differences for regional and whole body muscle mass. Skeletal muscle mass relative to body weight was 38% in men and 31% in women. In relation to muscle distribution, the differences were greater for skeletal muscle mass in the upper body (40% less muscle in women) than in the lower body (33% less muscle). In this population, the loss of muscle mass with age began in the fifth decade (45 years), a finding that agrees with other observations such as fiber cross sectional area and isometric and isokinetic strength, which are reported to change substantially only after 45 years of age. Due to the recent evolution of sarcopenia as a recognizable syndrome, there is still not much agreement in relation to its prevalence in aging populations [38, 39]. Baumgartner et al. [34], based on a definition of sarcopenia as appendicular skeletal muscle mass <2 standard deviations below the sex-specific young-normal mean for estimates of skeletal muscle mass, found a prevalence of sarcopenia of 24.1% in Hispanic women and 23.1% in non-Hispanic white women aged <70 years. The prevalence in men <70 years old was lower, with 16.9% in Hispanic men and 13.5% in non-Hispanic white men. Another study [39], conducted to confirm the sarcopenia rates reported by Baumgartner et al. [34], used body muscle mass measurements and reported a prevalence of sarcopenia of 22.6% in women and 26.8% in men ≥65 years. A more recent study [38] conducted in Spain evaluated healthy elderly participants aged >70 years. The observed prevalence of sarcopenia was 33% in women and 10% in men, differing from those described in the USA and other geographical areas. Ethnicity as well as other characteristics, such as health status and age, could explain these observed differences.

The prevalence of sarcopenia generally increases with age. Baumgartner et al. [34] observed an increase in the prevalence of sarcopenia after 80 years that reached >50% of individuals. Iannuzzi-Sucich et al. [39] also described an increase in the prevalence of sarcopenia in a subgroup of the studied population (80 years or older), reaching 31% in women and 52.9% in men. In reference to the relationship between testosterone levels and physical performance in older men, the Framingham Offspring study [40] described a significant association between serum free testosterone levels, walking speed, and short performance physical battery (SPPB) results. Men with low baseline free testosterone had 57% higher odds of reporting incident mobility limitation and 68% higher odds of worsening mobility limitations. Total testosterone and SHBG were not significantly associated with mobility limitation, subjective health, or physical performance measures.

The prevalence of sarcopenia varies from one study to another and these differences can be explained by different definitions of sarcopenia, differences in the studied populations and their reference (control) populations, sample sizes, and methods used to measure skeletal muscle mass. The unification of criteria to diagnose sarcopenia as well as the methods used to assess it will certainly aid in a better knowledge of the prevalence of this syndrome.

Pathophysiology: Another unresolved issue of sarcopenia is the pathophysiology of this syndrome. Because aging affects multiple organs, sarcopenia has been proposed to be the result of a multifactorial process affecting muscle, motor units, inflammatory cytokines, anabolic hormones, and nutritional intake in the elderly [41, 42].

Muscle mass is determined by a balance between protein synthesis and breakdown. It has been established that with advancing age, there is a decrease in whole body protein turnover [43]. In contrast to what happens in cachexia, where both skeletal muscle mass and fat mass are decreased, in the elderly the loss of muscle mass is accompanied by gains in fat mass [44]. Examination of the synthesis rate of particular proteins in skeletal muscle has shown that there is a particular synthesis rate, at least for each cell compartment in the skeletal muscle. The synthesis rate of mitochondrial and myosin heavy chain (MHC) proteins declines with age, whereas the synthesis rate of the sarcoplasmic protein pool was unchanged [43]. Ferrington et al. (1998) [45] have shown changes in other key skeletal muscle compartments, such as the sarcoplasmic reticulum, in aged rats. The turnover rate of SERCA pumps and ryanodine receptors decreased, whereas calsequestrin showed no changes. Studies about other key contractile elements in aging muscle, such as the α-actin protein, are recently available [46], and it was shown that in the vastus lateralis muscles of middle-aged *vs* elderly individuals, an isoform switch occurred with a decrease in skeletal muscle α-actin and an increase in the cardiac isoform of α-actin. This change is in accordance with the idea of a fast-to-slow transformation process during aging in the skeletal muscle. In other atrophy models, such as prolonged bed rest, the loss of thin contractile filaments (actin) was larger than that of thick contractile filaments (myosin) [47].

In addition to changes in skeletal muscle mass, there are changes in the motor units innervating the muscles. In humans, there is a decrease in the number of functional motor units with age. These changes have been confirmed in aged rats, where a reduction in the number of muscle fibers innervated per motor axon [41] was evident. These changes will lead to a decreased skeletal muscle fiber/motor neuron interaction that can further explain the decline in coordinated muscle action.

Other elements involved in the development of sarcopenia may be the loss of anabolic factors including neural growth factors, growth hormone, androgens and estrogens, and physical activity. An increase in oxidative stress and inflammatory cytokines such as interleukin 6 (IL-6) and tumor necrosis factor-α (TNF-α), and a decrease in food intake with aging have also been implicated [41, 48]. Cross-sectional and longitudinal studies have demonstrated that testosterone levels decrease with normal aging. Serum testosterone levels below the lower limit of normal, has a prevalence of 5% in healthy young men, up to 20% in the sixth decade, and increasing to 40–90% in men over 80 years [49]. Epidemiologic studies have demonstrated a relationship between levels of bioavailable testosterone and fat-free mass as well as muscle strength [49, 50]. These data correlated with physical performance tests. In the Framingham Offspring Study, men with low baseline of free testosterone concentrations showed a higher risk of incident or worsening mobility limitations [40]. In a study conducted in healthy young men to further elucidate the role of testosterone in the maintenance of skeletal muscle mass reported by Mauras et al. [6], a transient pharmacological hypogonadism was induced, decreasing fat-free mass, muscle strength, and fractional muscle protein synthesis in the volunteers. Despite this evidence, there are other studies, mainly that by Travison et al. [51], that have failed to show a clear association between testosterone concentration and physical function. This might be explained by certain aspects of the design of the study, including the selection of a younger population, a basal high physical activity level, mainly normal testosterone concentrations, and minimally demanding physical tests [50].

In short, testosterone has shown a tight association with skeletal muscle mass and a reasonable relationship with muscle strength, but no clear association with physical performance [50, 52]. The pathophysiology of sarcopenia appears, in conclusion, to be explained in part by intrinsic skeletal muscle changes associated with aging, but extrinsic causes also exist, and there are factors that aid in the development of sarcopenia or influence the degree of the attrition in skeletal muscle mass seen in the elderly.

Treatment options and impact of testosterone administration: Considering that protein breakdown and muscle atrophy is the hallmark of sarcopenia, many interventions have aimed to block the increased muscle catabolism seen in this syndrome. Among them, treatment with anabolic hormones, vitamin D, nutrition, and exercise have been studied. Controversial results have been obtained with all of the above-mentioned interventions, but 2 of them, testosterone and exercise, have been more successful. As was the case in relation to testosterone and the pathophysiology of sarcopenia, clinicians must discriminate between the endpoints of the studies that supplement older men with testosterone. In fact, the action of testosterone can be different when looking at muscle mass, strength, power, and whole-body functional probes. The anabolic effect of testosterone in aging men tends to be similar of that observed in young men but in a lesser extent. In general, studies have reported increases in lean body mass and decreases in fat mass, with varying responses concerning strength. Some studies have reported changes in grip strength but no increases in lower body strength [53, 54]. Others do report significant improvements in leg strength [49, 55]. Considering that sarcopenia is a syndrome that affects quality of life and risk of falls, changes in leg strength must be a desirable effect of the selected treatment. The factors that might lead to results showing little improvement in physical function after testosterone treatment in elderly men remains to be investigated. Critical points that should be revisited are basal testosterone levels of the selected population and testosterone concentrations reached during androgen treatment. The rigor of the selected physical probes ideally will present a real challenge in order to avoid an early ceiling effect on the sensitivity of the test.

Physical activity is always associated with a general well being outcome that stimulates cardiovascular, respiratory, and skeletal muscle systems. Endurance and resistance exercise has been shown to improve the rate of decline in muscle mass and strength that occurs with age, although resistance exercise have proven to be more effective increasing muscle mass and strength in older men [54]. There is controversy in the literature regarding the extent of the muscle response induced by exercise in the elderly. Some authors indicate that resistance exercise in older people produces smaller strength increases in absolute terms, but similar in relative terms, to younger people [55]. On the other hand, similar increases in percent muscle strength were found in healthy older individuals and in young people in a prospective investigation that also assessed changes at the satellite cell level following a heavy resistance strength training period [56].

It seems that a key feature of skeletal muscle, its plasticity, is retained even in very old individuals. Muscle cross sectional area, muscle strength, and physical performance have been shown to improve in very old nursing home residents [57] and in community residents [58] engaged in progressive resistance exercise training. The intensity of the resistance exercise required to obtain positive changes is also still under debate. The majority of studies suggest that a high intensity resistance exercise (70–90% of 1 repetition maximum) is needed in order to obtain the desired improvements in muscle mass and strength [59]. As little as 1 resistance training session per week has demonstrated positive strength changes [60]. This recent issue may be an interesting point to explore in order to attract interest of more individuals to participate in strength training programs that will aid in the prevention and treatment of sarcopenia.

In conclusion, understanding sarcopenia as a multifactorial syndrome also involves the potential discovery of a great number of therapeutic targets. So far, testosterone, but more clearly, exercise, have been the more successful therapeutic options. More studies with the newest therapies and/or improved exercise and hormone replacement therapies should be performed in order to gain advances against this quality of life (QOL)-threatening syndrome.

2.3. Metabolic syndrome

Definition: Metabolic syndrome is the collection of a number of metabolic abnormalities that lead to increased risk of cardiovascular disease and diabetes mellitus (DM) [61]. The definition of metabolic syndrome varies among international consensus groups. Four groups have proposed diagnostic criteria, the World Health Organization (WHO), the Study Group for Insulin Resistance (EGIR), the National Cholesterol Education Program Adult Treatment Panel III (NCEP ATP III), and the International Diabetes Federation (IDF). In general, all of these groups maintain similar criteria, but differ in their measurements and cut off points. The IDF and NCEP ATP III are currently the most used. The latter requires the presence of at least 3 of the following 5 criteria for diagnosis: central obesity, elevated triglycerides, low HDL cholesterol (HDL-C), hypertension, and impaired fasting glucose (greater than 110 mg/dL), without categories among the factors. Subsequently, the American Heart Association/National Heart, Lung, and Blood Institute (AHA/NHLBI) suggested considering 100 mg/dL as the cut off for glucose, while the International Diabetes Federation (IDF) established as a basic requirement the presence of central obesity confirmed by abdominal circumference measurement [62, 63]. Despite the great diversity of clinical criteria for diagnosing metabolic syndrome, the central issue is to recognize that its presence means an increased cardiovascular risk for the diagnosed patient, and to take action to counteract its consequences.

Epidemiology: Depending on the criteria used, age, gender, and race, the prevalence of metabolic syndrome varies markedly. However, the prevalence increases with age independently of the other criteria used, and it is higher in males when using the criteria of the WHO and EGIR. With the WHO criteria, the prevalence for men and women under 55 years is 14% and 4%, respectively, and 31% and 20% in the older age [62, 63]. In United States, using NCEP ATP III criteria, the overall prevalence is 24%, and increases directly with age and body mass index. In young Americans ages 12 to 19 years the prevalence is 4.2%, and it exceeds 40% by 65 to 69 years. A meta-analysis encompassing 172,573 patients concluded that there is a risk of cardiovascular death that is significantly higher in people with metabolic syndrome and that this is not only explained by its components separately [64].

Pathophysiology: Body fat is an important component of metabolic syndrome because adipose tissue is insulin-resistant in obesity, which increases free fatty acid (FFA) levels in the plasma. This has a direct effect on insulin target organs including liver and muscle, through specific actions that block the intracellular signaling of the insulin receptor. Moreover, in patients with metabolic syndrome, the adipose tissue was predominantly abdominal and associated with increased visceral fat as compared with peripheral distribution. Adipocytes in visceral fat are more metabolically active, releasing more FFA and inflammatory cytokines that drain directly to the liver via the portal circulation. This phenomenon, known as lipotoxicity, will be responsible for insulin resistance in these organs and the pancreas and unregulated high blood glucose. Lipo-toxicity also affects the cardiovascular system. In addition, FFA are able to increase oxidative stress, encourage a pro-inflammatory environment, and reduce systemic vascular reactivity, which are all factors negatively affecting cardiac cells. In association with these negative changes in adipose tissue, low testosterone levels worsen the clinical setting in the metabolic syndrome. Decreased androgen levels are associated with obesity, mainly with visceral fat accumulation. Epidemiological studies have demonstrated statistically significant correlations between plasma levels of testosterone and adipose tissue distribution, insulin sensitivity, lipoprotein metabolism, and the hemostatic system, among others. All of these cardiovascular risk factors impact endothelial function. It should be noted that these effects of testosterone vary according to sex and age. In normal men, plasma testosterone levels are correlated directly with HDL-C and inversely with triglycerides, LDL-cholesterol (LDL-C), fibrinogen, and plasminogen activator inhibitor type 1 (PAI-1). In addition, testosterone levels have correlated inversely with body mass index (BMI), waist circumference, visceral fat accumulation, insulin, and FFA. It is postulated that in men, low testosterone becomes a new element of the metabolic syndrome [61, 65].

Testosterone regulates the deposition of triglycerides in the abdominal fat tissue by lipoprotein lipase enzymes and a hormone sensitive lipase. Testosterone has an anticoagulant and profibrinolytic action, and by decreasing fibrinogen and PAI-1, it also has a pro-aggregatory effect through decreased platelet cyclooxygenase activity. During eugonadism, testosterone stimulates hormone-sensitive lipase and lipolysis. Thus, in testosterone deficiency, lipolysis is inhibited, favoring the accumulation of adipose tissue [6], which is reversed by testosterone administration. In addition, it has been reported that in hypogonadal patients, the deposition of visceral adipose tissue leads in turn to a further decrease in testosterone concentrations via conversion to estradiol by the aromatase. This leads to further abdominal fat deposition and a higher testosterone deficiency [4, 66]. In parallel, hyperinsulinemia is associated with decreased SHBG production, which decreases plasma total testosterone [67]. To date, the question of whether hypogonadism influences insulin resistance by increased abdominal obesity or whether obesity favors the reduction of plasma testosterone concentrations is still debated. However, insulin resistance leads to increased risk factors including increased triglycerides, lower HDL, and predominance of LDL-C. To these lipoprotein factors are added intolerance to carbohydrates, high blood pressure, and pro-coagulant and antifibrinolytic states [68]. Clinical studies show that men exhibit higher susceptibility to atherosclerosis than pre-menopausal women. The available data indicate that the evolution of atherosclerosis is more rapid in males, independent of dyslipidemia or evidence of endothelial damage, than in females [69]. The actual evidence indicates that low androgen concentrations are strongly associated with increases in cardiovascular risks including atherogenic lipid profile, insulin resistance, obesity, and metabolic syndrome [70, 71].

Impact of testosterone administration: Clinical studies generally show that the effects of exogenous testosterone on cardiovascular risk factors differ considerably depending on the dose, route of administration, and duration of treatment, as well as by age and condition of the patient. The findings most frequently observed are a decrease in HDL-C, a slight decrease in LDL-C, with sustained stability of the relationship between them, and moderation of insulin resistance leading to a decrease in triglyceride levels and visceral fat mass. Other less marked effects of androgen therapy are reduced levels of atherothrombotic lipoprotein Lp(a) and fibrinogen. According to current evidence, androgen therapy may exert beneficial or deleterious effects on various factors involved in the pathogenesis of atherosclerosis, and therefore further studies are required in order to determine optimal testosterone supplementation.

2.4. Considerations regarding clinical studies dealing with testosterone supplementation in sarcopenia and metabolic syndrome

Figure 2 emphasizes some of the determinants that should be considered when analyzing clinical studies working with androgen replacement therapy in sarcopenia and metabolic syndrome. It is important to bear in mind the level of testosterone that is sought with the proposed treatment and from this starting point, other important considerations must be made, including age of the individuals, in order to place the conclusions in an adequate context according to the population seeking treatment.

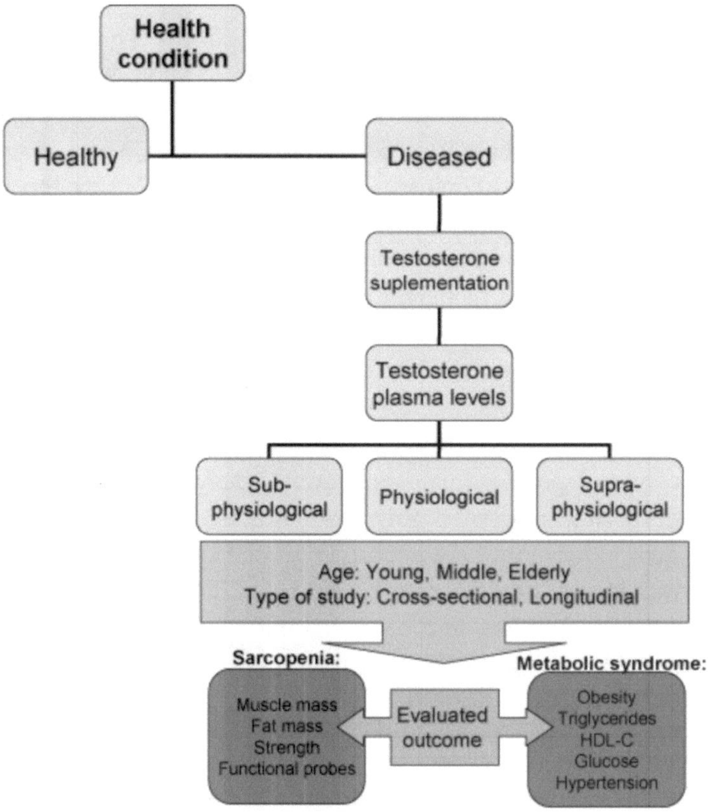

Figure 2. Highlight of some key considerations in studies of testosterone supplementation for sarcopenia and metabolic syndrome. The process starts with the diagnosis of the disease. From this point, therapy will be initiated and varying testosterone levels can be reached, normal, sub-, or supra-physiologic. Once in this condition, the type of study and the age of the studied sample will influence the results. Most importantly, the expected outcome should be clearly stressed in order to avoid any ambiguity.

2.5. Spinal and bulbar muscular atrophy (Kennedy's disease)

Definition: Spinal and bulbar muscular atrophy (SBMA), or Kennedy's disease, is an infrequent hereditary X-linked neurodegenerative disease that affects approximately 1/40,000 men, typically from age 30 years [72, 73]. It is characterized by slow degeneration and loss of motor neurons in the medulla and spinal cord [74, 75]. Patients exhibit progressive weakness, atrophy of facial, bulbar, and limb muscles, sensory disturbances, and hyper-creatine kinase (hyperCKemia), together with signs of androgen insensitivity [76]. Heterozygous and homozygous females are asymptomatic [77, 78], and the latter may have a subclinical phenotype [73]. The clinical signs are manifested initially as postural and perioral tremor, and progress to proximal or distal weakness of the limbs, dysarthria, dysphagia, hanging jaw, fasciculations, and muscle cramps [76, 79]. Muscle biopsies show changes associated with denervation, such as increased fiber size variability, atrophic fibers, and clumping of sarcolemmal nuclei and necrotic fibers [80, 81]. Nerve biopsy may show reduction of large myelinated fibers [82]. The disease usually progresses irreversibly and most patients die of pneumonia associated with dysphagia and disorders of the pharyngeal and laryngeal musculature, and some may require mechanical ventilation during the course of the disease [74, 83].

Etiology: The disease is caused by the expansion of a polymorphic tandem repeat sequence of the triplet CAG in exon 1 of the androgen receptor gene (AR) located on the X-chromosome (locus Xq11–12). The normal number of repeats is 9 to 36 [84, 85] and in the case of SBMA the number of repeats identified is 40 to 62 [85, 86]. The CAG encodes the amino acid glutamine (Q), so that the AR is expressed with a polyglutamine (poliQ) sequence in the amino terminal transactivation segment [87]. SBMA is considered 1 of the 9 hereditary polyglutamine neurodegenerative diseases [75]. It has been shown that the greater number of repeats in the polyglutamine sequence, the receptor activity is decreased. Thus, in SBMA the AR has limited or null activity. This AR mutant resides in the cytoplasm as apoAR associated with heat shock proteins (Hsps) and accessory proteins until it binds its ligand (testosterone and dihydrotestosterone). The hormone binding induces the exposure of the bipartite nuclear localization signal [88, 89] and translocation to the nucleus, where it is partially degraded by nuclear proteasome [90]. The AR mutation is not able to bind coactivators and corepressors, and its classical androgenic action is not performed [69]. The patient shows signs of androgen insensitivity such as asymmetric gynecomastia, reduced fertility, testicular atrophy, oligospermia, azoospermia, erectile dysfunction, and reduced libido or diabetes [72]. The poli-Q expanded AR deregulates transcription by interfering with several transcriptional coregulators. The number of the repeats is negatively correlated with age disease onset and directly with the severity and progression of the disease [72, 76].

Pathophysiology: The precise mechanism of the disease is still unknown, but there is growing evidence that the poli-Q-expanded AR is not adequately degraded, resulting in the accumulation of fragments of the poli-Q amino terminal fragment [73, 91]. These are accumulated in the nucleus of motor neurons, dorsal root ganglia, or visceral cells, and exert toxic effects that cause dysfunction and loss of neurons [79, 88, 92]. Aggregation requires the presence of androgens, migration of the mutated AR to the nucleus, and inhibition of gene expression of essential factors for the viability of affected neurons [88]. Once it joins the ligand, either testosterone or dihydrotestosterone (DHT), the poli-Q expanded AR migrates to the nucleus and due to misfolding [84], does not perform its genomic functions in the androgen response elements (ARE), but instead forms nuclear aggregates [92]. The nuclear aggregates (neuronal intranuclear inclusions) contain fragments of mutated AR, ubiquitin proteasome system (UPS) (ubiquitin and 19S and 20S proteasome core components), and heat shock proteins (Hsp40, Hsp70 and Hsp90) [93]. Segments with poli-Q expansions form antiparallel beta strands, and by hydrogen bonds the strands form a beta sheet structure, resulting in aggregation of these misfolded proteins as intranuclear inclusions, either as oligomers or larger aggregates [94]. The mutated ARs in the nucleus undergo partial proteolysis due to misfolding, resulting in the production of truncated forms of the poli-Q-expanded AR oligomers. The accumulation of mutant AR aggregates is regarded as protective [95, 96], while diffuse accumulation in the nucleus is considered toxic [92]. These aggregates are observed at light microscopy as inclusions in the nucleus and cytoplasm of affected motor and sensory neurons and those with no apparent signs of damage [92]. It has been found that the number of aggregates was not correlated with toxicity [88]. In addition, this same type of aggregate is seen in other tissues including scrotal skin and abdominal viscera [73]. There is clear evidence that mutated AR aggregation leads to transcriptional dysregulation in affected neurons [97]. Intermediate gene products have been described that reduce the expression of TFG-β receptor type II (TβRII), dynactin 1, and VEGF. Transgenic mice expressing a mutated AR with 97 glutamine repeats (AR-97Q) exhibited muscle atrophy and neurodegeneration similar to that of SBMA in studies, and this was associated with reduced transcription of TβRII [97]. Moreover, in a similar model of transgenic mice, AR-97Q was associated with early decrease in the expression of the p150 (*Glued*) subunit of dynactin (dynactin 1), and this was related to inadequate retrograde axonal transport resulting in the distal accumulation of neurofilaments, axonopathy with subsequent degeneration of motor neurons, and the onset of characteristic signs of SBMA, which was partially reversed by castration [98]. Overexpression of C terminus of heat shock cognate protein 70-interacting protein (CHIP) in double-transgenic mice significantly reduced the SBMA phenotype by promoting the degradation of the mutated receptor by way of ubiquitin proteasome system (UPS) and significantly reduced the appearance of nuclear aggregates of mutant AR [93], indicating that proper breakdown of mutated protein reduces the negative effects of poli-Q-expanded AR. Interestingly, over-expression of skeletal muscle tissue-specific normal AR induced a phenotype similar to SBMA in transgenic animals, mimicking the effects of poli-Q-expanded AR [75], which suggest that muscle dysfunction may at least partly be behind the pathology of motor neurons and is due to overexpression of the AR in the presence of androgens inducing decreased expression of VEGF, which is critical in maintaining the neuromuscular junction and the viability of motor neurons [75].

Treatment options: Clinical deprivation of androgens by various strategies has been tested, including the use of the competitive AR blocker flutamide, which was ineffective in animal models. The efficacy to prevent the peripheral conversion of testosterone to dihydrotestosterone (DHT) by blocking the enzyme 5-α-reductase using dutasteride has also been tested, and proved to be ineffective to prevent the progression of the disease [99]. The most promising strategy has been the use of leuprorelin, which is a LHRH analogue that reduces androgen secretion to undetectable levels in plasma and has proven effective in preventing toxic accumulation of mutated AR and neurodegeneration in human patients [100, 101]. Other experimental strategies are based on preventing the deregulation of transcription induced by the mutated AR, since it has been shown to inhibit the histone acetyltransferase (HAT) activity of nuclear proteins like Sp1 and cAMP response element-binding protein-binding protein (CBP) [102], which has been shown to induce a phenotype of SBMA and which has been prevented by histone-deacetylase inhibitors, such as sodium butyrate, in animal studies [100]. The strategy of increasing the degradation of mutated AR via the UPS or by induction of autophagy to reduce the presence of nuclear and cytoplasmic poli-Q AR has also been explored [88, 93], but to date the most effective mechanism to prevent progression of the disease is to reduce circulating androgen concentrations, thereby preventing migration of the mutated AR to the nucleus and its subsequent toxic effects.

http://dx.doi.org/10.5772/53080

3. Molecular basis of influence of high levels of testosterone on skeletal and cardiac muscle

High blood levels of androgens, above the physiological range, are produced by exogenous administration of testosterone or its synthetic derivatives. These hormones have been used by athletes to improve performance by increasing muscle mass and strength. Hypertrophy is the more recognized among the numerous documented hormonal effects of long-term use of androgens.

Muscle mass is regulated by the normal balance between synthesis and degradation of muscle proteins. There is consensus that the use of testosterone leads to hypertrophy by increasing net protein synthesis over protein degradation, however the pathways responsible for this effect, and this dependence of intracellular androgen receptor, have not been fully described to date. Moreover, testosterone activates skeletal muscle satellite cell and mesenchymal stem cell differentiation, which also accounts for the clinical effect of this hormone on body composition [103, 104]. Side effects related to use of anabolic steroids are focused especially on the cardiovascular system [105]. It is known that there are increases in blood pressure and peripheral arterial resistance [105-108], and there are also effects on the heart muscle, primarily left ventricular hypertrophy with restricted diastolic function [109-111]. Severe cardiac complications (heart failure, atrial fibrillation, myocardial infarction or sudden cardiac death) in strength athletes with acute anabolic/androgenic steroid abuse have also been reported [112, 113].

The anabolic actions of androgens enhance muscle strength and increase muscle size clinically [6, 7, 114]. *In vivo*, androgens increase skeletal muscle mass and induce cardiac hypertrophy [10, 109]. The effect of androgens may occur through either the classically described intracellular androgen receptor pathway (genomic pathway) or via a fast, non-genomic pathway. In contrast to the genomic pathway (minutes to hours), the non-genomic pathway has measurable effects in seconds to minutes. It is elicited by hormones, the effects of which cannot be abrogated by transcriptional inhibitors, and may occur without requiring the hormone to bind the intracellular receptors or the receptor to bind DNA [115].

As noted, hypertrophy processes involve changes in gene expression controlled by intracellular androgen receptor-mediated pathways, and recent studies have demonstrated an alternative rapid intracellular androgen receptor-independent mode of testosterone action. The establishment of the testosterone-androgen receptor complex acts as a transcriptional factor for the expression of different genes and proteins necessary for protein synthesis, energy production, and cell growth, which are also crucial for hypertrophic growth. Now, aside from the classical action mechanism of testosterone, non-classical effects have also been implicated in the growth of the muscle cell. Hypertrophy in both skeletal and cardiac muscle is an adaptive response of the cell to increase force and contractile activity. Although initially beneficial, the prolonged activation of muscle cells by hypertrophic stimuli may produce detrimental effects. Unlike that in cardiac muscle, hypertrophy of skeletal muscle cell is a reversible process.

Several pro-hypertrophic stimuli activate common pathways in the muscle cell [116]. Among pathways activated by these stimuli, key regulators are phosphatidylinositol-3 kinase (PI3K)/Akt and mitogen-activated protein/extracellular signal-regulated kinase kinase (MEK/ERK1/2) pathways [117-119]. It has also been proposed that testosterone actions involve membrane receptors that stimulated early intracellular signaling pathways through interaction with G proteins in primary cultures of skeletal muscle cells [12] as well as cardiac myocytes [120]. Common to these early effects are the fast intracellular Ca^{2+} increase, activation of Ca^{2+}-dependent pathways, and second-messenger cascades. Ca^{2+} is one of the most diverse and important intracellular second messengers as well as a key element in the excitation-contraction coupling of muscle cells. Ca^{2+} has been related to hypertrophy because of its ability to promote the activation of the protein phosphatase calcineurin through the establishment of a Ca^{2+}/calmodulin complex [121]. Calcineurin promotes translocation of the nuclear factor of activated T cells (NFAT) from cytoplasm to nucleus. NFAT family proteins are responsible for the expression of the early fetal genes, which are expressed during fetal development. These are silenced in adult stages but are re-expressed during cardiac hypertrophy, and thus are considered as hypertrophic markers [119, 121, 122].

Interlinked signaling pathways are related to hypertrophy of the muscle cells. Moreover, it has been described that testosterone induces intracellular Ca^{2+} increase through a non-genomic action mechanism in skeletal muscle cells [12, 13] and cardiomyocytes [120]. Studies in cultured muscle cells show that through a nongenomic mechanism, testosterone is implicated in the activation of a membrane receptor coupled to a $G\alpha q$ protein, thus resulting in the production of IP_3 and release of Ca^{2+} from endoplasmic reticulum [12, 120]. These Ca^{2+} oscillations induce the activation of ERK 1/2, which in turn phosphorylates mammalian target of rapamycin (mTOR), promoting hypertrophic cardiac growth [15].

The PI3K/Akt pathway has been related to cell survival and proliferation in almost all cell types. However, the up-regulation of the pathway by several stimuli induces cardiac hypertrophy. One of the most common downstream targets of Akt is the protein kinase glycogen synthase kinase 3-β (GSK3-β) [123]. Activated GSK3-β phosphorylates several members of the NFAT family, which promotes their translocation from nucleus to cytoplasm. Akt phosphorylates and inhibits GSK3-β, which increases the residence of NFAT in the nucleus. Moreover, Akt has the ability to phosphorylate mTOR, another downstream target of the PI3K/Akt pathway. In muscle cells, protein synthesis is highly regulated by mTOR, which stimulates protein translation and ribosome biosynthesis [124]. The mTOR lies upstream of critical translation regulators such as the 40S ribosomal protein S6 kinase 1 (S6K1) and the eukaryotic initiation factor 4E-binding protein 1 (4E-BP1). Activation of the mTOR pathway is a critical step to induce cardiac hypertrophy by testosterone *in vitro* [15].

Thus, considering the current information available regarding androgen actions on muscle cells, it has been proposed that muscle hypertrophy induced by testosterone requires both androgen receptor activity and signal transduction pathways to control protein synthesis.

4. Perspectives of androgen-mediated physiological and pathological responses

The role of androgens in modulating both musculoskeletal and cardiovascular function is of the highest importance, especially considering that androgen deficiency is strongly associated with several medical conditions, including sarcopenia, metabolic syndrome, obesity, diabetes, hypertension and atherosclerosis. Testosterone deficiency, as observed in LOH, further deprives muscle of important anabolic effects of androgens in human males. The action mechanism of androgens involves both androgen receptor and signal transduction pathways, so, essential for the diagnosis, clinical and pharmacological intervention studies, a detailed knowledge of these pathways is required. As cardiovascular side effects of testosterone reduce its actual therapeutic use, research in this field is badly needed to have a detailed knowledge of the effects of androgen alterations in order to elaborate safe therapeutic replacement protocols that appear to have a broad potential for high incidence pathological conditions.

Acknowledgment

This work was supported by FONDECYT (grant 1120259 to M.E. and grant 1110467 to E.J.) and by ACT 1111 (E.J.). C.B. is a CONICYT doctoral fellow (AT 24091020).

Author details

Carla Basualto-Alarcón[1], Rodrigo Maass[2], Enrique Jaimovich[1] and Manuel Estrada[1]

1 Universidad de Chile, Facultad de Medicina, Instituto de Ciencias Biomédicas, Chile

2 Universidad de Valparaíso, Facultad de Medicina, Campus San Felipe, Chile

References

[1] Bhasin S, Storer TW, Berman N, Callegari C, Clevenger B, Phillips J, Bunnell TJ, Tricker R, Shirazi A, Casaburi R. The effects of supraphysiologic doses of testosterone on muscle size and strength in normal men. The New England Journal of Medicine 1996; 335, 1-7.

[2] Evans NA. Current concepts in anabolic-androgenic steroids. The American Journal of Sports Medicine 2004; 32, 534-42.

[3] Isidori AM, Greco EA, Aversa A. Androgen deficiency and hormone-replacement therapy. British Journal of Urology International 2005; 96, 212-6.

[4] Isidori AM, Giannetta E, Greco EA, Gianfrilli D, Bonifacio V, Isidori A, Lenzi A, Fabbri A. Effects of testosterone on body composition, bone metabolism and serum lipid profile in middle-aged men: a meta-analysis. Clinical Endocrinology (Oxf) 2005; 63, 280-93.

[5] Zitzmann M. Effects of testosterone replacement and its pharmacogenetics on physical performance and metabolism. Asian Journal of Andrology 2008; 10, 364-72.

[6] Mauras N, Hayes V, Welch S, Rini A, Helgeson K, Dokler M, Veldhuis JD, Urban RJ. Testosterone deficiency in young men: marked alterations in whole body protein kinetics, strength, and adiposity. The Journal of Clinical Endocrinology and Metabolism 1998; 83, 1886-92.

[7] Sinha-Hikim I, Roth SM, Lee MI, Bhasin S. Testosterone-induced muscle hypertrophy is associated with an increase in satellite cell number in healthy, young men. American Journal of Physiology - Endocrinology and Metabolism 2003; 285, E197-205.

[8] Beato M. Gene regulation by steroid hormones. Cell 1989; 56, 335-44.

[9] Hickson RC, Galassi TM, Kurowski TT, Daniels DG, Chatterton RT. Androgen and glucocorticoid mechanisms in exercise-induced cardiac hypertrophy. American Journal of Physiology – Heart and Circulatory Physiology 1984; 246, H761-7.

[10] Marsh JD, Lehmann MH, Ritchie RH, Gwathmey JK, Green GE, Schiebinger RJ. Androgen receptors mediate hypertrophy in cardiac myocytes. Circulation 1998; 98, 256-61.

[11] Simental JA, Sar M, Wilson EM. Domain functions of the androgen receptor. The Journal of Steroid Biochemistry and Molecular Biology 1992; 43, 37-41.

[12] Estrada M, Espinosa A, Muller M, Jaimovich E. Testosterone stimulates intracellular calcium release and mitogen-activated protein kinases via a G protein-coupled receptor in skeletal muscle cells. Endocrinology 2003; 144, 3586-97.

[13] Estrada M, Liberona JL, Miranda M, Jaimovich E. Aldosterone- and testosterone-mediated intracellular calcium response in skeletal muscle cell cultures. American Journal of Physiology – Endocrinology and Metabolism 2000; 279, E132-9.

[14] Wilson C, Maass, R, Estrada, M. Cardiovascular Effects of Androgens. Basic and Clinical Endocrinology Up-to-Date. InTech, 2011. http://www.intechopen.com/books/basic-and-clinical-endocrinology-up-to-date/cardiovascular-effects-of-androgens.

[15] Altamirano F, Oyarce C, Silva P, Toyos M, Wilson C, Lavandero S, Uhlen P, Estrada M. Testosterone induces cardiomyocyte hypertrophy through mammalian target of rapamycin complex 1 pathway. Journal of Endocrinology 2009; 202, 299-307.

[16] Vicencio JM, Estrada M, Galvis D, Bravo R, Contreras AE, Rotter D, Szabadkai G, Hill JA, Rothermel BA, Jaimovich E, Lavandero S. Anabolic androgenic steroids and intracellular calcium signaling: a mini review on mechanisms and physiological implications. Mini-Reviews in Medicinal Chemistry 2011; 11, 390-8.

[17] Bhasin S, Cunningham GR, Hayes FJ, Matsumoto AM, Snyder PJ, Swerdloff RS, Montori VM. Testosterone therapy in men with androgen deficiency syndromes: an Endocrine Society clinical practice guideline. The Journal of Clinical Endocrinology and Metabolism 2010; 95, 2536-59.

[18] Surampudi PN, Wang C, Swerdloff R. Hypogonadism in the aging male diagnosis, potential benefits, and risks of testosterone replacement therapy. International Journal of Endocrinology 2012; 625434.

[19] Wu FC, Tajar A, Beynon JM, Pye SR, Silman AJ, Finn JD, O'Neill TW, Bartfai G, Casanueva FF, Forti G, Giwercman A, Han TS, Kula K, Lean ME, Pendleton N, Punab M, Boonen S, Vanderschueren D, Labrie F, Huhtaniemi IT. Identification of late-onset hypogonadism in middle-aged and elderly men. The New England Journal of Medicine 2010; 363, 123-35.

[20] Ohlsson C, Wallaschofski H, Lunetta KL, Stolk L, Perry JR, Koster A, Petersen AK, Eriksson J, Lehtimaki T, Huhtaniemi IT, Hammond GL, Maggio M, Coviello AD, Ferrucci L, Heier M, Hofman A, Holliday KL, Jansson JO, Kahonen M, Karasik D, Karlsson MK, Kiel DP, Liu Y, Ljunggren O, Lorentzon M, Lyytikainen LP, Meitinger T, Mellstrom D, Melzer D, Miljkovic I, Nauck M, Nilsson M, Penninx B, Pye SR, Vasan RS, Reincke M, Rivadeneira F, Tajar A, Teumer A, Uitterlinden AG, Ulloor J, Viikari J, Volker U, Volzke H, Wichmann HE, Wu TS, Zhuang WV, Ziv E, Wu FC, Raitakari O, Eriksson A, Bidlingmaier M, Harris TB, Murray A, de Jong FH, Murabito JM, Bhasin S, Vandenput L, Haring R. Genetic determinants of serum testosterone concentrations in men. PLoS Genetics 2010; 7, e1002313.

[21] Araujo AB, Esche GR, Kupelian V, O'Donnell AB, Travison TG, Williams RE, Clark RV, McKinlay JB. Prevalence of symptomatic androgen deficiency in men. The Journal of Clinical Endocrinology and Metabolism 2007; 92, 4241-7.

[22] Nieschlag E, Behre HM, Bouchard P, Corrales JJ, Jones TH, Stalla GK, Webb SM, Wu FC. Testosterone replacement therapy: current trends and future directions. Human Reproduction Update 2004; 10, 409-19.

[23] Harman SM, Metter EJ, Tobin JD, Pearson J, Blackman MR. Longitudinal effects of aging on serum total and free testosterone levels in healthy men. Baltimore Longitudinal Study of Aging. The Journal of Clinical Endocrinology and Metabolism 2001; 86, 724-31.

[24] Myers JB, Meacham RB. Androgen replacement therapy in the aging male. Reviews in Urology 2003; 5, 216-26.

[25] Plymate SR, Tenover JS, Bremner WJ. Circadian variation in testosterone, sex hormone-binding globulin, and calculated non-sex hormone-binding globulin bound

testosterone in healthy young and elderly men. Journal of Andrology 1989; 10, 366-71.

[26] Feldman HA, Longcope C, Derby CA, Johannes CB, Araujo AB, Coviello AD, Bremner WJ, McKinlay JB. Age trends in the level of serum testosterone and other hormones in middle-aged men: longitudinal results from the Massachusetts male aging study. The Journal of Clinical Endocrinology and Metabolism 2002, 87, 589-98.

[27] Gray A, Berlin JA, McKinlay JB, Longcope C. An examination of research design effects on the association of testosterone and male aging: results of a meta-analysis. Journal of Clinical Epidemiology 1991; 44, 671-84.

[28] Mulligan T, Iranmanesh A, Kerzner R, Demers LW, Veldhuis JD. Two-week pulsatile gonadotropin releasing hormone infusion unmasks dual (hypothalamic and Leydig cell) defects in the healthy aging male gonadotropic axis. European Journal of Endocrinology 1999; 141, 257-66.

[29] Calof OM, Singh AB, Lee ML, Kenny AM, Urban RJ, Tenover JL, Bhasin S. Adverse events associated with testosterone replacement in middle-aged and older men: a meta-analysis of randomized, placebo-controlled trials. Journals of Gerontology Series A: Biological Sciences and Medical Sciences 2005; 60, 1451-7.

[30] Basaria S, Coviello AD, Travison TG, Storer TW, Farwell WR, Jette AM, Eder R, Tennstedt S, Ulloor J, Zhang A, Choong K, Lakshman KM, Mazer NA, Miciek R, Krasnoff J, Elmi A, Knapp PE, Brooks B, Appleman E, Aggarwal S, Bhasin G, Hede-Brierley L, Bhatia A, Collins L, LeBrasseur N, Fiore LD, Bhasin S. Adverse events associated with testosterone administration. The New England Journal of Medicine 2010; 363, 109-22.

[31] Marks LS, Mazer NA, Mostaghel E, Hess DL, Dorey FJ, Epstein JI, Veltri RW, Makarov DV, Partin AW, Bostwick DG, Macairan ML, Nelson PS. Effect of testosterone replacement therapy on prostate tissue in men with late-onset hypogonadism: a randomized controlled trial. Journal of the American Medical Association 2006; 296, 2351-61.

[32] Nigro N, Christ-Crain M. Testosterone treatment in the aging male: myth or reality? Swiss Medical Weekly 2012; 142, w13539.

[33] Goldenberg SL, Koupparis A, Robinson ME. Differing levels of testosterone and the prostate: a physiological interplay. Nature Reviews Urology 2011; 8, 365-77.

[34] Baumgartner RN, Koehler KM, Gallagher D, Romero L, Heymsfield SB, Ross RR, Garry PJ, Lindeman RD. Epidemiology of sarcopenia among the elderly in New Mexico. American Journal of Epidemiology 1998; 147, 755-63.

[35] Rosenberg IH. Sarcopenia: origins and clinical relevance. Journal of Nutrition 1997; 127, 990S-991S.

[36] Cruz-Jentoft AJ, Baeyens JP, Bauer JM, Boirie Y, Cederholm T, Landi F, Martin FC, Michel JP, Rolland Y, Schneider SM, Topinkova E, Vandewoude M, Zamboni M. Sar-

copenia: European consensus on definition and diagnosis: Report of the European Working Group on Sarcopenia in Older People. Age and Ageing 2010; 39, 412-23.

[37] Janssen I, Heymsfield SB, Wang ZM, Ross R. Skeletal muscle mass and distribution in 468 men and women aged 18-88 yr. Journal of Applied Physiology 2000; 89, 81-8.

[38] Masanes F, Culla A, Navarro-Gonzalez M, Navarro-Lopez M, Sacanella E, Torres B, Lopez-Soto A. Prevalence of sarcopenia in healthy community-dwelling elderly in an urban area of Barcelona (Spain). The Journal of Nutrition Health and Aging 2012; 16, 184-7.

[39] Iannuzzi-Sucich M, Prestwood KM, Kenny AM. Prevalence of sarcopenia and predictors of skeletal muscle mass in healthy, older men and women. Journals of Gerontology Series A: Biological Sciences and Medical Sciences 2002; 57, M772-7.

[40] Krasnoff JB, Basaria S, Pencina MJ, Jasuja GK, Vasan RS, Ulloor J, Zhang A, Coviello A, Kelly-Hayes M, D'Agostino RB, Wolf PA, Bhasin S, Murabito JM. Free testosterone levels are associated with mobility limitation and physical performance in community-dwelling men: the Framingham Offspring Study. The Journal of Clinical Endocrinology and Metabolism 2010; 95, 2790-9.

[41] Morley JE, Baumgartner RN, Roubenoff R, Mayer J, Nair KS. Sarcopenia. Journal of Laboratory and Clinical Medicine 2001; 137, 231-43.

[42] Sakuma K, Yamaguchi A. Sarcopenia and cachexia: the adaptations of negative regulators of skeletal muscle mass. Journal of Cachexia, Sarcopenia and Muscle 2012; 3, 77-94.

[43] Short KR, Nair KS. The effect of age on protein metabolism. Current Opinion in Clinical Nutrition and Metabolic Care 2000; 3, 39-44.

[44] Balagopal P, Rooyackers OE, Adey DB, Ades PA, Nair KS. Effects of aging on in vivo synthesis of skeletal muscle myosin heavy-chain and sarcoplasmic protein in humans. American Journal of Physiology 1997; 273, E790-800.

[45] Ferrington DA, Krainev AG, Bigelow DJ. Altered turnover of calcium regulatory proteins of the sarcoplasmic reticulum in aged skeletal muscle. The Journal of Biological Chemistry 1998; 273, 5885-91.

[46] Staunton L, Zweyer M, Swandulla D, Ohlendieck K. Mass spectrometry-based proteomic analysis of middle-aged vs. aged vastus lateralis reveals increased levels of carbonic anhydrase isoform 3 in senescent human skeletal muscle. International Journal of Molecular Medicine 2012; 30, 723-733.

[47] Riley DA, Bain JL, Thompson JL, Fitts RH, Widrick JJ, Trappe SW, Trappe TA, Costill DL. Disproportionate loss of thin filaments in human soleus muscle after 17-day bed rest. Muscle and Nerve 1998; 21, 1280-9.

[48] Lenk K, Schuler G, Adams V. Skeletal muscle wasting in cachexia and sarcopenia: molecular pathophysiology and impact of exercise training. Journal of Cachexia, Sarcopenia and Muscle 2010, 1, 9-21.

[49] Bhasin S. Testosterone supplementation for aging-associated sarcopenia. Journals of Gerontology Series A: Biological Sciences and Medical Sciences 2003, 58, 1002-8.

[50] Snyder PJ. Low testosterone must explain diminished physical performance in the elderly--right? The Journal of Clinical Endocrinology and Metabolism 2010; 95, 2634-5.

[51] Travison TG, Shackelton R, Araujo AB, Morley JE, Williams RE, Clark RV, McKinlay JB. Frailty, serum androgens, and the CAG repeat polymorphism: results from the Massachusetts Male Aging Study. The Journal of Clinical Endocrinology and Metabolism 2010; 95, 2746-54.

[52] Storer TW, Magliano L, Woodhouse L, Lee ML, Dzekov C, Dzekov J, Casaburi R, Bhasin S. Testosterone dose-dependently increases maximal voluntary strength and leg power, but does not affect fatigability or specific tension. The Journal of Clinical Endocrinology and Metabolism 2003; 88, 1478-85.

[53] Gruenewald DA, Matsumoto AM. Testosterone supplementation therapy for older men: potential benefits and risks. Journal of the American Geriatrics Society 2003; 51, 101-15.

[54] Burton LA, Sumukadas D. Optimal management of sarcopenia. Journal of Clinical Interventions in Aging 2010; 5, 217-28.

[55] Borst SE. Interventions for sarcopenia and muscle weakness in older people. Age and Ageing 2004; 33, 548-55.

[56] Roth SM, Martel GF, Ivey FM, Lemmer JT, Tracy BL, Metter EJ, Hurley BF, Rogers MA. Skeletal muscle satellite cell characteristics in young and older men and women after heavy resistance strength training. Journals of Gerontology Series A: Biological Sciences and Medical Sciences 2001; 56, B240-7.

[57] Fiatarone MA, O'Neill EF, Ryan ND, Clements KM, Solares GR, Nelson ME, Roberts SB, Kehayias JJ, Lipsitz LA, Evans WJ. Exercise training and nutritional supplementation for physical frailty in very elderly people. The New England Journal of Medicine 1994; 330, 1769-75.

[58] Liu CJ, Latham NK. Progressive resistance strength training for improving physical function in older adults. Cochrane Database of Systematic Reviews 2009, CD002759.

[59] Fielding RA, Katula J, Miller ME, Abbott-Pillola K, Jordan A, Glynn NW, Goodpaster B, Walkup MP, King AC, Rejeski WJ. Activity adherence and physical function in older adults with functional limitations. Medicine & Science in Sports & Exercise 2007; 39, 1997-2004.

[60] Taaffe DR, Duret C, Wheeler S, Marcus R. Once-weekly resistance exercise improves muscle strength and neuromuscular performance in older adults. Journal of the American Geriatrics Society 1999; 47, 1208-14.

[61] Eckel RH, Grundy SM, Zimmet PZ. The metabolic syndrome. The Lancet 2005; 365, 1415-28.

[62] Alberti KG, Zimmet P, Shaw J. The metabolic syndrome-a new worldwide definition. The Lancet 2005; 366, 1059-62.

[63] Ford ES, Giles WH, Dietz WH. Prevalence of the metabolic syndrome among US adults: findings from the third National Health and Nutrition Examination Survey. Journal of the American Medical Association 2002; 287, 356-9.

[64] Gami AS, Witt BJ, Howard DE, Erwin PJ, Gami LA, Somers VK, Montori VM. Metabolic syndrome and risk of incident cardiovascular events and death: a systematic review and meta-analysis of longitudinal studies. Journal of the American College of Cardiology 2007; 49, 403-14.

[65] Dandona P, Aljada A, Chaudhuri A, Mohanty P, Garg R. Metabolic syndrome: a comprehensive perspective based on interactions between obesity, diabetes, and inflammation. Circulation 2005; 111, 1448-54.

[66] Isidori AM, Caprio M, Strollo F, Moretti C, Frajese G, Isidori A, Fabbri A. Leptin and androgens in male obesity: evidence for leptin contribution to reduced androgen levels. The Journal of Clinical Endocrinology and Metabolism 1999; 84, 3673-80.

[67] Laaksonen DE, Niskanen L, Punnonen K, Nyyssonen K, Tuomainen TP, Valkonen VP, Salonen R, Salonen JT. Testosterone and sex hormone-binding globulin predict the metabolic syndrome and diabetes in middle-aged men. Diabetes Care 2004; 27, 1036-41.

[68] ohnson LW, Weinstock RS. The metabolic syndrome: concepts and controversy. Mayo Clinic Proceedings 2006; 81, 1615-20.

[69] Kaushik M, Sontineni SP, Hunter C. Cardiovascular disease and androgens: a review. International Journal of Cardiology 2010; 142, 8-14.

[70] Jones RD, Nettleship JE, Kapoor D, Jones HT, Channer KS. Testosterone and atherosclerosis in aging men: purported association and clinical implications. American Journal of Cardiovascular Drugs 2005; 5, 141-54.

[71] Kapoor D, Aldred H, Clark S, Channer KS, Jones TH. Clinical and biochemical assessment of hypogonadism in men with type 2 diabetes: correlations with bioavailable testosterone and visceral adiposity. Diabetes Care 2007; 30, 911-7.

[72] Dejager S, Bry-Gauillard H, Bruckert E, Eymard B, Salachas F, LeGuern E, Tardieu S, Chadarevian R, Giral P, Turpin G. A comprehensive endocrine description of Kennedy's disease revealing androgen insensitivity linked to CAG repeat length. The Journal of Clinical Endocrinology and Metabolism 2002; 87, 3893-901.

[73] Finsterer J. Perspectives of Kennedy's disease. Journal of the Neurological Sciences 2010; 298, 1-10.

[74] Ferrante MA, Wilbourn AJ. The characteristic electrodiagnostic features of Kennedy's disease. Muscle and Nerve 1997; 20, 323-9.

[75] Monks DA, Rao P, Mo K, Johansen JA, Lewis G, Kemp MQ. Androgen receptor and Kennedy disease/spinal bulbar muscular atrophy. Hormones and Behavior 2008; 53, 729-40.

[76] Suzuki K, Katsuno M, Banno H, Takeuchi Y, Atsuta N, Ito M, Watanabe H, Yamashita F, Hori N, Nakamura T, Hirayama M, Tanaka F, Sobue G. CAG repeat size correlates to electrophysiological motor and sensory phenotypes in SBMA. Brain 2008; 131, 229-39.

[77] Paradas C, Solano F, Carrillo F, Fernandez C, Bautista J, Pintado E, Lucas M. Highly skewed inactivation of the wild-type X-chromosome in asymptomatic female carriers of spinal and bulbar muscular atrophy (Kennedy's disease). Journal of Neurology 2008; 255, 853-7.

[78] Soraru G, D'Ascenzo C, Polo A, Palmieri A, Baggio L, Vergani L, Gellera C, Moretto G, Pegoraro E, Angelini C. Spinal and bulbar muscular atrophy: skeletal muscle pathology in male patients and heterozygous females. Journal of the Neurological Sciences 2008; 264, 100-5.

[79] Rhodes LE, Freeman BK, Auh S, Kokkinis AD, La Pean A, Chen C, Lehky TJ, Shrader JA, Levy EW, Harris-Love M, Di Prospero NA, Fischbeck KH. Clinical features of spinal and bulbar muscular atrophy. Brain 2009; 132, 3242-51.

[80] Kennedy WR, Alter M, Sung JH. Progressive proximal spinal and bulbar muscular atrophy of late onset. A sex-linked recessive trait. Neurology 1968; 18, 671-80.

[81] Nagashima T, Seko K, Hirose K, Mannen T, Yoshimura S, Arima R, Nagashima K, Morimatsu Y. Familial bulbo-spinal muscular atrophy associated with testicular atrophy and sensory neuropathy (Kennedy-Alter-Sung syndrome). Autopsy case report of two brothers. Journal of the Neurological Sciences 1988; 87, 141-52.

[82] Sperfeld AD, Karitzky J, Brummer D, Schreiber H, Haussler J, Ludolph AC, Hanemann CO. X-linked bulbospinal neuronopathy: Kennedy disease. Archives of Neurology 2002; 59, 1921-6.

[83] Atsuta N, Watanabe H, Ito M, Banno H, Suzuki K, Katsuno M, Tanaka F, Tamakoshi A, Sobue G. Natural history of spinal and bulbar muscular atrophy (SBMA): a study of 223 Japanese patients. Brain 2006; 129, 1446-55.

[84] Davies P, Watt K, Kelly SM, Clark C, Price NC, McEwan IJ. Consequences of polyglutamine repeat length for the conformation and folding of the androgen receptor amino-terminal domain. Journal of Molecular Endocrinology 2008; 41, 301-14.

[85] Tanaka F, Doyu M, Ito Y, Matsumoto M, Mitsuma T, Abe K, Aoki M, Itoyama Y, Fischbeck KH, Sobue G. Founder effect in spinal and bulbar muscular atrophy (SBMA). Human Molecular Genetics 1996; 5, 1253-7.

[86] La Spada AR, Wilson EM, Lubahn DB, Harding AE, Fischbeck KH. Androgen receptor gene mutations in X-linked spinal and bulbar muscular atrophy. Nature 1991; 352, 77-9.

[87] McEwan IJ, Lavery D, Fischer K, Watt K. Natural disordered sequences in the amino terminal domain of nuclear receptors: lessons from the androgen and glucocorticoid receptors. Nuclear Receptor Signal 2005; 5, e001.

[88] Montie HL, Merry DE. Autophagy and access: understanding the role of androgen receptor subcellular localization in SBMA. Autophagy 2009; 5, 1194-7.

[89] Parodi S, Pennuto M. Neurotoxic effects of androgens in spinal and bulbar muscular atrophy. Frontiers in Neuroendocrinology 2011; 32, 416-25.

[90] Walcott JL, Merry DE. Ligand promotes intranuclear inclusions in a novel cell model of spinal and bulbar muscular atrophy. The Journal of Biological Chemistry 2002; 277, 50855-9.

[91] Walcott JL, Merry DE. Trinucleotide repeat disease. The androgen receptor in spinal and bulbar muscular atrophy. Vitamins & Hormones 2002; 65, 127-47.

[92] Adachi H, Katsuno M, Minamiyama M, Waza M, Sang C, Nakagomi Y, Kobayashi Y, Tanaka F, Doyu M, Inukai A, Yoshida M, Hashizume Y, Sobue G. Widespread nuclear and cytoplasmic accumulation of mutant androgen receptor in SBMA patients. Brain 2005; 128, 659-70.

[93] Adachi H, Waza M, Tokui K, Katsuno M, Minamiyama M, Tanaka F, Doyu M, Sobue G. CHIP overexpression reduces mutant androgen receptor protein and ameliorates phenotypes of the spinal and bulbar muscular atrophy transgenic mouse model. Journal of Neuroscience 2007, 27, 5115-26.

[94] Jochum T, Ritz ME, Schuster C, Funderburk SF, Jehle K, Schmitz K, Brinkmann F, Hirtz M, Moss D, Cato AC. Toxic and non-toxic aggregates from the SBMA and normal forms of androgen receptor have distinct oligomeric structures. Biochimica et Biophysica Acta 2012; 1822, 1070-8.

[95] Palazzolo I, Nedelsky NB, Askew CE, Harmison GG, Kasantsev AG, Taylor JP, Fischbeck KH, Pennuto M. B2 attenuates polyglutamine-expanded androgen receptor toxicity in cell and fly models of spinal and bulbar muscular atrophy. Journal of Neuroscience Research 2010; 88, 2207-16.

[96] Taylor JP, Tanaka F, Robitschek J, Sandoval CM, Taye A, Markovic-Plese S, Fischbeck KH. Aggresomes protect cells by enhancing the degradation of toxic polyglutamine-containing protein. Human Molecular Genetics 2003; 12, 749-57.

[97] Katsuno M, Adachi H, Minamiyama M, Waza M, Doi H, Kondo N, Mizoguchi H, Nitta A, Yamada K, Banno H, Suzuki K, Tanaka F, Sobue G. Disrupted transforming

growth factor-beta signaling in spinal and bulbar muscular atrophy. The Journal of Neuroscience 2010; 30, 5702-12.

[98] Katsuno M, Adachi H, Minamiyama M, Waza M, Tokui K, Banno H, Suzuki K, Onoda Y, Tanaka F, Doyu M, Sobue G. Reversible disruption of dynactin 1-mediated retrograde axonal transport in polyglutamine-induced motor neuron degeneration. The Journal of Neuroscience 2006; 26, 12106-17.

[99] Fernandez-Rhodes LE, Kokkinis AD, White MJ, Watts CA, Auh S, Jeffries NO, Shrader JA, Lehky TJ, Li L, Ryder JE, Levy EW, Solomon BI, Harris-Love MO, La Pean A, Schindler AB, Chen C, Di Prospero NA, Fischbeck KH. Efficacy and safety of dutasteride in patients with spinal and bulbar muscular atrophy: a randomised placebo-controlled trial. The Lancet Neurology 2011; 10, 140-7.

[100] Banno H, Katsuno M, Suzuki K, Takeuchi Y, Kawashima M, Suga N, Takamori M, Ito M, Nakamura T, Matsuo K, Yamada S, Oki Y, Adachi H, Minamiyama M, Waza M, Atsuta N, Watanabe H, Fujimoto Y, Nakashima T, Tanaka F, Doyu M, Sobue G. Phase 2 trial of leuprorelin in patients with spinal and bulbar muscular atrophy. Annals of Neurology 2009; 65, 140-50.

[101] Katsuno M, Adachi H, Doyu M, Minamiyama M, Sang C, Kobayashi Y, Inukai A, Sobue G. Leuprorelin rescues polyglutamine-dependent phenotypes in a transgenic mouse model of spinal and bulbar muscular atrophy. Nature Medice 2003; 9, 768-73.

[102] Dunah AW, Jeong H, Griffin A, Kim YM, Standaert DG, Hersch SM, Mouradian MM, Young AB, Tanese N, Krainc D. Sp1 and TAFII130 transcriptional activity disrupted in early Huntington's disease. Science 2002; 296, 2238-43.

[103] Dubois V, Laurent M, Boonen S, Vanderschueren D, Claessens F. (2012) Androgens and skeletal muscle: cellular and molecular action mechanisms underlying the anabolic actions. Cellular and Molecular Life Sciences 2012; 69, 1651-67.

[104] Kadi F. Cellular and molecular mechanisms responsible for the action of testosterone on human skeletal muscle. A basis for illegal performance enhancement. British Journal of Pharmacology 2008; 154, 522-8.

[105] Sullivan ML, Martinez CM, Gennis P, Gallagher EJ. The cardiac toxicity of anabolic steroids. Progress in Cardiovascular Diseases 1998; 41, 1-15.

[106] Fogari R, Preti P, Zoppi A, Fogari E, Rinaldi A, Corradi L, Mugellini A. Serum testosterone levels and arterial blood pressure in the elderly. Hypertension Research 2005; 28, 625-30.

[107] Freed DL, Banks AJ, Longson D, Burley DM. Anabolic steroids in athelics: crossover double-blind trial on weightlifters. British Medical Journal 1975; 2, 471-3.

[108] Lenders JW, Demacker PN, Vos JA, Jansen PL, Hoitsma AJ, van 't Laar A, Thien T. Deleterious effects of anabolic steroids on serum lipoproteins, blood pressure, and liver function in amateur body builders. International Journal of Sports Medicine 1988; 9, 19-23.

[109] De Piccoli B, Giada F, Benettin A, Sartori F, Piccolo E. Anabolic steroid use in body builders: an echocardiographic study of left ventricle morphology and function. International Journal of Sports Medicine 1991; 12, 408-12.

[110] Pearson AC, Schiff M, Mrosek D, Labovitz AJ, Williams GA. Left ventricular diastolic function in weight lifters. American Journal of Cardiology 1986; 58, 1254-9.

[111] Urhausen A, Holpes R, Kindermann W. One- and two-dimensional echocardiography in bodybuilders using anabolic steroids. European Journal of Applied Physiology and Occupational Physiology 1989; 58, 633-40.

[112] Nieminen MS, Ramo MP, Viitasalo M, Heikkila P, Karjalainen J, Mantysaari M, Heikkila J. Serious cardiovascular side effects of large doses of anabolic steroids in weight lifters. European Heart Journal 1996; 17, 1576-83.

[113] Thiblin I, Lindquist O, Rajs J. Cause and manner of death among users of anabolic androgenic steroids. Journal of Forensic Sciences 2000; 45, 16-23.

[114] Bhasin S, Woodhouse L, Casaburi R, Singh AB, Bhasin D, Berman N, Chen X, Yarasheski KE, Magliano L, Dzekov C, Dzekov J, Bross R, Phillips J, Sinha-Hikim I, Shen R, Storer TW. Testosterone dose-response relationships in healthy young men. American Journal of Physiology - Endocrinology and Metabolism 2001; 281, E1172-81.

[115] Simoncini T, Genazzani AR. Non-genomic actions of sex steroid hormones. European Journal of Endocrinology 2003; 148, 281-92.

[116] Bolster DR, Jefferson LS, Kimball SR. Regulation of protein synthesis associated with skeletal muscle hypertrophy by insulin-, amino acid- and exercise-induced signalling. Proceedings of the Nutrition Society 2004; 63, 351-6.

[117] Fluckey JD, Knox M, Smith L, Dupont-Versteegden EE, Gaddy D, Tesch PA, Peterson CA. Insulin-facilitated increase of muscle protein synthesis after resistance exercise involves a MAP kinase pathway. American Journal of Physiology - Endocrinology and Metabolism 2006; 290, E1205-11.

[118] Frey N, McKinsey TA, Olson EN. Decoding calcium signals involved in cardiac growth and function. Nature Medicine 2000; 6, 1221-7.

[119] Frey N, Olson EN. Cardiac hypertrophy: the good, the bad, and the ugly. Annual Review of Physiology 2003; 65, 45-79.

[120] Vicencio JM, Ibarra C, Estrada M, Chiong M, Soto D, Parra V, Diaz-Araya G, Jaimovich E, Lavandero S. Testosterone induces an intracellular calcium increase by a non-genomic mechanism in cultured rat cardiac myocytes. Endocrinology 2006; 147, 1386-95.

[121] Heineke J, Molkentin JD. Regulation of cardiac hypertrophy by intracellular signalling pathways. Nature Reviews Molecular Cell Biology 2006; 7, 589-600.

[122] Frey N, Olson EN. Modulating cardiac hypertrophy by manipulating myocardial lipid metabolism? Circulation 2002; 105, 1152-4.

[123] Antos CL, McKinsey TA, Frey N, Kutschke W, McAnally J, Shelton JM, Richardson JA, Hill JA, Olson EN. Activated glycogen synthase-3 beta suppresses cardiac hypertrophy in vivo. Proceedings of the National Academy of Sciences USA 2002; 99, 907-12.

[124] Proud CG. (2004) Ras, PI3-kinase and mTOR signaling in cardiac hypertrophy. Cardiovascular Research 2004; 63, 403-13.